Telerehabilitation

Editors

DAVID X. CIFU
BLESSEN C. EAPEN

PHYSICAL MEDICINE AND REHABILITATION CLINICS OF NORTH AMERICA

www.pmr.theclinics.com

Consulting Editor
SANTOS F. MARTINEZ

May 2021 • Volume 32 • Number 2

ELSEVIER

1600 John F. Kennedy Boulevard ● Suite 1800 ● Philadelphia, Pennsylvania, 19103-2899

http://www.theclinics.com

PHYSICAL MEDICINE AND REHABILITATION CLINICS OF NORTH AMERICA Volume 32, Number 2
May 2021 ISSN 1047-9651, 978-0-323-83594-7

Editor: Lauren Boyle
Developmental Editor: Diana Grace Ang

Reprints. For copies of 100 or more of articles in this publication, please contact the Commercial Reprints
Department, Elsevier Inc., 360 Park Avenue South, New York, NY 10010-1710. Tel.: 212-633-3874; Fax:
212-633-3820; E-mail: reprints@elsevier.com.

Physical Medicine and Rehabilitation Clinics of North America (ISSN 1047-9651) is published quarterly by
Elsevier Inc., 360 Park Avenue South, New York, NY 10010-1710. Months of issue are February, May,
August, and November. Business and Editorial Offices: 1600 John F. Kennedy Blvd., Suite 1800, Philadelphia,
PA 19103-2899. Customer Service Office: 3251 Riverport Lane, Maryland Heights, MO 63043. Periodicals post-
age paid at New York, NY and additional mailing offices. Subscription price per year is $322.00 (US individuals),
$879.00 (US institutions), $100.00 (US students), $366.00 (Canadian individuals), $923.00 (Canadian institutions), $100.00 (Canadian students), $463.00 (foreign individuals), $923.00 (foreign institutions), and $210.00
(foreign students). Foreign air speed delivery is included in all *Clinics* subscription prices. All prices are subject
to change without notice. **POSTMASTER:** Send address changes to *Physical Medicine and Rehabilitation
Clinics of North America*, Customer Service Office: Elsevier Health Sciences Division, Subscription Customer
Service, 3251 Riverport Lane, Maryland Heights, MO 63043. **Customer Service: 1-800-654-2452 (US).
From outside of the United States, call 314-447-8871. Fax: 314-447-8029. E-mail: JournalsCustomer
Service-usa@elsevier.com (for print support); JournalsOnlineSupport-usa@elsevier.com (for online
support).**

Physical Medicine and Rehabilitation Clinics of North America is indexed in *Excerpta Medica, MEDLINE/
PubMed (Index Medicus), Cinahl,* and *Cumulative Index to Nursing and Allied Health Literature.*

Contributors

CONSULTING EDITOR

SANTOS F. MARTINEZ, MD, MS
Diplomate of the American Academy of Physical Medicine and Rehabilitation, Certificate of
Added Qualification Sports Medicine, Assistant Professor, Department of Orthopaedics,
Campbell Clinic Orthopaedics, University of Tennessee, Memphis, Tennessee

EDITORS

DAVID X. CIFU, MD
Associate Dean for Innovation and Systems Integration, Virginia Commonwealth
University School of Medicine; Herman J. Flax, MD Professor and Chairman, Department
of Physical Medicine and Rehabilitation, Virginia Commonwealth University School of
Medicine, Richmond, Virginia; Senior TBI Specialist, US Department of Veterans Affairs,
Washington, DC; Principal Investigator, Long-term Impact of Military Relevant Brain Injury
Consortium, Central Virginia Veterans Affairs Health System, Richmond, Virginia

BLESSEN C. EAPEN, MD
Chief, VA Greater Los Angeles Health Care System; Associate Clinical Professor, Division
of Physical Medicine and Rehabilitation, Department of Medicine, David Geffen School of
Medicine at UCLA, Los Angeles, California

AUTHORS

RYAN EDWARD ALANO, MD, MPH
Resident Physician, Department of Physical Medicine and Rehabilitation, VA Greater Los
Angeles Healthcare System, Los Angeles, California

THIRU M. ANNASWAMY, MD, MA
Physical Medicine and Rehabilitation Service, VA North Texas Healthcare System,
Department of Physical Medicine and Rehabilitation, UT Southwestern Medical Center,
Dallas, Texas

DIXIE ARAGAKI, MD
Professor, Department of Medicine, Division of Physical Medicine and Rehabilitation, David
Geffen School of Medicine at UCLA, Program Director, Physical Medicine and Rehabilitation
Residency, VA Greater Los Angeles Healthcare System, Los Angeles, California

ARASH ASHER, MD
Director, Wellness, Resilience and Survivorship, Associate Clinical Professor of Medicine,
Department of Physical Medicine and Rehabilitation, Cedars-Sinai Samuel Oschin
Comprehensive Cancer Institute, Los Angeles, California

DANIEL BARROWS, LCSW, MHA, FACHE
Telehealth Program Analyst, Spinal Cord Injuries and Disorders, National Program Office,
Veterans Health Administration, Washington, DC

DOUGLAS E. BIDELSPACH, MPT
Department of Veterans Affairs, Lebanon, Pennsylvania

ALEKS BORRESEN, MD
Department of Physical Medicine and Rehabilitation, The University of Alabama at Birmingham, Birmingham, Alabama

KATHLEEN BURGESS, MD, MS
Director, Regional Multiple Sclerosis Program, VA Puget Sound Healthcare System, Clinical Associate Professor of Rehabilitation Medicine, University of Washington, Seattle, Washington

KEERTHANA CHAKKA, BS
UT Southwestern Medical School, Dallas, Texas

ANNE H. CHAN, DPT, MBA
Administrator, Department of Physical Medicine and Rehabilitation, Virginia Commonwealth University, Richmond, Virginia

LYNN ELIZABETH CHANG, DO, MS
Department of Physical Medicine and Rehabilitation, VA Greater Los Angeles Healthcare System, Los Angeles, California

PHILIP CHANG, DO
Staff Physician, Department of Physical Medicine and Rehabilitation, Cedars-Sinai Samuel Oschin Comprehensive Cancer Institute, Los Angeles, California

BABAK DARVISH, MD
Director, Cardiopulmonary Telehealth Service, Physical Medicine and Rehabilitation Service, VA Greater Los Angeles Healthcare System, Los Angeles, California

PAUL DUKARM, PhD, ABPP-CN
Assistant Professor, Department of Physical Medicine and Rehabilitation, Virginia Commonwealth University Health System, Richmond, Virginia

BARRY GOLDSTEIN, MD, PhD
Deputy Executive Director, Spinal Cord Injuries and Disorders, National Program Office, Veterans Health Administration, Washington, DC; Professor, Department of Rehabilitation Medicine, University of Washington, Seattle, Washington

MARK A. HAVRAN, DPT
Department of Veterans Affairs, Rehabilitation and Extended Care, VA Central Iowa Healthcare System, Des Moines, Iowa

ILEANA M. HOWARD, MD
Outpatient Medical Director, Rehabilitation Care Services, VA Puget Sound Healthcare System, Associate Professor of Rehabilitation Medicine, University of Washington, Seattle, Washington

NANCY HSU, PsyD, LCP
Assistant Professor, Department of Physical Medicine and Rehabilitation, Virginia Commonwealth University Health Sciences, Richmond, Virginia

SEETAL PREET KAUR CHEEMA, MD
Department of Anesthesia, VA Greater Los Angeles Healthcare System, Los Angeles, California

NINAD KHARGONKAR, MS
Department of Computer Science, The University of Texas at Dallas, Richardson, Texas

JESSICA KIECKER, OTR/L
Department of Physical Medicine and Rehabilitation, TREWI Program Coordinator, Minneapolis VA Healthcare System, Minneapolis, Minnesota

HENRY L. LEW, MD, PhD
Professor and Chair, Department of Communication Sciences and Disorders, University of Hawai'i at Mānoa, John A. Burns School of Medicine, Honolulu, Hawaii; Department of Physical Medicine and Rehabilitation, Virginia Commonwealth University School of Medicine, Richmond, Virginia

JERRY LUO, MD
Resident Physician, Department of Physical Medicine and Rehabilitation, VA Greater Los Angeles Healthcare System/David Geffen School of Medicine at UCLA, Los Angeles, California

SAMUEL J. MARTIN, DO
HonorHealth Rehabilitation Hospital, Scottsdale, Arizona

MARY E. MATSUMOTO, MD
Department of Physical Medicine and Rehabilitation, Minneapolis VA Healthcare System, Assistant Professor, Department of Rehabilitation Medicine, University of Minnesota, Minneapolis, Minnesota

CINDY McGEARY, PhD, ABPP
Associate Professor, Department of Psychiatry, The University of Texas Health Science Center, San Antonio, Texas

DON McGEARY, PhD, ABPP
Associate Professor and Vice Chair for Research, Department of Rehabilitation Medicine, The University of Texas Health Science Center, San Antonio, Texas

ANA MILLS, PsyD
Assistant Professor, Department of Physical Medicine and Rehabilitation, Virginia Commonwealth University, Richmond, Virginia

EUGENIO MONASTERIO, MD
Associate Professor, Department of Physical Medicine and Rehabilitation, Virginia Commonwealth University Health Sciences, Children's Hospital of Richmond at VCU, Richmond, Virginia

RASHMI S. MULLUR, MD
Associate Clinical Professor, Department of Medicine, Chief of Telehealth, VA Greater Los Angeles Healthcare System, David Geffen School of Medicine at UCLA, Los Angeles, California

UDAI NANDA, DO
Director, Headache Center of Excellence, Attending Physician, Interventional Pain Service, Department of Physical Medicine and Rehabilitation, VA Greater Los Angeles

Healthcare System, Clinical Instructor, Division of Physical Medicine and Rehabilitation, Department of Medicine, David Geffen School of Medicine at UCLA, Los Angeles, California

MOOYEON OH-PARK, MD, MS
Professor, Department of Rehabilitation Medicine, Department of Neurology, Albert Einstein College of Medicine, Montefiore Health System, Chief Medical Officer, Senior Vice President, Burke Rehabilitation Hospital, White Plains, New York

SANJOG PANGARKAR, MD
Director, Inpatient and Interventional Pain Service, Department of Physical Medicine and Rehabilitation, VA Greater Los Angeles Healthcare System, Professor of Medicine, Division of Physical Medicine and Rehabilitation, Department of Medicine, David Geffen School of Medicine at UCLA, Los Angeles, California

QUYNH GIAO PHAM, MD
Program Director, Pain Medicine Fellowship Training Program, Clinical Professor, Department of Medicine, Division of Physical Medicine and Rehabilitation, Greater Los Angeles VA Healthcare System, David Geffen School of Medicine at UCLA, Los Angeles, California

MELISSA E. PHUPHANICH, MD, MS
Resident Physician, Department of Physical Medicine and Rehabilitation, Greater Los Angeles VA Healthcare System, Los Angeles, California

BALAKRISHNAN PRABHAKARAN, PhD
Department of Computer Science, The University of Texas at Dallas, Richardson, Texas

GAURAV N. PRADHAN, PhD
Biomedical Informatics, Mayo Clinic College of Medicine, Scottsdale, Arizona

PREETI RAGHAVAN, MD
Director, Center of Excellence for Treatment, Recovery and Rehabilitation, Sheikh Khalifa Stroke Institute, Associate Professor of Physical Medicine and Rehabilitation and Neurology, Johns Hopkins University School of Medicine, Baltimore, Maryland

OLIVIER ROLIN, MD, PhD
Assistant Professor, Department of Physical Medicine and Rehabilitation, Virginia Commonwealth University Health Sciences, Children's Hospital of Richmond at VCU, Richmond, Virginia

KUNAL R. SINHA, MD
Resident Physician, Department of Physical Medicine and Rehabilitation, Greater Los Angeles VA Healthcare System, Los Angeles, California

JESSE STOKKE, DO
HonorHealth Rehabilitation Hospital, Scottsdale, Arizona

BRUNO S. SUBBARAO, DO
Physical Medicine and Rehabilitation Department, Phoenix Veterans Healthcare System, Phoenix, Arizona

REBECCA TAPIA, MD
South Texas Veterans Healthcare System, Assistant Professor, Department of Rehabilitation Medicine, UT Health San Antonio, San Antonio, Texas

MICHAEL TRUONG, BS candidate
University of California, San Diego, San Diego, California

JOSEPH WEBSTER, MD
Professor, Department of Physical Medicine and Rehabilitation, Virginia Commonwealth University, Staff Physician, Central Virginia VA Healthcare System, Richmond, Virginia

ELIZABETH WEINER, MD
Physical Medicine and Rehabilitation Residency (PGY-2), VA Greater Los Angeles Healthcare System, Los Angeles, California

MARY J. WELLS, PhD
Assistant Professor, Department of Physical Medicine and Rehabilitation, Virginia Commonwealth University Health System, Richmond, Virginia

GRACE C. WILSKE, OTR/L
Department of Physical Medicine and Rehabilitation, Minneapolis VA Healthcare System, Minneapolis, Minnesota

QUINN WONDERS, PharmD, BCPS
Clinical Pharmacy Specialist, Department of Pharmacy, Department of Physical Medicine and Rehabilitation, VA Greater Los Angeles Healthcare System, Los Angeles, California

PATRICIA YOUNG, MSPT, CP
Amputation System of Care, National Program Manager, Office of Connected Care, National Telerehabilitation Lead, VA Central Office, Washington, DC

GRACE ZHANG, MD
Physical Medicine and Rehabilitation Residency (PGY-2), VA Greater Los Angeles Healthcare System, Los Angeles, California

Contents

> Telehealth reduces disparities that result from physical disabilities, difficulties with transportation, geographic barriers, and scarcity of specialists, which are commonly experienced by individuals with spinal cord injuries and disorders (SCI/D). The Department of Veterans Affairs (VA) has been an international leader in the use of virtual health. The VA's SCI/D System of Care is the nation's largest coordinated system of lifelong care for people with SCI/D and has implemented the use of telehealth to ensure that Veterans with SCI/D have convenient access to their health care, particularly during the restrictions that were imposed by the COVID-19 pandemic.

> With the rapid shift to telemedicine brought on by the COVID-19 pandemic, physiatrists must get accustomed to the new technology and learn how to optimize their evaluations. For those practitioners managing patients with acquired brain injuries, which include stroke and traumatic brain injury, this can seem a daunting task given potential physical and cognitive barriers. However, as the authors discuss techniques to optimize visits, the aim is to illustrate how telehealth appointments can not only be comparable to in-person examinations but also may help increase outreach, compliance, and even satisfaction among this unique population.

> Amyotrophic lateral sclerosis and multiple sclerosis are neurodegenerative diseases requiring interdisciplinary rehabilitation services to maximize function, manage symptoms, prevent complications, and promote higher quality of life. Distance and disability may pose barriers to access of sub-specialized care. Telehealth is one solution to facilitate access and was rapidly expanded during the COVID-19 pandemic. This article details the utility of telehealth services across the disease spectrum-including to establish a diagnosis, monitor progression for ongoing management, and identify and manage symptoms and provide therapy interventions.

The challenges and promise of telehealth services for clinical care and research will be explored.

Patients with amputation have unique characteristics and needs that must be considered when services are being provided through a virtual platform. The types of amputation rehabilitation services that can be provided virtually are numerous and vary from a full clinical team evaluation to individual therapy services. Whether services are being provided in person or through a virtual platform, rehabilitation of the person with amputation ideally involves a collaborative interdisciplinary team. The potential benefits of providing amputation rehabilitation care through a virtual platform include enhanced access to specialized services, reduced travel burden, and improved continuity of care.

Cardiopulmonary telerehabilitation is a safe and effective alternative to traditional center-based rehabilitation. It offers a sustainable solution to more conveniently meet the needs of patients with acute or chronic, pre-existing or newly acquired, cardiopulmonary diseases. To maximize success, programs should prioritize basic, safe, and timely care options over comprehensive or complex approaches. The future should incorporate new strategies learned during a global pandemic and harness the power of information and communication technology to provide evidence-based patient-centered care. This review highlights clinical considerations, current evidence, recommendations, and future directions of cardiopulmonary telerehabilitation.

Telemedicine has clear benefits to the cancer population, including reducing the risk of contracting communicable disease, reaching remote populations, and added convenience. With adequate preparation, cancer rehabilitation telemedicine can serve as a suitable substitute for in-person encounters in several situations. There are limits with technologic deficits, reimbursement questions, and the inability to conduct hands-on physical examinations. It is important to appropriately triage patients to the most suitable visit type, whether telemedicine or in person, with aims of reducing unnecessary risks, monitoring for potential complications, and having productive encounters.

Advancements in medical science and technology, along with global increases in life expectancy, are changing the way health care services are delivered to the aging society. Telerehabilitation refers to rehabilitation services involving evaluation and treatment. It is an attractive option for older adults who may have multiple comorbidities. Limited access to in-person services and the concern about potential exposure to severe acute respiratory syndrome coronavirus-2 during this pandemic accelerated the implementation of telerehabilitation. This article review the scope, need, and implementation of telehealth and telerehabilitation in the aging population from the perspective of clinicians, patients, and caregivers.

Pediatric rehabilitation focuses on optimizing function and quality of life of children through a holistic and transdisciplinary patient-centered team approach. This article describes the incorporation of telehealth in pediatric rehabilitation and its growth over the past decade. It also reviews the experience of practitioners using telehealth by necessity during the 2020 COVID-19 pandemic. Evidence suggests many applications where telehealth can appropriately substitute for traditional in-person visits, and there are many potential applications of telehealth to be explored as a means to enhance connectivity of the interdisciplinary rehabilitation team and the outreach to patients in remote and underserved areas.

Telehealth visits result in high-quality care, with high patient and provider satisfaction. Strong evidence suggests that virtual physical therapy is non-inferior to conventional face-to-face physical therapy for a variety of musculoskeletal disorders. Postoperative telerehabilitation has a strong positive effect on clinical outcomes, and the increased intensity telerehabilitation programs offer is a promising option for patients. Studies demonstrate effective virtual postoperative management. The novel coronavirus disease 2019 pandemic has led to improved reimbursement for telehealth visits and accelerated widespread implementation of telemedicine. This article establishes experience and evidence-based practice guidelines for conducting telemedicine visits, with emphasis on the virtual physical examination.

Telerehabilitation for pain management uses communication technology to minimize geographic barriers. Access to such technology has proven critically important during the coronavirus disease-2019 pandemic and has been useful for patients with chronic pain disorders unable to travel. The evaluation and treatment of such disorders requires a whole health approach that individualizes treatment options and delivers care through a biopsychosocial approach. The goals of care are unchanged from an in-person patient-provider experience. Telerehabilitation can be successfully implemented in pain management with appropriate consideration for

demonstrated to provide functional improvements and satisfaction for the consumer and provider, and is applicable in various physical therapy treatment diagnostic areas. Research and technology enhancements will continue to offer new and innovative means to provide physical therapy. This article further provides points to make virtual PT successful and highlights some recommended equipment and outcome recommendations. The future is bright for providing virtual PT.

As a result of the COVID-19 public health emergency, the Centers for Medicare & Medicaid Services expanded its telehealth benefit on a temporary and emergency basis. Effective March 6, 2020, Medicare will pay for Medicare telehealth services at the same rate as regular, in-person visits. Medicare has prescribed specific guidance on the billing and coding of such services, having an impact on reimbursement for qualified providers. Additional guidance also exists on acceptable telehealth communication platforms and patient privacy.

This article discusses the use of physical and biometric sensors in telerehabilitation. It also discusses synchronous tele-physical assessment using haptics and augmented reality and asynchronous physical assessment using remote pose estimation. The article additionally focuses on computational models that have the potential to monitor and evaluate changes in kinematic and kinetic properties during telerehabilitation using biometric sensors such as electromyography and other wearable and noncontact sensors based on force and speed. And finally, the article discusses how virtual reality environments can be facilitated in telerehabilitation.

Telerehabilitation is an evolving modality for the delivery of rehabilitation care. It allows for innovative approaches for delivery of care in different locations and using different technology based on the patient's needs, clinical judgment of the provider, access to technology, and existing infrastructure of the health care system. Technology continues to evolve to expand the scope of care that can be provided over telerehabilitation, particularly to home. The COVID-19 pandemic has led to accelerated adoption of telerehabilitation with potential to expand access, improve interdisciplinary collaboration, and customize patient-centered care to an unprecedented degree.

PHYSICAL MEDICINE AND REHABILITATION CLINICS OF NORTH AMERICA

Foreword

Innovation and Adaptation

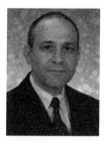

S.F. Martinez, MD, MS
Consulting Editor

The spectrum of medical delivery systems is widening with opportunities to meet and solve accessibility for patients. Even before the recent surge of online patient menu options, many offices had incorporated patient portals in their practices, which has generally been a favorable experience. Granted, not all circumstances are appropriate for the telemedicine landscape, but what an opportunity for our field to expand and evolve. Confidentiality, medicolegal exposure, availability, and compatibility of technology just mention a few unanswered concerns. There may also be license limitations on offering telemedicine for patients crossing state and country boundaries. Certainly, there are many questions to be answered, but I am optimistic that this recent trend will facilitate collaboration and offer more for our patients and their families.

S.F. Martinez, MD, MS
Physical Medicine and Rehabilitation
Campbell Clinic
Department of Orthopaedic Surgery
University of Tennessee School of Medicine
Memphis, TN 38104, USA

E-mail address:
smartinez@campbellclinic.com

Phys Med Rehabil Clin N Am 32 (2021) xv
https://doi.org/10.1016/j.pmr.2021.02.002
1047-9651/21/© 2021 Published by Elsevier Inc.

Preface

A Note from the Editors

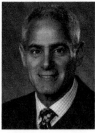 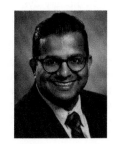

David X. Cifu, MD   Blessen C. Eapen, MD
Editors

Welcome to the twenty-first century of Physical and Rehabilitation Medicine! Virtual health care is no longer a vision of the future or a designer approach to care, it now represents an integral aspect of most clinicians' practices. This issue is dedicated entirely to the art and science of Telerehabilitation, which had been slowly increasing in use for more than a decade and has now skyrocketed with the advent of innovative platforms, approaches, and the urgencies brought on by the worldwide pandemic. The COVID-19 pandemic has rapidly elevated telehealth rehabilitation services from an interesting adjuvant to care that has had good research evidence of efficacy, to a primary service delivery approach for most individuals with acute and chronic disabling conditions. While the explosion of virtual health care is likely to dissipate to some degree with enhanced control of the virus, given the positive experiences that many clinicians, individuals with disability, their families, and the funders of care have been having with telehealth rehabilitation services, it seems inevitable that the traction achieved over the past year will continue and keep these innovations integrated into care. Importantly, a number of health care providers and systems have been using basic (eg, telephonic) and advanced (eg, wearable biometric data streams linked with electronic health records) approaches for a decade or more, and these health care providers and researchers have identified excellent acceptance by individuals with disability (and their families), with specific emphasis on convenience, timeliness, and real-world utility, and similar good clinical efficacy of services and treatment. On the other hand, many clinicians have identified challenges with virtual health care that have ranged from technological challenges to provider-patient disconnection. For this cutting-edge issue, we have brought together the nation's leaders in the practical use of virtual rehabilitation health care to produce a clinic-ready resource for a wide range of practitioners, across the main diagnoses and settings, and including the logistics for implementation and keys for success. We have brought together a range of experienced specialists across diagnoses, technology, and populations to

Phys Med Rehabil Clin N Am 32 (2021) xvii–xviii
https://doi.org/10.1016/j.pmr.2021.02.001
1047-9651/21/© 2021 Published by Elsevier Inc.

provide a practical resource for all users, from the beginner to the advanced practitioner. While there are many elements of Telerehabilitation usage that are common across platforms, diagnosis groups, and practices, the authors have also identified many of the unique elements and nuances of virtual care. This issue covers a wide range of common and focused rehabilitation diagnoses, including spinal cord injury, brain injury, cancer, amputation, cardiac and pulmonary dysfunction, multiple sclerosis, amyotrophic lateral sclerosis, pain management, headache, orthopedics, and musculoskeletal injuries. In addition, the unique approaches to specific patient populations of geriatric and pediatric individuals, and the delivery of a treatments, including wellness and integrative medicine, psychology, and physical therapy, are addressed. Last, articles covering telehealth documentation, reimbursement and privacy regulations, the use of telehealth biometric technology, and innovative approaches to telehealth offer both practical and thought-provoking reviews and updates to support the optimal use of virtual health care. While technologies will further advance and approaches will improve, this issue offers a broad-based foundation from which to initiate, build, and expand a diverse and effective virtual rehabilitation practice to complement and supplement traditional clinical care. The reader of these articles is, thus, able to apply both the basic elements of virtual health across a wide range of patient diagnoses to either get started or feel more comfortable in using them, and the cutting-edge, innovative approaches and recommendations to provide an even greater diversity and quality of rehabilitation care. Most importantly, virtual health care offers a readily available complement to in-person health care delivery that offers the opportunity for even more personalized and patient-centric services, providing the right care, at the right time, to the right person and in the right way.

David X. Cifu, MD
Department of Physical Medicine & Rehabilitation
Virginia Commonwealth University School of Medicine
1223 E. Marshall St.
Richmond, Virginia 23284, USA

Blessen C. Eapen, MD
Physical Medicine and Rehabilitation Service
11301 Wilshire Blvd.
Los Angeles, CA, 90073, USA

E-mail addresses:
dcifu@vcu.edu (D.X. Cifu)
blessen.eapen2@va.gov (B.C. Eapen)

Virtual Care in the Veterans Affairs Spinal Cord Injuries and Disorders System of Care During the COVID-19 National Public Health Emergency

Daniel Barrows, LCSW, MHA[a,1], Barry Goldstein, MD, PhD[a,b,*]

KEYWORDS

- Telehealth • Virtual health • Spinal cord injuries and disorders (SCI/D)
- Veterans Administration (VA) • Veterans Health Administration (VHA) • COVID-19

KEY POINTS

- Video-based telehealth and other forms of delivering care virtually are useful tools in the provision of care to individuals with spinal cord injuries and disorders (SCI/D).
- A wide range of services can be virtually delivered by SCI/D interdisciplinary team members, including education, counseling, reinforcement, monitoring, and information gathering.
- The Veterans Administration increased the use of virtual health during the COVID-19 National Health Emergency so that continuity of care could be maintained for Veterans with SCI/D.
- Telehealth supports care delivery to Veterans with SCI/D in a manner that is convenient and efficient.

INTRODUCTION

The Veterans Health Administration (VHA) is an international leader in the use of virtual health, including live video telehealth, asynchronous store-and-forward telehealth, remote patient monitoring, and mobile health. There are more than 9 million Veterans enrolled in the Department of Veterans Affairs (VA) health care system, and of those, approximately 6 million receive health care at VA medical centers and community-based outpatient clinics throughout the United States each year.[1] Among these users

[a] Spinal Cord Injuries and Disorders, National Program Office, Veterans Health Administration, 810 Vermont Avenue NW, Washington, DC 20571, USA; [b] Department of Rehabilitation Medicine, University of Washington, 325 9th Avenue, Box 359612, Seattle, WA 98104, USA
[1] Present address: 150 Muir Road (R-1, 117), Martinez, CA 94553.
* Corresponding author. 4820 Northeast 106th Street, Seattle, WA 98125.
E-mail address: barry.goldstein@va.gov

Phys Med Rehabil Clin N Am 32 (2021) 207–221
https://doi.org/10.1016/j.pmr.2021.01.007
1047-9651/21/Published by Elsevier Inc.

pmr.theclinics.com

of VA health care, 1.6 million Veterans (27.2%) received some type of virtual health care, and more than 4.8 million virtual visits were conducted between October 1, 2019 and September 30, 2020 (FY2020). Although this volume reflects higher use than in previous years, likely because of the COVID-19 pandemic, the VA has seen a steady and significant increase in the delivery of virtual care since 2009, when it aggressively implemented telehealth as part of the VA's Transformation 21 (T-21) Initiative, an effort aimed at modernizing VA care. The growth of virtual care services is illustrated in **Fig. 1**, which shows the percentage of VA's overall patient population served through virtual care modalities over the past 5 years.

Although the VA's T-21 Initiative ushered in the VA's modern age use of telehealth, the use of virtual care was not new to VA. As the nation's largest integrated health care system, the VA was an early adopter and innovator in implementing the use of telehealth technologies to expand access to health care services to Veterans across the country. For example, in collaboration with the University of Nebraska in 1968, neurologic and psychiatric services were provided by a 2-way closed-circuit television system to VA patients located at VA Medical Centers (VAMC) in Omaha, Lincoln, and Grand Island, Nebraska.[2] In 1970, a microwave bidirectional television system was set up between Massachusetts General Hospital and the Bedford VA Medical Center's psychiatric ward to deliver video-based care.[3] These early efforts were reflective of the VA's commitment to technological innovation in enhancing care to Veterans. The potential value of this increased access is important for many individuals and groups, including the most vulnerable Veterans. Virtual care can reduce disparities that result from physical disabilities, difficulties with transportation, geographic barriers, and scarce specialists. In using virtual care to address disparities and access barriers, a particularly important subgroup to consider is Veterans with spinal cord injuries and disorders (SCI/D) owing to the severity of disabilities associated with severe neurologic impairments, scarcity of knowledgeable SCI/D experts, and long distances to access care in VA SCI/D centers.

VETERANS ADMINISTRATION SPINAL CORD INJURIES AND DISORDERS SYSTEM OF CARE AND VIRTUAL CARE

VA has the largest integrated, comprehensive, single network of SCI/D care in the nation, providing a full range of primary and specialty care to Veterans with SCI/D.

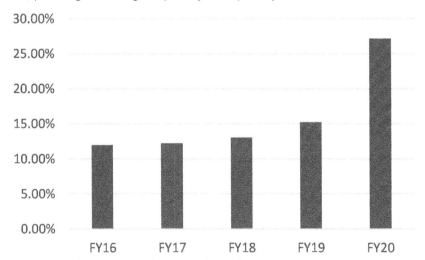

Fig. 1. Percent of VA patients who received virtual care services.

More than 25,000 (FY20: 25,187 in the SCI/D Registry) eligible Veterans receive health care and services within the VA SCI/D System of Care, which is designed to provide lifelong care for all eligible Veterans with SCI/D. This SCI/D System of Care is focused on the provision of care from initial spinal cord injury, or onset of spinal cord disease, throughout the entire lifespan and includes health care management, health promotion and disease prevention, sustaining care, management of new health problems, and long-term care. In addition, the VA's SCI/D System of Care is geographically dispersed throughout the nation, while maintaining integrated services and information systems. This dispersity allows continuity of care to be maintained even when Veterans move around the country, whether temporarily or permanently. At times, non-Veterans also receive care in the VA. For instance, rehabilitation is provided in the VA SCI/D System of Care to active-duty military service members with SCI/D, as established by a memorandum of agreement between the VA and Department of Defense.[4]

In the VA Spinal Cord Injury System of Care, the population served includes individuals with traumatic injuries and several nontraumatic spinal cord disorders, including multiple sclerosis, motor neuron disease, transverse myelitis, severe spondylotic cervical myelopathy, and spinal cord tumor. People with all levels of injury and severity are followed in the SCI/D System of Care, including individuals that are ventilator dependent and that need end-of-life care.[5]

The VA SCI/D System of Care is organizationally designed as a "hub-and-spokes" model in which 25 regional SCI/D centers (hubs), strategically located throughout the country, provide comprehensive primary and highly specialized care tailored to the needs of Veterans with SCI/D. Each of the regional SCI/D centers provides a full continuum of services, including acute rehabilitation, sustaining medical/surgical treatment, primary and preventive care, including annual evaluations, mental health services, provisions for prosthetics and durable medical equipment, and unique SCI/D care, such as ventilator management, respite care, and end-of-life care. Interconnected SCI/D programs and activities coordinate and extend care into the community, including SCI/D home care and other noninstitutional extended care programs. SCI/D centers are staffed by interdisciplinary teams (IDTs) of highly trained SCI/D health care clinicians, which include but are not limited to physicians; physician assistants; nurse practitioners; nurses; physical, occupational, recreation, and kinesiotherapists; psychologists; social workers; pharmacists; dietitians; and vocational counselors.

Each SCI/D center works with VAMC within a geographic catchment that does not have SCI/D centers, called VA SCI/D Spokes; smaller SCI/D teams in those VAMCs are called VA SCI/D Patient Aligned Care Teams. Approximately 110 spokes have dedicated SCI/D teams to deliver primary and basic SCI/D specialty care, and they work collaboratively with the respective SCI/D center to ensure that Veterans with SCI/D receive comprehensive care to address their diverse and complex needs. A spoke is often geographically closer and more accessible to a Veteran's place of residence.

Services in the VA SCI/D System of Care span clinical settings, including inpatient, outpatient, long-term, home, and telehealth care. There are also unique dedicated institutional SCI/D long-term care units at 6 of the VA SCI/D centers. An SCI/D National Program Office provides operational, programmatic, administrative, management, and strategic oversight to the SCI/D System of Care and is organizationally aligned in VA Central Office.

In addition to the VA SCI/D System of Care infrastructure and services, there is an organized and accurate registry of Veterans with SCI/D. Standardized information about demographics, services and utilization, and outcomes is specified and collected for purposes of clinical care, operations, benchmarking, quality improvement, and research. The VA SCI/D registry is a standardized, automated database, which contains aggregated data created at the point of care. There are strict registry inclusion criteria, and the resultant data have been validated throughout the SCI/D System of Care. Using the registry, operational reports are created and made available through the VHA Support Service Center. A registry-based telehealth utilization report provides detailed reporting on telehealth usage among the VA's SCI/D patient population.

Although this comprehensive network of physical locations and infrastructure is in place to provide SCI/D care, health care delivery to this population is complicated by barriers related to underlying physical disabilities, complex comorbid conditions, sparse SCI/D specialty services in most communities, and the rural residence of many Veterans with SCI/D. The use of SCI/D virtual care allows for Veterans with SCI/D to have more frequent contact and communications with SCI/D specialists, especially when large geographic distances limit access to specialty care. Many benefits of virtual care extend to individuals with SCI/D, including improved access, better coordinated patient care, closer follow-up, improved access to specialists, and increased patient satisfaction with care, whereas other benefits, such as prevention of secondary conditions, reduction in emergency room utilization, and cost savings, are less certain.[6–10]

Health care access provided to Veterans in the VA SCI/D System of Care is significantly enhanced using a wide range of virtual care modalities. These modalities include synchronous modalities, such as live video telehealth, asynchronous activities, such as store-and-forward telehealth, interactive remote patient monitoring, secure messaging, and a variety of mobile applications designed to promote Veteran health through self-care coaching. Telehealth within the SCI/D System of Care is supported by the SCI/D National Program Office with a dedicated Telehealth Program Analyst responsible for oversight, program and policy development, training, and supporting field-based telehealth staff in the SCI/D System of Care.

Spinal Cord Injuries and Disorders Telehealth Coordinators

As part of the T-21 Initiative in 2009, VA telehealth was expanded to further develop people-centric, results-driven, and forward-looking systems. As part of this initiative, each of the VA's 25 SCI/D centers (hubs) was staffed with an SCI/D telehealth nurse coordinator, responsible for the implementation, oversight, expansion, and ongoing support of telehealth programs for the respective SCI/D center and its affiliated spokes. In most cases, the SCI/D Telehealth Coordinator is an experienced registered nurse, trained in the care of people with SCI/D as well as being technologically and telehealth proficient. These coordinators are responsible for establishing virtual care programs and ensuring that SCI/D virtual care modalities are effective and used efficiently by other members of the SCI/D IDT. Beyond the technical support and administrative oversight of telehealth operations, there are advantages in having a registered nurse function in this role. Because of their clinical expertise, the SCI/D telehealth coordinators are often involved in the direct provision of telehealth-based care to Veterans with SCI/D. For instance, some maintain a panel of Veterans with SCI/D that they regularly communicate with using video for follow-up care, education, and health maintenance. Other SCI/D telehealth coordinators monitor and coordinate care for patients who are participating in telehealth-based chronic disease management programs for conditions such as hypertension and diabetes. As members of the SCI/D clinical team, the telehealth coordinators participate in treatment planning and advance telehealth-based options to optimize patient care.

Utilization and Workload (Before and After the COVID National Public Health Emergency)

The implementation of telehealth use throughout the SCI/D System of Care has been an evolving process, particularly during the past 10 years. The use of telehealth and other virtual health modalities is not simply a case of what can or cannot be performed virtually. From the perspective of the health care clinician, initial adoption of telehealth was challenging, as it involved a cultural shift in the way care was delivered. Clinicians, especially those who work with complex patient populations, value in-person visits and sometimes question if high-quality care will be compromised without "hands-on" encounters with patients. Acute rehabilitation following the new onset of SCI/D remains an inpatient encounter rather than an attempt to do so virtually. There are many discrete clinical interactions with SCI/D patients that require an in-person, hands-on encounter, such as the detailed and standardized International Standards for Neurological Classification of Spinal Cord Injury. New onset of specific symptoms (eg, neurologic loss, fever, respiratory symptoms) continues to be evaluated in face-to-face visits rather than virtual visits.

Besides these specific examples, the use of telehealth is now used to supplement and support almost all aspects of delivering clinical care to Veterans with SCI/D. All SCI/D disciplines have used virtual care and telehealth to communicate with Veterans, particularly during the COVID pandemic. The virtual annual evaluation highlights evaluations by the SCI/D IDT. Because most SCI/D outpatient clinics closed during the early months of the pandemic, annual evaluations were often performed virtually. SCI/D providers, nurses, therapists, social workers, psychologists, dieticians, and pharmacists have conducted their portion of the annual evaluation using telehealth. More generally, virtual health has been effective in providing patient education, counseling, reinforcement, monitoring, straightforward observations, and information gathering.

During the COVID pandemic, there have been unique interactions that demonstrate the value of virtual health. A standardized, nationally approved SCI/D COVID-19 screen template was developed in the early months of the pandemic and has been used by SCI/D center and spokes teams to reach out to Veterans with SCI/D. Various SCI/D team members use telephone and telehealth to contact the Veteran and ask questions, including the primary qualifying SCI/D diagnosis, living setting, caregiver status, if the patient has new concerns, and if there are new or additional symptoms. Many sites proactively contacted all Veterans on their respective SCI/D registries.

SCI/D clinicians are using telehealth to problem solve and triage new problems. Evaluating new equipment problems, reviewing progress and/or new concerns with pressure injuries, and addressing medication issues are examples of the usefulness of telehealth in addressing new concerns. Telehealth has also been used for continuity, management of chronic problems, and/or continuing treatment, such as weight management, mental health counseling, diabetes follow-up, and a variety of educational programs.

The use of clinical video telehealth is especially useful to enhance encounters made by SCI/D home care nurses during their in-person visits with Veterans living in the community. During a home visit, the SCI/D nurse sometimes needs input from a provider; a simple video connection can bring in any type of specialist for consultation. In addition, store-and-forward telehealth is used during SCI/D home visits to transmit images of pressure injuries to consulting providers and ensure efficient care management. Often, this eliminates the need for travel, which is complicated if weight-bearing on the pressure injury is contraindicated. The VA has recently engaged in a pilot to enhance SCI/D home care using wearable technology that allows the transmission of vital signs, such as oxygen levels, heart rate, blood pressure, and temperature, allowing providers to virtually monitor a patient's condition and provide interventions when necessary.

An additional challenge to telehealth implementation is that Veterans with SCI/D often value the opportunity to come to the SCI/D center to see their providers and other Veterans in person. Many Veterans have been receiving care in the SCI/D System of Care for decades, and they develop trusting relationships with care providers. Veterans establish friendships and close relationships with peers. Although virtual care may offer convenience, improved access, lower costs and may be an appropriate modality for many SCI/D-related services, some Veterans still choose to have in-person visits for these other reasons.

The COVID-19 pandemic resulted in a monumental shift in both utilization and attitudes toward telehealth among providers and Veterans. Especially during the initial months of the pandemic, telehealth use became a fundamental tool in maintaining continuity of care for Veterans with SCI/D served by the VA. As illustrated in **Figs. 2–4**, there has been a remarkable increase in the number of Veterans with SCI/D who have participated in telehealth visits during FY2020. This increase is not surprising given that most routine outpatient in-person visits were canceled during the early months of the pandemic, and visits were shifted to virtual care. **Fig. 2** shows the percentage of Veterans listed on the SCI/D registry who have received telehealth services. The figure demonstrates the steady adoption of telehealth use within the SCI/D system of care in FY2016 to FY2019 and the dramatic increase experienced during the COVID-19 pandemic during FY20.

Fig. 3 shows the total number of telehealth visits provided to Veterans with SCI/D during the past 5 years, also illustrating the gradual increase in telehealth utilization in the previous 4 years, which greatly accelerated during FY20. In comparing FY2019 to FY20, there was more than a 400% increase in telehealth visits. This increase in telehealth utilization during the COVID pandemic reflects the SCI/D System of Care effective response to the pandemic and new constraints on face-to-face visits because Veterans with SCI/D are at extremely high risk of complications following respiratory disease. People who live with SCI/D often develop respiratory complications and/or are at risk of complications, hospitalizations, or death from respiratory

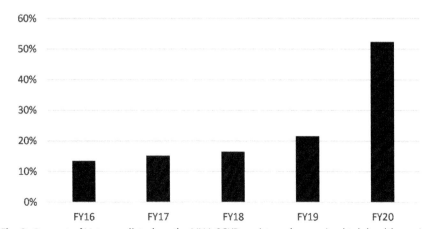

Fig. 2. Percent of Veterans listed on the VHA SCI/D registry who received telehealth services.

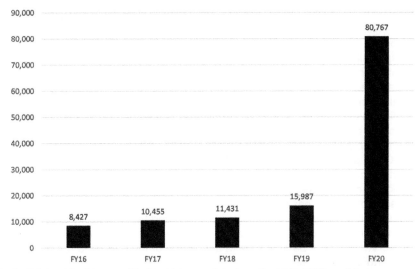

Fig. 3. Telehealth visits provided to Veterans listed on the VHA SCI/D registry.

illnesses. Burns and colleagues[11] recently published research concerning a higher mortality for Veterans with SCI/D (19%) than the general Veteran population (7.7%) enrolled for VHA health care; both populations have a similar proportion of individuals aged 65 years or greater. The SCI/D Veteran case fatality rate with COVID-19 is 2.4 times the rate observed in the non-SCI/D Veteran population, with an absolute rate that is 11% greater (95% confidence interval: 5%–19%; Z score = 4.8; $P < .0002$). Because of the high risk for COVID-related complications, hospitalizations, and death, there were aggressive efforts to contact Veterans with SCI/D by clinicians using telehealth to avoid in-person visits, and to screen Veterans with SCI/D for symptoms of COVID or other respiratory problems.

When telehealth usage among Veterans with SCI/D is analyzed at the individual patient level, as illustrated in **Fig. 4**, Veterans who participated in telehealth received an average of 3 telehealth visits per year between FY2016 and FY2019. In FY20, that

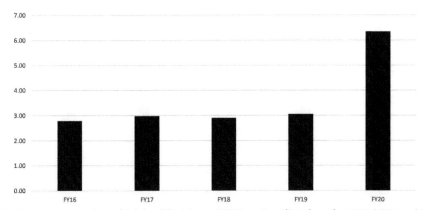

Fig. 4. Average number of telehealth visits per SCI/D patient listed on the VHA SCI/D registry who received telehealth.

doubled to approximately 6 visits per year, reflecting increased use during the COVID-19 pandemic.

One of the original goals of telehealth implementation in VA was to increase access, especially for Veterans who live in rural areas and need to travel long distances to a clinic or medical center. Long distance travel is particularly difficult for people with disabilities, including SCI/D. However, there are issues that can make telehealth use challenging for rural Veterans. Connectivity, through cellular broadband, wired, or satellite-based Internet, is limited in rural areas of the country. In late FY20, the VA implemented a new program called "Digital Divide," which provides an assessment of the "technology gaps" that might prevent a Veteran from participating in telehealth. Once gaps are identified, solutions can be offered to the Veteran, which may include a referral to the Federal Communication Commission Lifeline program to subsidize home Internet service and provide devices such as smartphones or tablets. In addition, the VA has a program to loan broadband-enabled iPads to Veterans who lack such devices. As technology advances and the availability of high-speed Internet options expands to more rural communities across the nation, it is expected that more Veterans will be able to take advantage of the improved access offered through virtual modalities.

Although one might expect that rural Veterans would be the primary users of VA telehealth services, urban Veterans also took advantage of virtual care services. In FY19, 21.98% of Veterans listed on the SCI/D registry and designated as "rural" took advantage of telehealth services, whereas 19.02% of those designated as "urban" did the same, reflecting a modest difference between the 2 groups. In FY20, as illustrated in **Fig. 5**, there was a small shift, likely because of the COVID-19 pandemic, with 46.1% of "rural" Veterans receiving telehealth services compared with 52.7% of their urban-residing counterparts. During the pandemic, other factors likely unrelated to geography prevented or discouraged Veterans with SCI/D from seeking in-person care, including closure of many SCI/D clinics, limiting admissions to inpatient SCI/D center beds, delaying elective procedures, and reluctance by Veterans with SCI/D to go in to clinics and medical centers.

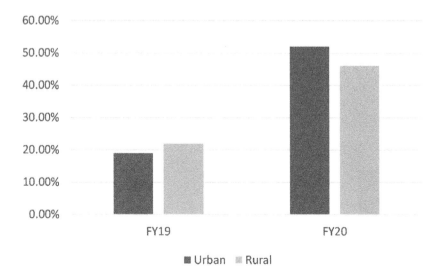

Fig. 5. Percent of SCI/D Veterans receiving telehealth services based on geography.

In addition to the need to accurately identify the VA SCI/D population, which is provided by the SCI/D registry described earlier, tracking telehealth utilization is highly dependent on accurate and specific coding of SCI/D telehealth encounters. When telehealth was initially introduced throughout the SCI/D System of Care years ago, tracking implementation and utilization were complicated by the absence of a coding system to easily differentiate telehealth visits from in-person visits, and visits provided by SCI/D providers versus other VA providers. Differentiating between provider types was remedied with the development of an SCI/D-specific telehealth workload coding system, which now provides accurate tracking of workload, including the location and provider of care. The system requires providers to accurately code the encounter in the VA's electronic medical record system.

Although Veterans with SCI/D are often provided both SCI/D-specific primary and specialty care services by SCI/D-trained clinicians within the SCI/D System of Care, some Veterans with SCI/D receive care in non-SCI/D settings by non-SCI/D clinicians (eg, primary care, mental health services). **Fig. 6** illustrates that 57% of telehealth services provided to Veterans with SCI/D were SCI/D-specific, whereas the remaining 43% of the services they received were provided in settings outside the SCI/D System of Care. In addition, Veterans with SCI/D may be enrolled and receive services from a VA facility's remote home monitoring program to manage chronic diseases, such as hypertension and diabetes, which is managed by nurses who may not be solely dedicated to SCI/D care.

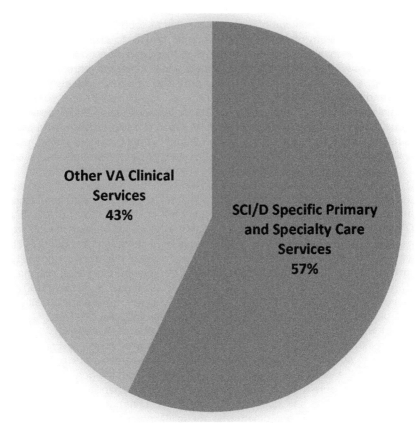

Fig. 6. VHA telehealth services delivered to Veterans with SCI/D in FY20.

The establishment of more effective workload tracking, combined with the ability to more accurately identify the VA's SCI/D patient population using the SCI/D registry, places the VA in a better position to use data more effectively to better understand the current state, establish improvement goals and performance benchmarks, and expand use of telehealth within the SCI/D Veteran population.

In summary, when comparing the VA's SCI/D cohort with the overall population of Veterans served by the VA, a greater percentage of Veterans with SCI/D (52.3%) took advantage of VA telehealth services compared with 27.9% of the overall VA patient population.

Performance Measurement

The VHA is the largest integrated health system in the United States. In 1995, under the leadership of the VHA Undersecretary for Health, Kenneth Kizer, MD, MPH, a major initiative was launched that included a focus on achievement of performance-based outcomes. This initiative has been evolving for years and has resulted in recognition of VA for leadership in clinical informatics and data-driven performance improvement. To best serve Veterans, the alignment of strategic direction, business operations, technology, and data must be methodically designed, aggregated, and managed to deliver the right information to the right people at the right place and time. During this same period, there have been significant efforts to increase the use of performance-based metrics for telehealth in VA. Beginning in FY11, performance expectations were set for all VHA facilities to achieve delivery of virtual care-based services to a minimum percentage of Veterans enrolled at each VA facility. At the same time, the SCI/D System of Care set performance targets to align with VA's goals and to increase telehealth utilization. As a result of these and other implementation efforts, steady growth in the use of telehealth has been seen over the years, as illustrated earlier in **Fig. 1**. Establishing standards and providing accurate data identified best practices and potential areas of improvement.

Maintaining relevant and achievable targets for telehealth use and expansion has faced challenges related to the competition for resources and provider time as well as the need to have adequate and cooperative buy-in from providers to incorporate telehealth use into their practice. The SCI/D System of Care has made a concerted effort to ensure that the establishment of performance metrics includes input from SCI/D subject matter experts in the field. Recently, this has been accomplished through the establishment of "think tanks" made up of field-based clinicians to address a wide variety of issues related to the care of Veterans with SCI/D. In the SCI/D Registry and Outcomes Think Tank, a performance measurement workgroup defines metrics to drive the enhancement and quality of services in the SCI/D System of Care. Recognizing the importance of virtual modalities in maintaining continuity of care and improving access to specialty services for Veterans with SCI/D during the COVID-19 pandemic, this group established an FY2021 goal to achieve 100% of outpatient SCI/D providers with capabilities to provide video-based telehealth services to patients in their home or other non-VA sites using the VA Video Connect (VVC) Platform. This goal aligns with a larger VA-wide goal to ensure that all primary care providers have this capability. Recognizing the importance of providing convenient access to specialty care for Veterans with SCI/D regardless of where they live and to address the varied needs that arise in this population, the goal in SCI/D goes a step further to ensure that all SCI/D clinicians have the capability to deliver virtual care, including physical and occupational therapists, pharmacists, social workers, mental health practitioners, and others who are delivering outpatient care to Veterans with SCI/D. The goal is to ensure that all SCI/D IDT clinicians are able to provide care, and Veterans with SCI/D have the choice to receive in-person or virtual care. In looking forward, the Think Tank workgroups are considering volume-based targets, which will aim to drive expanded use of telehealth to a larger percentage of Veterans with SCI/D and to ensure that facilities continue to offer telehealth-based services as a routine component of care for Veterans with SCI/D.

Technological Considerations

The initial implementation of telehealth within VA involved connecting 2 VA care sites by video. Within the SCI/D System of Care, this allowed Veterans with SCI/D to participate in visits, being present at the clinic or the SCI/D center. Telehealth visits between two VA care sites was particularly important for transitions of care. It also allowed Veterans to travel to a closer SCI/D spoke site location and still receive services from SCI/D specialists located at a distant SCI/D center in collaboration with the SCI/D spoke team. The technology and special telehealth equipment involved in these encounters are housed at VA clinics and SCI/D centers, operated by specially trained Telehealth Clinical Technicians and SCI/D Telehealth Coordinators. There are great coordinative advantages in these synchronous real-time video appointments between VA facilities and include activities such as discharge planning; specialty consultations, including pressure injury, neurogenic bladder, and pain management; preoperative planning; and wheelchair seating assessments. In general, Veterans and clinicians value these telehealth encounters, but coordination of the clinic-based telehealth visits is difficult, particularly when several clinicians participate. Challenges with clinic-to-clinic live video telehealth include coordination of appointments, equipment, space, and staff between 2 geographically separated teams.

Recognizing the potential to reach directly in to the Veterans' homes, VA has more recently released an application known as VVC, which allows Veterans to participate in virtual visits with a clinician using any video-enabled device, including a smartphone, tablet, or personal computer. VVC eliminates the need for the Veteran to travel and allows for direct conversation with the clinician. It also simplifies coordination for the visit in comparison with clinic-based telehealth. However, in implementing this program, challenges included a lack of technology, knowledge, and skills, especially for older Veterans, to participate in these types of visits. To solve this, the VA funded a program to loan Apple iPads, mentioned earlier, to Veterans who lacked their own devices. During the last quarter of calendar year 2020, the VA provided 57,000 of these devices to Veterans, and an additional 18,000 are on order. The program to provide tablets to Veterans solved many problems. However, Veterans with SCI/D may still have challenges or barriers in using iPads, particularly when hand function is impaired. A variety of strategies, tools, and modifications to use the devices have been used as needed by each individual Veteran with SCI/D. For instance, some Veterans require the activation of accessibility features built into the Apple iOS software to control the device with voice or a stylus. Simplification of multiple steps required to join an appointment has also been helpful for many Veterans with SCI/D. Devices can be set up in a mode known as "single use," which disables many of the features of an iPad in order to simplify its use for 1 application and minimizing multiple steps that normally would have to be taken to access the VVC application. In normal use, a Veteran receives an e-mail reminder about their upcoming video appointment, which contains a link to join the virtual meeting. However, some Veterans have been challenged with multiple steps required to join a VVC meeting, including use of a password to unlock the iPad, opening an e-mail application, finding the particular e-mail with their appointment, clicking the link to join the appointment, and then going through multiple steps to join the appointment. This challenge has been resolved with system modifications, which allow a provider to call the Veteran's specific device through the VVC application, only requiring a single click on the screen of the iPad by the Veteran.

The SCI/D Telehealth Coordinators and other SCI/D IDT members are invaluable in addressing barriers, training, education, positioning, adaptive equipment (eg, grips, stands, and styluses), and modifications of software settings to enable Veterans with SCI/D to more easily use VVC. Although the VA has set up a help desk hotline that operates on a 24-hour, 7-day-a-week schedule for Veterans who need assistance in setting up and using their VVC application, one of the limitations is that the technicians who staff the hotline are not trained to understand the unique physical limitations and challenges that are relevant to the use of technology by a person with SCI/D. Efforts are underway to address these limitations through increased training.

A more recent development, a mobile app called MyVA Images, is an example of the rapid advancement of virtual health apps that have tremendous potential for interactive asynchronous modalities. MyVA Images allows Veterans and/or their caregivers to securely submit still images or short video clips, in response to requests entered by providers to aid in evaluation and treatment. For example, a provider may request a photograph of an area of pressure injury for further evaluation and treatment. A gait video clip may be requested to further assess walking, mobility, and balance. Photographs of the environment may be requested to evaluate safety, accessibility, and barriers in the home. The MyVA Images App is in the pilot phase with expected wide rollout during 2021. Other mobile applications in use by VA provide self-management for pressure injuries, management of posttraumatic stress disorder, pain management, and coaching during quarantine and isolation during the COVID pandemic.

DISCUSSION

During the past several years, virtual health technologies have expanded rapidly, increasing access to health care in ways that were never before possible. For people with SCI/D and other severe disabilities, there is great potential in using telehealth to address needs and unique barriers to care. In addition, virtual health can be used during local, national, or international emergencies, when travel, access, systems, infrastructure, and in-person visits are affected.

The VA SCI/D System of Care has seen the unprecedented use of virtual health technologies during the COVID-19 health emergency. Because in-person visits were restricted, many disciplines from the SCI/D IDT used direct telehealth communication with Veterans with SCI/D to address a variety of needs and functions, including outreach to check on the status of each Veteran on the SCI/D Registry during the COVID pandemic; contact with Veterans with SCI/D to encourage flu vaccinations; follow-up of SCI/D complications (eg, pressure injuries, neurogenic bladder, and chronic pain); monitoring of chronic conditions, such as diabetes mellitus and hypertension; acute and subacute rehabilitation following onset of SCI/D by various members of the SCI/D IDT; medication reconciliation by SCI/D pharmacists; and annual evaluations.

Before and during the COVID-19 pandemic, many virtual health modalities have been used in the VA SCI/D System of Care. The greatest growth and use have been direct synchronous telehealth from clinicians to Veterans with SCI/D in their homes. Given the mobility challenges and vulnerability of Veterans with SCI/D to clinical complications, minimizing exposure during the COVID National Public Health Emergency to health threats experienced during in-person health care visits using telehealth in the home was and remains a top priority.

The advancement of technology during the past few years has also allowed expansion of virtual health to most Veterans with SCI/D, even in extremely rural environments, and expands the ability to provide what the Veteran needs at the right time while staying at home. During and following the pandemic, it is likely that continued rapid development and implementation of virtual health modalities and tools will occur.

There have been previous studies and articles about the use of telehealth in people with spinal cord injury.[7] Many of the studies were feasibility, observational, or pilot studies with small samples, primarily using telehealth communication directly to the consumer. Diverse questions were studied, and various outcome measures were used, most of which focused on the postrehabilitation period following an acute spinal cord injury. Other studies examined various modalities, often using asynchronous telehealth, including store-and-forward images of pressure injuries, Web-based treatments, and interactive home monitoring. In general, and anecdotally, there is wide acceptance of virtual health by many patients, consumers, caregivers, and clinicians. Nevertheless, there has been little systematic study of the use of virtual care modalities in the SCI/D population. Much work is needed to determine the relative benefits, effectiveness, costs, and obstacles to the wide use of virtual health as compared with face-to-face health care by the SCI/D community.

There is no doubt that virtual care will be part of the evolution of health care throughout the world for years to come. Many aspects of these technological advances have the potential to solve many access problems shared across disability groups. Changes have already begun. Data published by the Centers for Medicare and Medicaid Services demonstrated similar changes as evidenced in VA and in the SCI/D System of Care. Between 2014 and 2016, there was a 37.7% increase in the number of beneficiaries with disabilities using telehealth and a 53.7% increase in the total services used by these same beneficiaries.[12]

The COVID-19 pandemic has transformed health care as well as society and the economy. This current article focuses on the use of virtual health by Veterans with SCI/D during the COVID-19 National Public Health Emergency. A description of utilization and virtual modalities is provided comparing the current year with previous years of concerted efforts to provide virtual care to Veterans with SCI/D. This global health emergency has presented unprecedented challenges to in-person health care visits and catalyzed the rapid development of virtual care to meet and move beyond those challenges. During the COVID pandemic, VA telehealth and other virtual care modalities have been used to connect Veterans with SCI/D and IDT clinicians to maintain health, prevent complications, and address new issues because access to the VA SCI/D System of Care was significantly curtailed. In all likelihood, this situation will continue for several months or perhaps years. At the time of this writing, there is another surge that has resulted in record high numbers and rates for new daily cases, hospitalizations, and deaths. Reliance on virtual health modalities during the COVID pandemic will remain a priority in the VA SCI/D System of Care.

During the COVID-19 pandemic, there have been many advantages in the use of telehealth and other virtual modalities. Virtual care has provided a means of consistent communication, access, and continuity of care that overcome physical barriers during a time when in-person services were discontinued, "stay-at-home" orders were established, and physical distancing measures were used to reduce community and nosocomial spread. Secondary benefits included the conservation of personal protective equipment and decreased use of beds for other purposes to expand COVID units and to allow flexibility and adaptability to physical or geographic boundaries where there are surges.

Although the future utilization of VA SCI/D virtual care following the COVID-19 pandemic is unknown, telehealth use will probably be greater than prepandemic levels, now that a significant number of providers and Veterans have experienced its advantages. As with other technologic advancements, there is great potential for use of virtual health modalities by people with disabilities. Nevertheless, there remain broad questions about the development of virtual health and its application for people with disabilities. There is recent evidence that the digital divide remains large between Americans with and without a disability. The Pew Research Center recently found that disabled Americans are about 3 times as likely as those without a disability to say they never go online (23% vs 8%), One-in-four disabled adults say they have high-speed Internet at home, a smartphone, a desktop or laptop computer, *and* a tablet, compared with 42% of those who report not having a disability. Regardless of age, disabled Americans are adopting technology at lower rates, although the divide is even greater with older disabled Americans.[13] In the VA SCI/D System of Care, the average age of Veterans on the SCI/D Registry is 63 years of age, underscoring the complexities involved in a population of severely disabled that is in many cases older adults.

There are broad issues related to the development of virtual health for people with disabilities. There is a moral imperative to ensure that innovations in virtual care are available and accessible to people with disabilities. Although there is face validity to the potential benefits of virtual care for disabled Americans, advances in the field can paradoxically further heighten health and social disparities. Involving people with disabilities on the development, implementation, and study of virtual health is of the utmost importance.

There is much work left to do. There are still fundamental questions about effectiveness of virtual health, optimizing virtual care in the SCI/D community, addressing barriers, rigorously addressing satisfaction by Veterans and clinicians, and examining costs. Because Veterans with SCI/D is a well-defined population and there is a well-organized infrastructure for care, the VA SCI/D System of Care is an ideal setting to examine many of these questions.

CLINICS CARE POINTS

- Virtual health increases access and offers advantages for people with severe disabilities, such as spinal cord injuries and disorders.

- Virtual health increases access during periods of natural disasters and other public health emergencies, such as the COVID-19 pandemic.

- Telehealth offers advantages to prospectively contact people living in the community at high risk for complications, such as Veterans with spinal cord injuries and disorders during the COVID-19 pandemic.

- The Veterans Health Administration is an international leader in the use of virtual health and has greatly increased use of telehealth during the COVID National Public Health Emergency in the Spinal Cord Injuries and Disorders System of Care.

- There are some aspects of the spinal cord injuries and disorders examination that cannot be performed virtually, including the International Standards for Neurological Classification of Spinal Cord Injury.

- In the spinal cord injuries and disorders population, there are still fundamental questions about effectiveness of virtual health, how best to optimize care, limitations of telehealth, and how best to address barriers, rigorously addressing satisfaction by Veterans and clinicians and examining costs.

DISCLOSURE

The authors have nothing to disclose.

REFERENCES

1. How many Veterans receive healthcare at VA each year?. Available at: https://www.va.gov/health/aboutvha.asp#: ~ :text=The%20Veterans%20Health%20Administration%20(VHA,Veterans%20enrolled%20in%20the%20VA. Accessed December 15, 2020.
2. Wittson CL, Benschoter MS. Two-way television: helping the medical center reach out. Am J Psychiatry 1972;129(5):624–7.
3. Dwyer TF. Telepsychiatry: psychiatric consultation by interactive television. Am J Psychiatry 1973;130(8):865–9.
4. Memorandum of Agreement between Department of Veterans Affairs and Department of Defense for medical treatment provided to active duty service members with spinal cord injury, traumatic brain injury, blindness, or polytraumatic injuries (2009).
5. VHA Directive 1176(2): Spinal cord injuries and disorders system of care, September 30, 2019 (Revised February 7, 2020).
6. Careau E, Dussault J, Vincent C. Development of interprofessional care plans for spinal cord injury clients through videoconferencing. J Interprof Care 2010;24(1):115–8.
7. Irgens I, Rekand T, Arora M, et al. Telehealth for people with spinal cord injury: a narrative review. Spinal Cord 2018;56:643–55.
8. Woo C, Seton JM, Washington M, et al. Increasing specialty care access through use of an innovative home telehealth-based spinal cord injury disease management protocol (SCI DMP). J Spinal Cord Med 2016;39(1):3–12.
9. Coulter EH, McLean AN, Hasler JP, et al. The effectiveness and satisfaction of web-based physiotherapy in people with spinal cord injury: a pilot randomized controlled trial. Spinal Cord 2017;55:383–9.
10. Houlihan BV, Brody M, Everhart-Skeels S, et al. Randomized trial of a peer-led, telephone-based empowerment intervention for persons with chronic spinal cord injury improves health self-management. Arch Phys Med Rehabil 2017;98:1067–76.
11. Burns SP, Eberhart AC, Sippel JL, et al. Case-fatality with coronavirus disease 2019 (COVID-19) in United States Veterans with spinal cord injuries and disorders. Spinal Cord 2020;58(9):1040–1.
12. CMS. Information on Medicare telehealth report. Centers for Medicare & Medicaid Services. 2018. Available at: https://www.cms.gov/About-CMS/Agency-Information/OMH/Downloads/Information-on-Medicare-Telehealth-Report.pdf. Accessed December 15, 2020.
13. Pew Research Center. Disabled Americans are less likely to use technology. 2017. Available at: https://www.pewresearch.org/fact-tank/2017/04/07/disabled-americans-are-less-likely-to-use-technology/. Accessed December 15, 2020.

Telerehabilitation in Acquired Brain Injury

Bruno S. Subbarao, DO[a],*, Jesse Stokke, DO[b], Samuel J. Martin, DO[b]

KEYWORDS

- Telemedicine • Telerehabilitation • Telehealth • Acquired brain injury • Stroke
- Traumatic brain injury

KEY POINTS

- Telehealth visits for patients with acquired brain injuries and their caregivers can ease the burden of transportation, improve compliance, and increase overall satisfaction.
- Management strategies are largely unaffected in the telehealth setting, and telerehab options have been found to be equal or superior to in-person therapy to treat many associated deficits.
- Telehealth evaluations can be reliable and often equivalent to in-person examinations but remember to ensure safety when asking a patient to perform any challenging or complex physical examination maneuvers.
- Because of the limitations of the telemedicine physical examination, a thorough history is invaluable and will help focus on your assessments.
- Trust your gut. If you suspect any red flag symptoms, no matter how subtle, error on the side of safety and have the patient be evaluated in person or through the emergency department.

INTRODUCTION

With the rapid shift to telemedicine brought on by the COVID-19 pandemic, providers in all specialties have been required to adapt to caring for individuals remotely. As a patient population, those with acquired brain injuries, which include stroke and traumatic brain injury (TBI), most often require long-term care and follow-up but face unique physical, mental, and psychological challenges in consistently attending in-office visits. Thus, telemedicine provides an opportunity not only to keep those individuals safe but to improve outreach and ensure compliance with a rehabilitation plan. As there are journals already dedicated to in-depth strategies for the rehabilitation of patients with acquired brain injuries (please see *Physical Medicine and Rehabilitation Clinics of North America: Traumatic Brain Injury Rehabilitation and Physical Medicine*

[a] Physical Medicine and Rehabilitation Department, Phoenix Veterans Healthcare System, Building 34, 650 E Indian School Rd, Phoenix, AZ 85012, USA; [b] HonorHealth Rehabilitation Hospital, 8850 E Pima Center Pkwy, Scottsdale, AZ 85258, USA
* Corresponding author.
E-mail address: brunopmrdoc@gmail.com

Phys Med Rehabil Clin N Am 32 (2021) 223–238
https://doi.org/10.1016/j.pmr.2021.01.001
1047-9651/21/Published by Elsevier Inc.

and *Rehabilitation Clinics of North America: Stroke Rehabilitation*), this article focuses on optimal techniques and special considerations for effective management in a tele-rehabilitation setting.

BACKGROUND

Acquired brain injury (ABI) continues to be one of the leading causes of long-term adult disability worldwide.[1,2] Two of the leading causes of ABI are TBI and stroke. It is estimated that more than 69 million individuals suffer a TBI each year[3]; and, of those hospitalized for a TBI in the United States, greater than 40% go on to develop long-term disability.[4] As many as 3.17 million people in the United States live with a long-term disability related to a TBI.[5] Strokes are the largest contributors to long-term disability globally.[1,2] The annual incidence of strokes in the United States is 795,000.[6]

TBIs are traditionally classified as either mild, moderate, or severe. Multiple classification schema exists to determine the severity of a TBI. One such example is from the VA/DoD[7] and classifies the severity of TBIs based on structural imaging, loss of consciousness (LOC), alterations of consciousness (AOC), posttraumatic amnesia (PTA), and the Glasgow Coma Scale (GCS). Of note, the DoD has suggested against using only the GCS to diagnose TBIs.[8] Importantly, 75% to 90% of all TBIs are classified as mild.[9,10] Applying the VA/DoD criteria, TBIs are mild if structural imaging is within normal limits, LOC occurs for no longer than 30 min, AOC and PTA resolve within 24 hours, and the patient scores no lower than 13 on the GCS.

Strokes are classified as either ischemic or hemorrhagic. Ischemic strokes may result from thrombosis, embolism, and/or hypoperfusion, whereas hemorrhagic strokes may result from intracerebral or subarachnoid hemorrhage. Ischemic strokes are by far the most common, accounting for up to 87% of total strokes in the United States.[6]

The sequelae following an ABI can be variable and often depend on the extent of the initial injury. Although some impairments resolve within the first few months following the injury, others may persist for years.[11-15] A thorough history is invaluable to elicit these common symptoms, especially when you are limited with your physical examination.

ADVANTAGES AND DISADVANTAGES OF TELEMEDICINE

The advantages and disadvantages to telemedicine for this unique population may have some overlap with other conditions found throughout this book. However, a quick review is warranted when faced with a decision of whether or not a telehealth visit is appropriate for the provider and the patient. Ideally, in all cases, at least the first visit will be face to face, and a thorough, comprehensive physical examination is performed to help guide future follow-up visits. Consider also having the patient return for a face-to-face visit if any significant changes to their health arise or once per year.

Advantages

- Can evaluate the patient in their home, assess how they perform activities of daily living in their own environment, and identify any barriers that exist.
- Can have quick access to speak with family and/or caregivers with the patient's permission.
- Improve access to care for those in a rural setting and those whose access to transportation is limited or impaired due to, for example, paresis, seizures, or visual dysfunction. In fact, one study demonstrated that a similar group of patients, ones with Parkinson disease, using telemedicine for care, on average, saved 100 miles of travel and 3 hours of time.[16]

- Limits missed appointments. Considering cognitive dysfunction in many patients with ABI, if the patient forgets an appointment, a phone call can be made, and the individual can quickly jump on to the telemedicine visit.

Disadvantages

- Limited ability to effectively assess for issues such as tone/spasticity.
- Poor audio/video quality. This pertains to some individuals in remote areas with poor signal but can also apply to individuals who are wheelchair bound or hemiparetic for example and have difficulty maneuvering their camera for appropriate assessment.
- There is a lack of human touch/connection, which can be significant in these individuals who already may feel depressed and isolated secondary to their acquired disabilities.
- Challenges with technology given brain injury and resultant cognitive dysfunction. Consider also that cerebrovascular accidents more commonly affect older individuals who may not be as adept with newer technologies.
- Effects of bright video screens or prolonged screen time can lead to headaches, fatigue, and visual complaints in this population.

TAKING HISTORY THROUGH TELEHEALTH

Obtaining a history should be very similar to that of an office visit, with a few caveats:

- At the beginning of the visit, always obtain a call-back number from the patient in the event the connection is poor.
- Have the patient confirm their home address or current location in case of emergency.
- Unlike an office visit, the practitioner is limited to a confined view of the patient. Ask the patient if they are currently alone and/or in a setting in which they feel comfortable discussing their medical history.
- Before the visit, center your image on your camera so that the patient can see you clearly. It can be difficult to have personal conversations and develop rapport virtually. Ensure that your patient feels you are giving them your full attention and that your visit is private.

Beyond a detailed investigation of the inciting event and their recovery process up to this point, in the subacute to chronic setting focus shifts to any possible sequelae that may impede community reintegration. As with all patients, using a holistic approach to history taking is optimal, keeping in mind that many symptoms that occur after ABIs can be managed with a focus on lifestyle changes. Do not forget to review medications, dive into social history, and inquire about premorbid conditions. A symptom-based approach is otherwise warranted, and the following section can serve as a quick reference guide.

- Mental health
  - Depression screening
    - Depression is highly prevalent following a TBI, regardless of severity.[17,18]
    - Approximately one-third of stroke survivors experience depression following their initial recovery.[19,20]
    - Consider routinely asking if the patient is feeling down or depressed, as many other symptoms can be addressed by first treating depression.[21]
  - Mood
    - Mood can be labile following an ABI; the patient should be asked if they have been experiencing any increases or changes in the following:

- Agitation
- Aggression
- Anxiety
- Paranoia
- Emotional lability
- Apathy
- Impulsivity
- Cognition
  - Cognitive impairment is one of the most common sequelae following an ABI.[11,14,22] More importantly, cognitive impairment is a risk factor for poor rehabilitation outcomes.[11,22]
  - Long-term cognitive sequelae following a TBI occur in as many as 15% of mild TBI cases and 65% of moderate-to-severe cases.[11] Research has shown that 43% of these individuals experience disability secondary to these sequelae.[11]
  - Patients should be asked if they have experienced changes in any of the following:
    - Memory
    - Attention
    - Concentration
    - Decision-making
- Headaches
  - Posttraumatic headaches (PTH) are the most common, persistent, physical symptom identified after a TBI.[12,13] PTHs typically resolve within weeks after injury but may persist for months to years.[12]
  - The patient should be asked the following regarding their headaches:
    - Character
    - Frequency
    - Intensity
    - Duration
    - Location
    - Relieving/worsening factors (triggers, if known)
    - Current medication regimen
- Sleep
  - Sleep disturbances create persistent, disabling complications for patients following a TBI.[23,24]
  - Patients should be asked if they are experiencing any of the following:
    - Excessive daytime sleepiness
    - Increased sleep need
    - Insomnia
    - Disrupted/fragmented sleep
    - Fatigue
      - Poststroke fatigue may be present in up 75% of cases.[25]
- Pain
  - Pain after stroke (PAS) is common and can manifest as various pain syndromes.[26] PAS has been found to worsen both depression and cognitive impairments in stroke survivors.[26]
  - The following potential pain generators should be discussed with the patient:
    - Spasticity
      - Velocity-dependent increase in muscle tone that displays increased resistance to passive stretching.
    - Complex regional pain syndrome

- Chronic pain, usually affecting an arm or leg, which can occur after an injury or stroke but is out of proportion to the initial injury. It is often accompanied by a variety of associated symptoms such as swelling, atrophy, and skin color changes.
- Poststroke shoulder pain
  - Shoulder subluxation secondary to motor weakness occurs in up to 84% of stroke cases.[27] Should also consider tendinitis and heterotopic ossification on the differential.
- Vertigo and dizziness
  - Posttraumatic dizziness has been found to be an independent predictor of failure to return to work following a TBI.[28]
    - Ask the patient if they have been experiencing dizziness or vertigo following their injury.
    - Ask about any recent falls and any current assistive devices they are using.
- Cranial nerve (CN) injuries
  - CN injuries after ABI most commonly involve the olfactory, facial, or oculomotor nerves.[29]
    - Ask the patient if they have been experiencing any of the following:
      - Anosmia/hyposmia
      - Diplopia or other visual changes or vision loss
      - Facial pain or paresthesia
- Neuromotor function
  - Motor dysfunction and paresis are hallmarks of a stroke. Increased muscle tone may also be present in 30% to 40% of cases.[30]
    - The following should be discussed with the patient:
      - Current physical therapy
        - If not in therapy, what are their barriers to participation
      - Changes in:
        - Strength
        - Balance
        - Coordination
        - Sensation
        - Gait
      - Falls/dropping objects
      - Ability to perform activities of daily living and instrumental activities of daily living
      - Dysphagia
        - Dysphagia is a major risk factor for aspiration pneumonia.[31]
        - Difficulty swallowing specific food or drink
        - Coughing while eating
        - Ask if they have had a formal swallow evaluation
        - Ask if they have previously had speech therapy
      - Changes in spasticity/increased tone
      - Wounds
      - Incontinence

PHYSICAL EVALUATION THROUGH TELEHEALTH

Conducting a physical examination via telehealth presents a unique set of challenges. In fact, the physical examination itself was previously identified by physicians as one of the most commonly reported factors inhibiting further implementation of telehealth to care for patients with mild TBI.[32] The following will be a guide to optimize your examination and help avoid any pitfalls during these visits. General considerations during the examination include the following:

- Have patience and remember to be flexible. There are times when a video connection cannot be made, and a phone visit will have to suffice. In these cases, have a low threshold for requesting a face-to-face visit for the near future.
- Trust your gut and understand the limitations of telemedicine. If you have any clinical concerns regarding the patient or see red flag signs, do not hesitate to recommend a face-to-face visit or to ask the patient to go directly to the emergency department.
- Always ensure patient safety. For example, consider fall risk when asking patients to stand or evaluating gait.
- Adjust volume so you can clearly hear the patient and inquire if they can hear you as well.
- Consider lighting, camera positioning, and patient positioning for adequate observation.[32]

RED FLAGS

Red flags in patients with brain injury encompass mainly neurologic symptoms but can also include additional at-risk systems. Findings that should prompt further emergent evaluation:

- Sudden change/decline in behavior, cognition, alertness, speech, strength, gait, sensation, or bowel/bladder function
- New-onset CN dysfunction, anisocoria, loss of vision, double vision, or seizures
- Numbness or weakness on one side of the body, slurred speech, confusion, vision change
- Unilateral swelling, especially along with tachypnea or respiratory distress
- A headache, nausea, vomiting, dizziness, or drowsiness that does not resolve[33,34]

PHYSICAL EXAMINATION

Many aspects pertinent to the examination of patients with ABI are accomplished through simple, yet close and detailed observations. Telehealth visits will not vary much from an in-person visit in that sense, but it may help to have a family member or a caregiver present during the examination for some select tests. Remember, subtle issues in the physical examination may be difficult to assess over video telehealth. It is critical to keep in mind the patient's history because of these limitations, as the history can often clue you in to these subtleties. And it bears repeating, maintain a low threshold for recommending a face-to-face visit or a visit to the emergency department for any serious concerns.

- Normal examination observations of all systems should be commented on, but focus will mainly concern the neurologic, musculoskeletal, and psychological systems.
- *Skin*
  ○ Observe if percutaneous endoscopic gastrostomy/tracheostomy/foley in place, nonerythematous. Observe surgical scars such as from craniotomy or endarterectomy. Evaluate any suspected or gross wounds or decubitus ulcers.
- HEENT (head, eyes, ears, nose, and throat)

- ○ If suspect or known visual neglect, ask the patient to draw a line across a piece of paper and bisect it by drawing a line in the middle.[35]
- Cardiovascular
  - ○ Lower extremity edema, and if present ask about warmth, erythema, or tenderness, as deep vein thrombosis occurrence is increased in this population.[36]
- Musculoskeletal
  - ○ Prompt patients through range-of-motion (ROM) exercises, with demonstration if needed, for upper and lower extremities
  - ○ Consider performing these tests if indicated through history
    - ▪ *Spurling maneuver*: evaluation for cervical radiculopathy for those who suffered whiplash concurrent with their TBI.[37] Patient extends neck then rotates side to side, "Look straight up, then to the left corner, now back just a bit more" and same thing to the right. A positive finding is the verbalization of radicular symptoms that go beyond the shoulder.[38]
    - ▪ *Sulcus sign*: this sign is apparent with shoulder subluxation, a common finding after stroke with resultant hemiparesis. To elicit it, ask the patient to be seated in an upright position, shoulder relaxed, and elbow resting in lap. Instruct patient to apply downward traction at elbow. If positive, a visible groove will be created at the shoulder.
- Neurologic
  - ○ Mental status
    - ▪ Conducting a Mini-Mental Status Examination (MMSE) has been shown to be an equivalent assessment regardless of telehealth versus in-person.[39,40]
      - • Have objects nearby and ready (pencil, watch, etc.)
      - • Choose words with easier pronunciation and speak clearly. "Quarter" has been found to be difficult to understand over video[40]
    - ▪ Recent studies have demonstrated superiority in sensitivity with the Montreal Cognitive Assessment's (MoCA) visuoexecutive subtests in patients with transient ischemic attack/stroke as compared with MMSE.[41,42] More information on the MoCA can be found here (www.mocatest.org). Of note, similar to the MMSE, MoCA administration via telehealth has been found to be reliable, accurate, and similar to in-person administration.[43]
  - ○ Speech
    - ▪ Describe rate, fluency, comprehension, repetition, volume, and tone
  - ○ CNs
    - ▪ CN I (olfactory)
      - • Ask the patient to confirm they can smell coffee or food.[44]
    - ▪ CN II (optic)
      - • Ask the patient about vision. If decreased or concerned, instruct patient to cover one eye at a time to evaluate vision by describing yourself, holding objects or pictures up, or counting number of fingers.
      - • Consider referring to the American Association of Ophthalmology Website (HYPERLINK "https://www.aao.org/eye-health/tips-prevention/home-eye-test-children-adults" \o "https://www.aao.org/eye-health/tips-prevention/home-eye-test-children-adults"https://www.aao.org/eye-health/tips-prevention/home-eye-test-children-adults) for Snellen charts and instructions for self-examination.[45,46]
      - • Ask the patient to move closer to screen to visualize pupil size.
    - ▪ CN III, IV, and VI (oculomotor, trochlear, abducens)
      - • Comment on ptosis, proptosis, and ocular alignment

- Ask the patient to glance fully left to right, then up and down
  - CN V (trigeminal)
    - Ask patients to touch all 3 divisions and if sensations are equal
    - Open and close mouth, bite down to clench jaw
  - CN VII (facial)
    - Ask the patient to smile, wrinkle their forehead, close their eyes, comment if nasolabial folds symmetric
  - CN VIII (vestibulocochlear)
    - Comment if the patient asks to have you repeat questions frequently
    - Ask the patient to rub their fingers together by each ear and see if they can hear the sound equally on either side
  - CN IX and X (glossopharyngeal and vagus)
    - Comment on any dysarthria and quality of speech
  - CN XI (accessory)
    - Ask the patient to shrug their shoulders and rotate their neck left and right
  - CN XII (hypoglossal)
    - Ask the patient to stick their tongue out
- Coordination
  - Demonstrate and ask the patient to perform rapid alternating movements including pronation-supination wrist slaps, alternating finger taps, heel-to-shin, and perform finger-to-nose-to-camera (remind to have camera positioned just beyond a full reach)
- *Proprioception*: always ensure patient safety. If a high concern for fall risk exists and no other person present, consider recommending face-to-face visit for evaluation. Otherwise, ask the patient to stand in front of their bed or couch to improve safety.
  - Romberg and tandem walking[44]
- *Reflexes:* user reliability and clinical significance may be limited but can walk patients through checking reflexes with the edge of a smartphone or spatula[47]
- Sensory
  - Ask the patient if they are having paresthesia. If so, have the patient outline the area of numbness for a better idea of distribution
  - Ask the patient to use pencil with eraser to test side-to-side sharp and dull sensations[44]
- *Motor:* because of the nature of telehealth physical examinations, the focus must shift to a more macro evaluation. For example, assessing for antigravity strength helps to appreciate where functional limitations may lie, even if more mild or subtle complaints of weakness are not clearly assessable.
  - *Upper extremity:* test antigravity shoulders abduction, elbow, wrist, and finger flexion, to help determine asymmetry thumb and forearm rolling[48]
  - *Lower extremity:* test antigravity hip flexion, knee extension, and dorsiflexion
  - Spasticity:
    - Ask the patient about weakness and stiffness and observe for abnormal posture or ROM[49]
    - See if the patient has difficulty opening their hand, extending arm, reaching for object, spreading knees apart, or raising foot
    - If a caregiver is present, you can instruct and demonstrate how to perform Modified Ashworth Assessment[49]
  - Gait

Table 1
Managing the sequelae of acquired brain injury

Symptoms	Nonpharmacologic Management	Pharmacologic Management	Telehealth Consideration
Mood (Anxiety/ Depression)	CBT, neuropsychology,[51] exercise & diet, breathing/relaxation techniques, Acupuncture	SSRI, SNRI, atypical antidepressants, TCA, serotonin modulators, MOAs	Patients with anxiety/depression shown to prefer telehealth visits vs F2F.[52] Cochrane database review found telerehab for depressive symptoms poststroke to be noninferior to in-person.[50]
Agitation/Irritability	Same as abovementioned, anger management, behavioral modification	Beta-blockers have best evidence for reducing agitation,[53–55] (propranolol best CNS penetration[56]) atypical antipsychotics,[57] (seroquel and olanzapine) mood stabilizing AEDs,[58] (valproic acid and carbamazepine)	Less likely to provoke patients with external stimuli. Increased safety for patient and provider. Video CBT shows significant and clinically meaningful reductions in anger.[59]
Posttraumatic Headaches	Physical therapy, ice/heat packs, CBT, biofeedback, massage therapy	Prophylaxis vs abortive, NSAIDs, APAP, ASA, triptans, beta-blockers, AEDs, TCAs	Please refer to the Don McGeary and Cindy McGeary's article, "Telerehabilitation for Headache Management," in this issue within this book.
Insomnia/Sleep	Sleep hygiene, sleep study to rule out OSA, CBT	Melatonin, hypnotics, antidepressants, antipsychotics, antihistamines	Assess bedroom with patient's permission to consider environment modifications. Tele-CBT shown to decrease insomnia severity index and be effective at improving sleep.[60]
Fatigue	Address sleep as abovementioned, aquatic therapy, exercise & diet, self-management strategies	Methylphenidate and modafinil,[61] melatonin[51]	Telehealth visits can save up to 3 h per visit.[16] Telerehab exercise programs show statistically significant improvements in fatigue.[62]

(continued on next page)

Table 1
(continued)

Symptoms	Nonpharmacologic Management	Pharmacologic Management	Telehealth Consideration
Cognitive Dysfunction	Neuropsychology evaluation,[51] speech therapy, compensatory strategies	Neurostimulant for attention, concentration, processing speed, initiation, orientation, verbalization (amantadine[63-66] and methylphenidate[57,58,63,67]), donepezil for memory[61]	Can reduce stress related to visit and save time from reduced transportation.[16] Systematic review found telecognitive rehabilitation to be effective when compared with in-person rehabilitation.[68]
Vestibular (Balance) Deficits	Vestibular rehabilitation, balance training, habituation techniques, DME (Cane, FWW)	Should avoid chronic use.[69] If needed acutely, antihistamines, anticholinergics, TCAs, SSRIs, and CCBs	Reduced fall risk. Can observe in home environment. Virtual reality rehab has been found to out-perform gait and balance training compared with conventional rehab.[70]
Visual Dysfunction	Neuro-ophthalmology referral, vision rehabilitation, visual scanning techniques, corrective eyewear		Ask if screen is causing any visual disturbance (headache, blurriness), consider phone visit if severe. Meta-analysis for screening for certain eye conditions found be effective using tele-ophthalmology services.[71]
Auditory Dysfunction	Audiology referral, hearing devices, white-noise generators, tinnitus CBT, environmental modifications, tinnitus retraining therapy		Can have patient wear headphones to modify volume and improve communication during visit or using text-based communication. Patients show high satisfaction in web-based services for hearing health.[72]
Motor Dysfunction/ Deficits	Both telerehab and in-person physical therapy, occupational therapy; orthotics/bracing, electrical stimulation	Antispasmodics, fluoxetine, or other SSRIs potentially,[73] botox	Systematic review of telerehab interventions for motor deficits after stroke were found to have equal or better effects when compared with in-person therapy.[74]

Abbreviations: ADLs, activities of daily living; AEDs, antiepileptic drugs; APAP, acetaminophen; ASA, aspirin; CBT, cognitive behavioral therapy; CCB, calcium channel blockers; DME, durable medical equipment; F2F, face-to-face visit; FWW, front wheel walker; MOA, monoamine oxidase inhibitor; NSAIDs, nonsteroidal anti-inflammatory drugs; OSA, obstructive sleep apnea; SNRI, serotonin norepinephrine reuptake inhibitor; SSRI, selective serotonin reuptake inhibitor; TCA, tricyclic antidepressant.

- As mentioned in the proprioception section, ensure safety before evaluation. Ask the patient to walk away from and toward the camera[47] to visualize entire gait phase as well as use of any assistive devices
- Psychological
  - Most observations in this section can be made throughout the visit. For a more comprehensive examination, please refer to the Mary J. Wells and colleageus' article, "Telehealth in Rehabilitation Psychology and Neuropsychology," in this issue within this book.
    - Observe patient's appearance: if dressed and groomed appropriately
    - Comment on if their affect is flat versus congruent with the topic of conversation
    - Evaluate their mood: if euthymic, agitated, anxious, or depressed
    - Rate of speech and tone: if pressured, hyperverbal, or conversant
    - Listen if patient's responses and comments are appropriate
    - Ask the patient about visual or auditory hallucinations
    - Comment on recall, insight, and judgment

TELEHEALTH MANAGEMENT OF ACQUIRED BRAIN INJURY

Table 1 provides a broad overview of management strategies for the most common sequelae of ABIs and telehealth considerations in their implementation. For more in-depth management strategies, the authors recommend referring to the following:

- Physical Medicine and Rehabilitation Clinics of North America: Traumatic Brain Injury Rehabilitation
- Physical Medicine and Rehabilitation Clinics of North America: Stroke Rehabilitation

It is also worth noting that the rehabilitation management of patients with ABI extend beyond just physician visits and that telerehabilitation services exist in most, if not all, associated services including physical therapy, occupational therapy, speech and language pathology, neuropsychology, and tele-support groups. Although research has only recently started into the efficacy of these services, the preliminary results seem promising. A recent Cochrane Review on telerehabilitation for stroke offered some comforting results for those anxious about the transition to telehealth management for this cohort. The study found no difference in regard to activities of daily living, balance outcomes, health-related quality of life, depressive symptoms, and upper limb function between telerehabilitation and usual care when treating patients in the sub-acute and chronic phases.[50]

SUMMARY

Although using telehealth technology to care for patients with ABIs can seem daunting at first, by using active listening, communicating well with your patients, and applying a bit of creativity for the physical examination, telehealth visits can become a preferred method for management in the long term. The advantages of telehealth can be numerous for this particular population, and satisfaction and compliance can increase when this option is available to them. However, knowing the limitations of this technology is key. Always trust your instincts and refer the patient for a face-to-face visit or to the emergency department if you have any concerns. If you are open and honest with your patients, there is no doubt that your telehealth visits will be successful ones.

CLINICS CARE POINTS

- Because of the limitations of the telemedicine physical examination, a thorough history is invaluable and will help focus on your assessments.
- Telehealth evaluations can be reliable and often equivalent to in-person examinations but remember to ensure safety when asking a patient to perform any challenging or complex physical examination maneuvers.
- Trust your gut. If you suspect any red flag symptoms, no matter how subtle, error on the side of safety and have the patient be evaluated in person or through the emergency department.
- Telehealth visits for this population and their caregivers can ease the burden of transportation, improve compliance, and increase overall satisfaction.
- Management strategies are largely unaffected in the telehealth setting, and telerehab options have been found to be equal or superior to in-person therapy to treat many associated deficits.

DISCLOSURES

The authors have nothing to disclose.

REFERENCES

1. GBD 2016 Neurology Collaborators. Global, regional, and national burden of neurological disorders, 1990-2016: a systematic analysis for the Global Burden of Disease Study 2016. Lancet Neurol 2019;18(5):459–80.
2. Krishnamurthi RV, Feigin VL, Forouzanfar MH, et al, GBD Stroke Experts Group. Global and regional burden of first-ever ischaemic and haemorrhagic stroke during 1990-2010: findings from the global burden of disease study 2010. Lancet Glob Health 2013;1(5):e259–81.
3. Dewan MC, Rattani A, Gupta S, et al. Estimating the global incidence of traumatic brain injury. J Neurosurg 2018;130(4):1080–97. Accessed Nov 2, 2020.
4. Selassie AW, Zaloshnja E, Langlois JA, et al. Incidence of long-term disability following traumatic brain injury hospitalization, United States, 2003. J Head Trauma Rehabil 2008;23(2):123–31.
5. Zaloshnja E, Miller T, Langlois JA, et al. Prevalence of long-term disability from traumatic brain injury in the civilian population of the United States, 2005. J Head Trauma Rehabil 2008;23(6):394–400.
6. Virani SS, Alonso A, Benjamin EJ, et al, American Heart Association Council on Epidemiology and Prevention Statistics Committee and Stroke Statistics Subcommittee. Heart disease and stroke statistics-2020 update: a report from the American heart association. Circulation 2020;141(9):e139–596.
7. STATEMENTS Q. VA/DoD clinical practice guideline for management of concussion/mild traumatic brain injury. J Rehabil Res Dev 2009;46(6):1–60.
8. Assistant Secretary of Defense. Traumatic brain injury: updated definition and reporting. Washington, DC: Department of Defense; 2015.
9. Kraus JF, McArthur DL. Epidemiologic aspects of brain injury. Neurol Clin 1996; 14(2):435–50.
10. Vos PE, Battistin L, Birbamer G, et al, & European Federation of Neurological Societies. EFNS guideline on mild traumatic brain injury: report of an EFNS task force. Eur J Neurol 2002;9(3):207–19.

11. Rabinowitz AR, Levin HS. Cognitive sequelae of traumatic brain injury. Psychiatr Clin North Am 2014;37(1):1–11.

12. Lucas S. Posttraumatic headache: clinical characterization and management. Curr Pain Headache Rep 2015;19(10):48.

13. Lew HL, Otis JD, Tun C, et al. Prevalence of chronic pain, posttraumatic stress disorder, and persistent postconcussive symptoms in OIF/OEF veterans: polytrauma clinical triad. J Rehabil Res Dev 2009;46(6):697–702.

14. Patel M, Coshall C, Rudd AG, et al. Natural history of cognitive impairment after stroke and factors associated with its recovery. Clin Rehabil 2003;17(2):158–66.

15. Yamamoto S, Levin HS, Prough DS. Mild, moderate and severe: terminology implications for clinical and experimental traumatic brain injury. Curr Opin Neurol 2018;31(6):672–80.

16. Dorsey ER, Venkataraman V, Grana MJ, et al. Randomized controlled clinical trial of "virtual house calls" for Parkinson disease. JAMA Neurol 2013;70:565–70.

17. Ouellet MC, Beaulieu-Bonneau S, Sirois MJ, et al. Depression in the first year after traumatic brain injury. J Neurotrauma 2018;35(14):1620–9.

18. Ponsford J, Alway Y, Gould KR. Epidemiology and natural history of psychiatric disorders after TBI. J Neuropsychiatry Clin Neurosci 2018;30(4):262–70.

19. Ferro JM, Caeiro L, Figueira ML. Neuropsychiatric sequelae of stroke. Nat Rev Neurol 2016;12(5):269–80.

20. Das J, G K R. Post stroke depression: the sequelae of cerebral stroke. Neurosci Biobehav Rev 2018;90:104–14.

21. Kruse RC, Li Z, Prideaux CC, et al. Pharmacologic treatment for depression at injury is associated with fewer clinician visits for persistent symptoms after mild traumatic brain injury: a medical record review study. PM R 2018;10(9):898–902.

22. Whyte E, Skidmore E, Aizenstein H, et al. Cognitive impairment in acquired brain injury: a predictor of rehabilitation outcomes and an opportunity for novel interventions. PM R 2011;3(6 Suppl 1):S45–51.

23. Duclos C, Dumont M, Wiseman-Hakes C, et al. Sleep and wake disturbances following traumatic brain injury. Pathol Biol (Paris) 2014;62(5):252–61.

24. Orff HJ, Ayalon L, Drummond SP. Traumatic brain injury and sleep disturbance: a review of current research. J Head Trauma Rehabil 2009;24(3):155–65.

25. Choi-Kwon S, Kim JS. Poststroke fatigue: an emerging, critical issue in stroke medicine. Int J Stroke 2011;6(4):328–36.

26. Delpont B, Blanc C, Osseby GV, et al. Pain after stroke: a review. Rev Neurol (Paris) 2018;174(10):671–4.

27. American Stroke Association. Questions about shoulder pain. 2018. www.stroke.org/. Accessed November 4, 2020.

28. Chamelian L, Feinstein A. Outcome after mild to moderate traumatic brain injury: the role of dizziness. Arch Phys Med Rehabil 2004;85(10):1662–6.

29. Coello AF, Canals AG, Gonzalez JM, et al. Cranial nerve injury after minor head trauma. J Neurosurg 2010;113(3):547–55.

30. Pundik S, McCabe J, Skelly M, et al. Association of spasticity and motor dysfunction in chronic stroke. Ann Phys Rehabil Med 2019;62(6):397–402.

31. Martino R, Foley N, Bhogal S, et al. Dysphagia after stroke: incidence, diagnosis, and pulmonary complications. Stroke 2005;36(12):2756–63.

32. Martinez RN, Hogan TP, Lones K, et al. Evaluation and treatment of mild traumatic brain injury through the implementation of clinical video telehealth: provider perspectives from the veterans health administration. PM R 2017;9(3):231–40.

33. Concussion danger signs. Centers for disease control and prevention. Available at: https://www.cdc.gov/headsup/basics/concussion_danger_signs.html. Accessed October 5, 2020.
34. Stroke signs and symptoms. Centers for disease control and prevention. Internet. Updated Aug 28, 2020. .Available at: https://www.cdc.gov/stroke/signs_symptoms.htm. Accessed October 5, 2020.
35. Robblee J. Conducting a telemedicine neurologic exam. American headache society video. Available at: https://americanheadachesociety.org/covid-19-resources/. Accessed October 21, 2020.
36. Cifu DX, Kaelin DL, Wall BE. Deep venous thrombosis: incidence on admission to a brain injury rehabilitation program. Arch Phys Med Rehabil 1996;77(11): 1182–5.
37. Thoomes EJ, van Geest S, van der Windt DA, et al. Value of physical tests in diagnosing cervical radiculopathy: a systematic review. Spine J 2018;18(1):179–89.
38. Tong HC, Haig AJ, Yamakawa K. The Spurling test and cervical radiculopathy. Spine (Phila Pa 1976) 2002;27(2):156–9.
39. McEachern W, Kirk A, Morgan DG, et al. Reliability of the MMSE administered in-person and by telehealth. Can J Neurol Sci 2008;35(5):643–6.
40. Ciemins Elizabeth, Holloway Barbara, Coon Patricia, et al. Telemedicine and the mini-mental state examination: assessment from a distance. Telemed J E Health 2009;15:476–8.
41. Shi D, Chen X, Li Z. Diagnostic test accuracy of the Montreal cognitive assessment in the detection of post-stroke cognitive impairment under different stages and cutoffs: a systematic review and meta-analysis. Neurol Sci 2018;39(4): 705–16.
42. Fu C, Jin X, Chen B, et al. Comparison of the mini-mental state examination and montreal cognitive assessment executive subtests in detecting post-stroke cognitive impairment. Geriatr Gerontol Int 2017;17(12):2329–35.
43. DeYoung N, Shenal BV. The reliability of the montreal cognitive assessment using telehealth in a rural setting with veterans. J Telemed Telecare 2019;25(4): 197–203.
44. Verduzco-Gutierrez M, Bean AC, Tenforde AS, et al. How to Conduct an Outpatient Telemedicine Rehabilitation or Prehabilitation Visit. PM R 2020;12:714–20.
45. Boes Christopher J, Leep Hunderfund Andrea N, Jennifer M, et al. A primer on the in-home teleneurologic examination A COVID-19 pandemic imperative. Neurol Clin Pract 2020. https://doi.org/10.1212/CPJ.0000000000000876. 10.1212/CPJ.0000000000000876.
46. Home eye test for children and adults. American academy of ophthalmology. Available at: https://www.aao.org/eye-health/tips-prevention/home-eye-test-children-adults. Accessed October 11, 2020.
47. Laskowski ER, Johnson SE, Shelerud RA, et al. The telemedicine musculoskeletal examination. Mayo Clin Proc 2020;95(8):1715–31. Erratum in: Mayo Clin Proc. 2020 Oct;95(10):2299. PMID: 32753146; PMCID: PMC7395661.
48. Nowak Dennis. The thumb rolling test: a novel variant of the forearm rolling test. Can J Neurol Sci 2011;38:129–32.
49. Harper KA, Butler EC, Hacker ML, et al. A comparative evaluation of telehealth and direct assessment when screening for spasticity in residents of two long-term care facilities. Clin Rehabil 2020;2. https://doi.org/10.1177/0269215520963845.
50. Laver KE, Schoene D, Crotty M, et al. Telerehabilitation services for stroke. Cochrane Database Syst Rev 2013;2013(12):CD010255. Update in: Cochrane

Database Syst Rev. 2020 Jan 31;1:CD010255. PMID: 24338496; PMCID: PMC6464866.

51. Cicerone KD, Langenbahn DM, Braden C, et al. Evidence-based cognitive rehabilitation: updated review of the literature from 2003 through 2008. Arch Phys Med Rehabil 2011;92(4):519–30.

52. Norden JG, Wang JX, Desai SA, et al. Utilizing a novel unified healthcare model to compare practice patterns between telemedicine and in-person visits. Digit Health 2020;6. 2055207620958528.

53. Fleminger S, Greenwood RRJ, Oliver DL. Pharmacological management for agitation and aggression in people with acquired brain injury. Cochrane Database Syst Rev 2006;(Issue 4):CD003299.

54. Brooke MM, Patterson DR, Questad KA, et al. The treatment of agitation during initial hospitalization after traumatic brain injury. Arch Phys Med Rehabil 1992; 73:917–21.

55. Mysiw WJ, Sandel ME. The agitated brain injured patient. Part 2: pathophysiology and treatment. Arch Phys Med Rehabil 1997;78:213–20.

56. Meyfroidt G, Baguley IJ, Menon DK. Paroxysmal sympathetic hyperactivity: the storm after acute brain injury. Lancet Neurol 2017;16(9):721–9. Erratum in: Lancet Neurol. 2018 Mar;17 (3):203. PMID: 28816118.

57. Talsky A, Pacione LR, Shaw T, et al. Pharmacological interventions for traumatic brain injury. Psychostimulants, antidepressants, and other agents may speed the recovery of patients suffering from the functional deficits that follow an insult to the brain. BCMJ 2010;53:26–31.

58. Effie Chew MD, Ross D, Zafonte DO. Pharmacological management of neurobehavioral disorders following traumatic brain injury—A state-of-the-art review. J Rehabil Res Dev 2009;46(6):851–78.

59. Morland LA, Greene CJ, Rosen CS, et al. Telemedicine for anger management therapy in a rural population of combat veterans with posttraumatic stress disorder: a randomized noninferiority trial. J Clin Psychiatry 2010;71(7):855–63.

60. Seyffert M, Lagisetty P, Landgraf J, et al. Internet-delivered cognitive behavioral therapy to treat insomnia: a systematic review and meta-analysis. PLoS One 2016;11(2):e0149139.

61. Zhang L, Plotkin RC, Wang G, et al. Cholinergic augmentation with donepezil enhances recovery in short-term memory and sustained attention after traumatic brain injury. Arch Phys Med Rehabil 2004;85(7):1050–5.

62. Galiano-Castillo N, Cantarero-Villanueva I, Fernández-Lao C, et al. Telehealth system: a randomized controlled trial evaluating the impact of an internet-based exercise intervention on quality of life, pain, muscle strength, and fatigue in breast cancer survivors. Cancer 2016;122(20):3166–74.

63. Levy M, Andrea B, Theresa C, et al. Treatment of agitation following traumatic brain injury: a review of the literature. NeuroRehabilitation 2005;20:279–306.

64. Hammond F, Allison KB, James HN, et al. Effectiveness of amantadine hydrochloride in the reduction of chronic traumatic brain injury irritability and aggression. J Head Trauma Rehabil 2014;29(5):391–9.

65. Leone H, Polsonetti BW. Amantadine for traumatic brain injury: does it improve cognition and reduce agitation. J Clin Pharm Ther 2005;30:101–4.

66. Nickels JL, Schneider WN, Dombovy ML, et al. Clinical use of amantadine in brain injury rehabilitation. Brain Inj 1994;8(8):709–18.

67. Hicks AJ, Clay FJ, Hopwood M, et al. The efficacy and harms of pharmacological interventions for aggression after traumatic Brain Injury—Systematic Review. Front Neurol 2019;10:1169.

68. Cotelli M, Manenti R, Brambilla M, et al. Cognitive telerehabilitation in mild cognitive impairment, Alzheimer's disease and frontotemporal dementia: a systematic review. J Telemed Telecare 2019;25(2):67–79.
69. Bronstein AM, Lempert T. Management of the patient with chronic dizziness [review]. Restor Neurol Neurosci 2010;28(1):83–90.
70. Lei C, Sunzi K, Dai F, et al. Effects of virtual reality rehabilitation training on gait and balance in patients with Parkinson's disease: a systematic review. PLoS One 2019;14(11):e0224819.
71. Kawaguchi A, Sharafeldin N, Sundaram A, et al. Tele-ophthalmology for age-related macular degeneration and diabetic retinopathy screening: a systematic review and meta-analysis. Telemed J E Health 2018;24(4):301–8.
72. Ratanjee-Vanmali H, Swanepoel W, Laplante-Lévesque A. Patient uptake, experience, and satisfaction using web-based and face-to-face hearing health services: process evaluation study. J Med Internet Res 2020;22(3):e15875.
73. Chollet F, Tardy J, Albucher JF, et al. Fluoxetine for motor recovery after acute ischaemic stroke (FLAME): a randomised placebo-controlled trial. Lancet Neurol 2011;10(2):123–30. Erratum in: Lancet Neurol. 2011 Mar;10(3):205. PMID: 21216670.
74. Sarfo FS, Ulasavets U, Opare-Sem OK, et al. Tele-rehabilitation after stroke: an updated systematic review of the literature. J Stroke Cerebrovasc Dis 2018; 27(9):2306–18.

Telehealth for Amyotrophic Lateral Sclerosis and Multiple Sclerosis

Ileana M. Howard, MD[a,b],*, Kathleen Burgess, MD, MS[a,b]

KEYWORDS

- Amyotrophic lateral sclerosis • Multiple sclerosis • Telehealth • Telemedicine

KEY POINTS

- Neurodegenerative diseases, such as amyotrophic lateral sclerosis (ALS) and multiple sclerosis (MS), require ongoing interdisciplinary team management to proactively adapt the plan of care based on anticipated disease progression.
- Providers caring for people living with MS or ALS are required to provide care that is flexible, responds to a changing medical state, and is patient-centered.
- Providing care for people with MS or ALS via various telehealth venues is feasible and effective.
- Telehealth studies addressing needs of people living with MS should continue to focus on improving the quality and rigor in their design.

INTRODUCTION

Neurodegenerative disorders (**Box 1**), such as amyotrophic lateral sclerosis (ALS) and multiple sclerosis (MS), present with unique disease trajectories, diagnostic considerations, and a complex array of secondary symptoms in comparison with other neuro-rehabilitation diagnoses. Using telehealth to care for people with neurologic disorders is not new and was first initiated with telestroke in 1999. Prior to the coronavirus pandemic, movement to incorporate telehealth for neurodegenerative disorders was hindered by lack of support from insurance carriers, lack of inexpensive technology, and lack of acceptance of a new technology by medical providers.

The coronavirus pandemic has accelerated the process of acceptance of telehealth by clients and providers. Prior to this time, telehealth medical visits were compared with a face to face visit. At that time, convenience and travel cost savings benefited

Neither of the authors have financial or other conflicts of interest to disclose.
[a] Rehabilitation Care Services, VA Puget Sound Healthcare System, 1660 South Columbian Way, Seattle, WA 98108, USA; [b] Department of Rehabilitation Medicine, University of Washington, 325 Ninth Avenue, Box 359612 Seattle, WA 98104, USA
* Corresponding author:
E-mail address: ileana.howard@va.gov

Box 1
Neurodegenerative disease
Alzheimer disease
ALS
Friedreich ataxia
Huntington disease
Lewy body disease
Multiple sclerosis
Parkinson disease
Spinal muscular atrophy

the client. Advances in technology such as the prolific spread of personal computer ownership with cameras, smart phones, and high-speed Internet were lowering barriers to use. However, since the coronavirus pandemic, the face-to-face visit now has the added potential to include exposure to the coronavirus with potential dire consequences for all parties involved. Consequently, both clients and medical providers have now embraced telehealth to the extent that the virtual medical room will most likely continue to play a much more significant role in medical visits long after the pandemic is over.

Additionally, increased access to and use of the Internet have allowed for more people to use telelehealth. Per the Pew Research Center, approximately 90% of Americans use the Internet.[1] Use is highest in the 18- to 29- year-old age group and lowest in those over the age of 65. Rural Americans use the Internet less than urban dwellers do 63% to 71%. Lower income, less education, and minority status may cause more reliance on cell phones alone compared with using broadband.

Both ALS and MS are appropriate neurodegenerative disorders to use as a framework for how to incorporate telehealth into the provider's matrix. ALS, also known as Lou Gehrig disease, is a neurodegenerative neuromuscular disorder and the most common motor neuron disease. Although the precise pathophysiology of this disease remains largely unclear, loss of motor neurons leads to loss of control of voluntary muscles. ALS can affect various muscles, leading to inability to walk, use arms/hands, speak, swallow, and breathe. In addition, there is growing recognition of extramotor manifestations of the disease, including cognitive impairment affecting more than half of patients with ALS[2] and autonomic nervous system dysfunction,[3] challenging the previous conception of ALS as a strictly motor neuron disease.

Physical decline with ALS is variable although tends to occur more rapidly than other neurodegenerative diseases like Parkinson, Huntington, or Alzheimer diseases. The average survival from onset to death is 2 to 5 years.[4] Consequently, health care providers who care for people living with ALS frequently are required to be flexible, be ready to address new physical deficits and possibly address palliative care issues early on in the client-provider relationship.

Once disability is significant, and mobility, fatigue, mechanical breathing support, and cognition are significantly impaired, travel to see a medical provider can be an ominous endeavor. Additionally, nearly half of people living with ALS in the United State live more than 50 miles from a multidisciplinary ALS clinic.[5] Add to this the fact that ALS specialists and interdisciplinary teams are typically in larger metropolis areas, and one can see that telehealth offers a unique opportunity to provide care to people living with ALS.

MS, another neurodegenerative disorder, is the most common immune-mediated disorder affecting the central nervous system. It is estimated to impact approximately 750,000 people in the United States[6] and is the number one cause of disability in young adults. Although the exact cause of destruction is unclear, altered T and B cells cause destruction to the myelin and axons in gray and white matter in the brain and spinal cord. This results in a variety of deficits including weakness in the arm and legs, sensory deficits, speech and swallow impairments, fatigue, bowel and bladder dysfunction, spasticity, visual changes, pain, and mood and cognitive alterations.

The disease course of MS is variable. Some people experience significant or mild relapses wherein their function is impaired for a certain period of time (24 hours to 30 days), but then they experience some degree of resolution of their symptoms, which can be partial or complete. Alternatively, a smaller percentage of people do not experience these relapses and tend to have a slow progression of their disability. Unlike ALS, people can live with MS and accompanying significant disability for many years. Overall, It is calculated that MS can take approximately 7 years off someone's life,[7] and progressing from diagnosis to death in a few short years, like ALS, is rare.

Consequently, health care providers caring for people living with MS may also need to adapt to a changing presentation in their patients. Similar to ALS, people living with MS may live rurally and have limited access to local professionals who specialize in MS. In 2007, Minden showed that at least 31% of people living with MS did not have access to specialty care.[8] Again, telehealth provides an alternative way to provide specialized health care to this patient population.

Because of their substantial physical, psychological and social needs, people living with ALS and MS may require frequent, specialized, and interdisciplinary care. The object of this article is to present a summary of how a rehabilitative approach to neurodegenerative disorders can be addressed through a telehealth framework.

Telehealth and telemedicine are terms used to describe providing health care services to patients through the use of technology. There is no 1 accepted definition. Service may be provided through a variety of modes including telephone, Web-based applications, face-to-face video telehealth, and store and forward mechanisms. For the purpose of this article, the authors will use telehealth to refer to services provided by physicians or other health care providers to clients through the use of technology.

TELEHEALTH FOR MULTIPLE SCLEROSIS
Background

MS has long been used to test the feasibility and impact of telehealth. However, studies have had their limitations. A Cochrane review in 2015[9] looked at randomized and controlled clinical trials that compared telerehabilitation intervention/s in people living with MS with a control intervention. Out of a possible 4030 articles, ultimately only 9 articles were reviewed. The methodological quality of the studies was found to be low, and evidence was low as well with regard to interventions causing improvement in short-term disability, improving function, or quality of life. Evidence on cost effectiveness was not found, and adverse events were not noted.

Yeroushalmi and colleagues in 2020[10] did a more recent comprehensive literature review of telemedicine and multiple sclerosis looking at articles through January 2018. They looked at peer-reviewed, full-text, English language studies and excluded single case studies, pediatric studies, poster and symposium abstracts and nonpeer-reviewed publications. They ultimately reviewed 28 articles. Because of the heterogeneity of the studies, they were unable to do a meta-analysis. They found that randomized controlled studies showed either no significant difference between telehealth and face-to-face visits or showed beneficial outcomes for people with MS. They opined that telemedicine was shown to be beneficial, cost-effective, and well-accepted by clients and providers in terms of symptom management and clinical examinations. Most of the studies were considered to be low cost. They commented that implementation of telemedicine can be restricted because of limited or no insurance coverage. They remarked some studies showed a lack of compliance and low engagement over time. Cognitive and neurologic impairments also posed certain challenges, especially when there was no caregiver to provide assistance.

Other researchers have shown that telehealth is well accepted by clients, caregivers, and providers[11,12] and is as effective as usual care.[13] A systematic review of telehealth delivered to people with disabilities living in rural areas was completed in 2019. This review did not look at a specific disease, age group, type of outcome, or geographic area. The researchers ultimately assessed 11 studies from peer-reviewed journals. Overall, they found that clients were satisfied with telehealth intervention, as well as caregivers and providers. They found that some studies were small, lacked controls, and did not offer comparisons with outcomes of traditional face-to-face interventions.[12]

Telehealth and Diagnosis of Multiple Sclerosis

There have been no studies looking at the reliability of diagnosing MS via a telehealth visit. Although the coronavirus pandemic has put immense pressure on both the client and the provider to avoid all unnecessary in person visits, there are times when a clinician simply cannot get enough data to make an accurate diagnosis via telehealth. In these cases, per the American Academy of Neurology (AAN), it is recommended to document the provider's impression along with limitations and recommend an in-person evaluation. The AAN recognizes that without specialized equipment or a competent medical aid on the client's end, a comprehensive eye examination, many components of the neuromuscular examination including reflexes, detailed assessment of tone and strength and vestibular testing are generally not able to be completed through video telehealth.[14]

Assessing Disease Progression Using Telehealth

Despite the limitations listed previously, there are enough aspects of the neuromuscular examination that can take place over video telehealth to make assessing disease progression viable in some instances. Bove and colleagues[15] demonstrated that the EDSS can be reliably performed over telehealth. Additionally, patient-reported outcome measures such as the Patient Determined Disease Steps (PDDS) have been developed specifically for MS and have been shown to strongly correlate with EDSS scores.[16] Other self-assessment forms such as the MSIS-29 can also be used to help the provider assess disease progression.[17]

Telehealth and Symptom Treatment

Providers who care for people living with MS understand the myriad ways MS can impact function. Various symptoms have been shown to be successfully addressed through telehealth.

Exercise and physical activity

Exercise has been shown to improve walking speed[18] and quality of life, decrease falls, improve function, decrease disease progression, and improve mood in people living with MS.[19,20] Plow and colleagues[21] showed that telephone-delivered physical activity intervention improved physical activity in people living with MS. Rintala and colleagues[22] completed a meta-analysis on technology-based distance physical rehabilitation interventions. Their analysis included studies that were Internet based, telephone based, or a combination of a telephone with a pedometer. Results showed that technology-based distant physical rehabilitation interventions had a statistically significant effect on physical activity compared with control groups, similar to control groups in terms of effect on walking, and had a significant impact on physical activity when compared with no treatment. There did not appear to be a significant difference in outcomes based on the mode of technology used. Additionally, behavioral intervention provided over telehealth has been shown to improve physical activity in people living with MS.[13,20]

Fatigue

Fatigue can be a major problem for people living with MS, and up to 90% of people report fatigue at some time.[23] In addition, fatigue is frequently reported by clients to be their most disabling symptom.[24] Fatigue in MS is likely multifactorial, resulting from the disease process of MS itself, medication effects, environmental factors, altered cognition, and/or depression. Behavioral interventions have been shown to be effective at reducing fatigue in people living with MS and have been shown to be valid when done remotely via telephone and video telehealth.[21,25,26]

Mood

MS can have a significant impact on mood. Etiology is likely multifactorial because of disease impacts on the brain, medication effects, impact of chronic disease, and disability. Egner and colleagues demonstrated that rehabilitative care addressing various concerns, including depression, can be successfully addressed via telephone or video telehealth.[27] Various treatments such as mindfulness,[28] cognitive behavioral therapy,[29] self-management,[25] exercise,[30,31] and psychotherapy[32] have been shown to be effective, decreasing depression in people living with MS, both via telephone and through video telehealth.

Symptom management

Various studies have shown multiple other aspects of MS care can be addressed via telehealth including video gaming to improve cognition,[33] medication monitoring,[34] online support groups,[35] cognitive assessments,[36] treatment of chronic pain,[25] and dietary interventions.[37] Although not in patients with multiple sclerosis, telehealth has been shown to be a reliable way to do home safety evaluations[38] and support caregivers.[39]

TELEHEALTH FOR AMYOTROPHIC LATERAL SCLEROSIS

ALS presents several unique challenges to the rehabilitation team. With a mean survival of 3 to 5 years, ALS often presents a model of relatively rapidly progressive disease that tests the limits of the telehealth system. The ALS interdisciplinary team must not only address the current functional limitations of the patient, but also anticipate future needs as the disease progresses. Quarterly visits with the interdisciplinary team are considered standard of care[40] because of the relatively rapid rate of progression in this disease.

Diagnosis and Monitoring Progression

Delays in diagnosis of ALS are common, with reported delays from 8 to 15 months.[41] Reasons for delay are multifactorial, but include limited access to neuromuscular specialists. In the absence of reliable disease biomarkers, ALS remains a clinical diagnosis, primarily based on careful history and physical examination and supported by laboratory and electrodiagnostic testing findings. Access to care is even more challenging for rural-dwelling individuals with limited access to subspecialist care. International teleconsultation for neuromuscular diagnoses has been described.[42] Consensus on optimizing the neuromuscular examination for telehealth is lacking, but there are early reports of means of carrying out this evaluation with available technology.[43]

Following diagnosis, several assessments are used routinely in the ALS clinic to monitor the burden of disease over time, including pulmonary function testing and standardized outcome measures, such as the ALS FRS-R. These outcome measures may be used to track disease progression and response to treatment, determine eligibility for clinical trials, or guide clinical interventions. Spirometry testing results may guide timing and help risk stratify feeding tube placement or eligibility for hospice services. Small handheld spirometers are available to provide measurements for forced vital capacity (FVC). During the COVID-19 pandemic, lack of access to spirometry impacted most NEALS consortium ALS sites.[44] Several other peripheral devices have been employed to track outcome measurements for ALS in the patient's home (**Box 2**).

Interdisciplinary Care for Amyotrophic Lateral Sclerosis by Telehealth

Once a diagnosis of ALS is established, quarterly multidisciplinary team visits are the standard of care. Fortunately, there is evidence to support equivalent outcomes with telehealth-delivered multidisciplinary care as compared to traditional face-to-face visits.[45] In addition, telehealth may lend itself well to more integrated interprofessional models (interdisciplinary and transdisciplinary care) out of necessity; these models are associated with higher satisfaction for both patient and health care professional.[46] While a patient may routinely come to the outpatient clinic for a lengthy interdisciplinary team visit spanning several hours, videoconferencing fatigue is pervasive[47] and may limit the length of time patients are able to tolerate sitting in front of the camera and device for a health care visit. Therefore, interdisciplinary clinic appointments should be compressed when possible to maximize efficiency and minimize the redundancy often present in the traditional multidisciplinary clinic visit. Team conferences may be carried out similarly by virtual conference. Patients report satisfaction with neurologic consultation, convenience of receiving care at home, and economic and time savings compared with traditional care.[48]

Care coordination is an important component of high-quality ALS care that often is performed remotely in most cases. Most care coordination already likely exists as

---

Box 2
Examples of peripheral devices for physical assessment in amyotrophic lateral sclerosis in conjunction with telehealth

Handheld spirometer

Pulse oximeter

Dynamometer

Physical activity monitor/accelerometer

Quantitative speech assessment by digital voice recording

GPS data from cellular phones

hybrid (virtual/traditional) models with a combination of telephone, secure email, and in-person visits. There is growing interest into the concept of incorporating peripheral equipment such as a pulse oximeter or mobile device applications to facilitate remote monitoring and triage of medical concerns by the coordinator.[49–51] Although the bulk of peripheral devices for the collection of outcomes data, such as accelerometers has been used for research purposes,[52] more work needs to be done to best understand how to incorporate these devices into clinical practice.

As mentioned earlier in this article, a main barrier to ALS care is geographic inaccessibility. Even when individuals are able to travel to the ALS specialty care team, they rely on their local care providers for follow-up and interval care needs. Telehealth provides opportunities to foster collaboration between the local providers and the subspecialty team in a way that might not be possible under a traditional care model. With group video appointments, a home health therapist or primary care provider has the potential to join in the video conference and exchange information with the subspecialist team.

The leading cause of death in ALS relates to aspiration pneumonia and respiratory failure.[53] Optimal management of the person with neuromuscular respiratory failure often requires not only provision of the appropriate equipment, but ongoing follow-up for training and troubleshooting to support adherence and optimal use of noninvasive mechanical ventilation and pulmonary hygiene. Telehealth has been employed to deliver this care; this intervention has been found to result in decreased health care utilization (emergency room visits and hospitalizations).[54,55] Telehealth care is well-received by individuals with ALS on noninvasive ventilation.[56]

Patients with ALS often require specialized therapy evaluations to make recommendations on durable medical equipment (DME) and other interventions appropriate to their current and future needs. Telehealth can connect the specialized therapist to a person with ALS who otherwise would not be able to access the ALS center and ensure that the most appropriate equipment is ordered that can adapt to expected progression of disability. These evaluations may require either a trained telepresenter or a local therapist equipped to perform physical measurements. Home safety evaluations can be provided through the means of telehealth, which is a great benefit to patients with ALS and their families to adapt the home to increase safety and accessibility. Alternatively, asynchronous telemedicine has been described to perform home-based evaluations by using a nurse to perform the home visit and videotaping and sending the content to the specialty team for review at a later time.[57]

Likewise, assistive technology evaluations provided by telehealth have the advantage of offering perspective into the patient's home and therefore may provide more relevant information to the clinician. Recommendations for environmental control units or home automation can provide increased independence despite functional impairments. Telehealth visits to the patient's home provide a unique insight into the individual's set up and use of his or her own personal computer equipment, which can facilitate computer access evaluation and adaptive equipment recommendations. Bulbar muscle weakness, which can interfere with communication, is a common feature in ALS and presents unique barriers to participation in telehealth visits. Fortunately, some AAC devices can also serve as the telehealth platform on the patient's end. In addition, typing into a chat box provides another option for communication for the patient who is unable to communicate by voice.

Advanced Care Planning and End of Life

Telehealth visits to home provide a unique window into the patient's environment and may provide a reasonable setting for advanced care planning discussions. Among the most common topics covered in tele-ALS visits were goals of care, representing 74% of visits in 1 study.[58] Telehealth may be a particularly valuable resource for providing end-of-life support.[59] This service provides a means of maintaining continuity of care for a person no longer able to travel to the medical center for his or her care, and provides valuable support from the specialty team to the home health and hospice caregivers.

SUMMARY

Telehealth is a powerful tool that can provide access to specialized health care services for individuals who would otherwise have barriers because of distance or disability. Among neurodegenerative disorders, literature supports the acceptability and efficacy of telehealth-based interventions to provide care to individuals with ALS and MS.

Because of the coronavirus pandemic,[60] most providers and patients now have first-hand experience as to the benefits of telehealth. However, despite the clear benefits, many barriers threaten the sustainability of this modality. These include limitations in access caused by the digital divide, as well as cognitive and physical disabilities, current limitations of the technology, and ongoing legal and reimbursement concerns.

More work is needed to ensure telehealth provides truly equitable access to care for all, despite disability or socioeconomic and racial differences. Physical, cognitive, and visual deficits can render the visit ineffective if caregiver assistance is unavailable. Limitations in access to broadband Internet and computers can still pose barriers between patients and health care providers in what has been known as the digital divide. These discrepancies were magnified during the COVID-19 pandemic.[61] Some ALS clinics reported a strong preference in their patient population for telephone rather than video visits during the pandemic.[48] In order to minimize inequities in access to the Internet, the US government has invested funds in the development of broadband infrastructure in rural areas. Several strategies may also be employed by clinicians to increase access for all individuals, including offering services by both telephone and video, as well as consideration of assistive technology for alternative computer access or communication devices for persons with disabilities.

The COVID-19 public health emergency changed the clinical landscape by permitting greater public access to telehealth through reduction of the financial and legal barriers. However, reciprocal licensing across states, reimbursement parity for physicians, and coverage for allied health services are important steps that would have great impact on the sustainability of this mode of care.[62] A recent systematic review of telehealth for ALS found that the main barriers to implementation relate to health care provider experience and perception regarding finance and legislation.[63] Reimbursement discrepancies between telephone and video visits, despite similar use of resources on the health care provider's end, also disincentivize use of these services. Finally, telehealth visits may require uncompensated administrative time or informatics support to ensure the client is able to access the technology.

Clinically, some questions remain regarding how to optimize telehealth modalities for care of these patient populations. Some parts of the physical examination may not be possible to be done remotely. Best practices for diagnostic subspecialty evaluations that require more detailed physical examination, for example, during initial diagnosis of ALS and MS, would add greatly to the field.

The shift to virtual encounters for research studies brings promise and additional challenges for patients with MS and ALS. The optimization of telehealth for research recruitment and enrollment may permit greater access to experimental therapies for individuals who otherwise may not have access.[64] However, the digital divide may further decrease diversity in study populations. In addition, proprietary tools for virtual functional assessment (eg, through wearable technology or digital voice recording) may add further cost and complexity compared with traditional in-clinic measures.[44]

Challenges in reimbursement and access to technology notwithstanding, meeting the needs related to provision of telehealth for the population of patients with ALS and MS has the potential to offer a universal design transformation for health care, making care accessible to individuals regardless of level of function or disability.

CLINICS CARE POINTS

- MS and ALS are neurodegenerative disorders with evidence of benefit from use of telehealth.
- Disease progression in MS and ALS can be monitored by telehealth; patient-reported outcome measures and peripheral devices, such as home spirometers or accelerometers, can be used as adjuncts to monitor disease progression.
- Telehealth has been used successfully to address secondary symptoms in MS (eg, fatigue, cognitive impairments, and mood disorders) and deliver physical therapy interventions.
- In addition, remote monitoring of pulmonary function and noninvasive ventilation by telehealth for patients with ALS correlates with decreased health care utilization.
- More work is needed to determine the role of telehealth in determining a diagnosis of MS and ALS.
- Telehealth and the use of technology for remote outcome measures may extend opportunities for participation in clinical trials for patients with ALS

REFERENCES

1. Pew Research Center. Internet/Broadband Fact Sheet. 2019. 2020. Available at: https://www.pewresearch.org/internet/fact-sheet/internet-broadband. Accessed November 1, 2020.
2. Ringholz GM, Appel SH, Bradshaw M, et al. Prevalence and patterns of cognitive impairment in sporadic ALS. Neurology 2005;65(4):586–90.
3. Baltadzhieva R, Gurevich T, Korczyn AD. Autonomic impairment in amyotrophic lateral sclerosis. Curr Opin Neurol 2005;18(5):487–93.
4. Mehta P, Kaye W, Raymond J, et al. Prevalence of amyotrophic lateral sclerosis - United States, 2015. MMWR Morb Mortal Wkly Rep 2018;67(46):1285–9.
5. Horton DK, Graham S, Punjani R, et al. A spatial analysis of amyotrophic lateral sclerosis (ALS) cases in the United States and their proximity to multidisciplinary ALS clinics, 2013. Amyotroph Lateral Scler Frontotemporal Degener 2018; 19(1–2):126–33.
6. Wallin MT, Culpepper WJ, Campbell JD, et al. The prevalence of MS in the United States: a population-based estimate using health claims data. Neurology 2019; 92(10):e1029–40.
7. Lunde HMB, Assmus J, Myhr KM, et al. Survival and cause of death in multiple sclerosis: a 60-year longitudinal population study. J Neurol Neurosurg Psychiatry 2017;88(8):621–5.
8. Minden SL, Frankel D, Hadden L, et al. Access to health care for people with multiple sclerosis. Mult Scler 2007;13(4):547–58.

9. Khan F, Amatya B, Kesselring J, et al. Telerehabilitation for persons with multiple sclerosis. Cochrane Database Syst Rev 2015;(4):CD010508.

10. Yeroushalmi S, Maloni H, Costello K, et al. Telemedicine and multiple sclerosis: a comprehensive literature review. J Telemed Telecare 2020;26(7–8):400–13.

11. Robb JF, Hyland MH, Goodman AD. Comparison of telemedicine versus in-person visits for persons with multiple sclerosis: a randomized crossover study of feasibility, cost, and satisfaction. Mult Scler Relat Disord 2019;36:101258.

12. Zhou L, Parmanto B. Reaching people with disabilities in underserved areas through digital interventions: systematic review. J Med Internet Res 2019; 21(10):e12981.

13. Adamse C, Dekker-Van Weering MG, van Etten-Jamaludin FS, et al. The effectiveness of exercise-based telemedicine on pain, physical activity and quality of life in the treatment of chronic pain: a systematic review. J Telemed Telecare 2018; 24(8):511–26.

14. American Academy of Neurology. AAN Telemedicine and Covid-19 implementation guide. 2020. Available at: https://www.aan.com/siteassets/home-page/tools-and-resources/practicing-neurologist–administrators/telemedicine-and-remote-care/20-telemedicine-and-covid19-v103.pdf. Accessed November 1, 2020.

15. Bove R, Bevan C, Crabtree E, et al. Toward a low-cost, in-home, telemedicine-enabled assessment of disability in multiple sclerosis. Mult Scler 2019;25(11): 1526–34.

16. Learmonth YC, Motl RW, Sandroff BM, et al. Validation of patient determined disease steps (PDDS) scale scores in persons with multiple sclerosis. BMC Neurol 2013;13:37.

17. Moccia M, Lanzillo R, Brescia Morra V, et al. Assessing disability and relapses in multiple sclerosis on tele-neurology. Neurol Sci 2020;41(6):1369–71.

18. Pearson M, Dieberg G, Smart N. Exercise as a therapy for improvement of walking ability in adults with multiple sclerosis: a meta-analysis. Arch Phys Med Rehabil 2015;96(7):1339–48.e7.

19. Stuifbergen AK, Blozis SA, Harrison TC, et al. Exercise, functional limitations, and quality of life: a longitudinal study of persons with multiple sclerosis. Arch Phys Med Rehabil 2006;87(7):935–43.

20. Turner AP, Knowles LM. Behavioral Interventions in Multiple Sclerosis. Fed Pract 2020;37(Suppl 1):S31–5.

21. Plow M, Finlayson M, Liu J, et al. Randomized controlled trial of a telephone-delivered physical activity and fatigue self-management interventions in adults with multiple sclerosis. Arch Phys Med Rehabil 2019;100(11):2006–14.

22. Rintala A, Hakala S, Paltamaa J, et al. Effectiveness of technology-based distance physical rehabilitation interventions on physical activity and walking in multiple sclerosis: a systematic review and meta-analysis of randomized controlled trials. Disabil Rehabil 2018;40(4):373–87.

23. Shah A. Fatigue in multiple sclerosis. Phys Med Rehabil Clin N Am 2009;20(2): 363–72.

24. Kraft GH, Freal JE, Coryell JK. Disability, disease duration, and rehabilitation service needs in multiple sclerosis: patient perspectives. Arch Phys Med Rehabil 1986;67(3):164–8.

25. Ehde DM, Elzea JL, Verrall AM, et al. Efficacy of a telephone-delivered self-management intervention for persons with multiple sclerosis: a randomized controlled trial with a one-year follow-up. Arch Phys Med Rehabil 2015;96(11):1945–58.e2.

26. Mohr DC, Hart S, Vella L. Reduction in disability in a randomized controlled trial of telephone-administered cognitive-behavioral therapy. Health Psychol 2007;26(5): 554–63.

27. Egner A, Phillips VL, Vora R, et al. Depression, fatigue, and health-related quality of life among people with advanced multiple sclerosis: results from an exploratory telerehabilitation study. NeuroRehabilitation 2003;18(2):125–33.

28. Cavalera C, Rovaris M, Mendozzi L, et al. Online meditation training for people with multiple sclerosis: a randomized controlled trial. Mult Scler 2019;25(4): 610–7.

29. Mohr DC, Hart SL, Julian L, et al. Telephone-administered psychotherapy for depression. Arch Gen Psychiatry 2005;62(9):1007–14.

30. Turner AP, Hartoonian N, Sloan AP, et al. Improving fatigue and depression in individuals with multiple sclerosis using telephone-administered physical activity counseling. J Consult Clin Psychol 2016;84(4):297–309.

31. Moss-Morris R, McCrone P, Yardley L, et al. A pilot randomised controlled trial of an Internet-based cognitive behavioural therapy self-management programme (MS Invigor8) for multiple sclerosis fatigue. Behav Res Ther 2012;50(6):415–21.

32. Proctor BJ, Moghaddam N, Vogt W, et al. Telephone psychotherapy in multiple sclerosis: a systematic review and meta-analysis. Rehabil Psychol 2018;63(1): 16–28.

33. Charvet LE, Yang J, Shaw MT, et al. Cognitive function in multiple sclerosis improves with telerehabilitation: results from a randomized controlled trial. PLoS One 2017;12(5):e0177177.

34. Turner AP, Roubinov DS, Atkins DC, et al. Predicting medication adherence in multiple sclerosis using telephone-based home monitoring. Disabil Health J 2016;9(1):83–9.

35. Leavitt VM, Riley CS, De Jager PL, et al. eSupport: feasibility trial of telehealth support group participation to reduce loneliness in multiple sclerosis. Mult Scler 2020;26(13):1797–800.

36. Settle JR, Robinson SA, Kane R, et al. Remote cognitive assessments for patients with multiple sclerosis: a feasibility study. Mult Scler 2015;21(8):1072–9.

37. Wingo BC, Rinker JR, Goss AM, et al. Feasibility of improving dietary quality using a telehealth lifestyle intervention for adults with multiple sclerosis. Mult Scler Relat Disord 2020;46:102504.

38. Gately ME, Trudeau SA, Moo LR. Feasibility of telehealth-delivered home safety evaluations for caregivers of clients with dementia. OTJR (Thorofare N J) 2020; 40(1):42–9.

39. Williams KN, Perkhounkova Y, Shaw CA, et al. Supporting family caregivers with technology for dementia home care: a randomized controlled trial. Innov Aging 2019;3(3):igz037.

40. Miller RG, Jackson CE, Kasarskis EJ, et al. Practice parameter update: the care of the patient with amyotrophic lateral sclerosis: multidisciplinary care, symptom management, and cognitive/behavioral impairment (an evidence-based review): report of the Quality Standards Subcommittee of the American Academy of Neurology. Neurology 2009;73(15):1227–33.

41. Paganoni S, Macklin EA, Lee A, et al. Diagnostic timelines and delays in diagnosing amyotrophic lateral sclerosis (ALS). Amyotroph Lateral Scler Frontotemporal Degener 2014;15(5–6):453–6.

42. Pearl PL, Sable C, Evans S, et al. International telemedicine consultations for neurodevelopmental disabilities. Telemed J E Health 2014;20(6):559–62.

43. Saporta MA, Granit V, Lewis R, et al. Yes, we can: neuromuscular examination by telemedicine. Muscle Nerve 2020;62(6):E83–5.
44. Andrews JA, Berry JD, Baloh RH, et al. Amyotrophic lateral sclerosis care and research in the United States during the COVID-19 pandemic: challenges and opportunities. Muscle Nerve 2020;62(2):182–6.
45. Selkirk SM, Washington MO, McClellan F, et al. Delivering tertiary centre specialty care to ALS patients via telemedicine: a retrospective cohort analysis. Amyotroph Lateral Scler Frontotemporal Degener 2017;18(5–6):324–32.
46. Howard I, Potts A. Interprofessional care for neuromuscular disease. Curr Treat Options Neurol 2019;21(8):35.
47. Wiederhold BK. Connecting through technology during the coronavirus disease 2019 pandemic: avoiding "zoom fatigue". Cyberpsychol Behav Soc Netw 2020; 23(7):437–8.
48. Capozzo R, Zoccolella S, Musio M, et al. Telemedicine is a useful tool to deliver care to patients with amyotrophic lateral sclerosis during COVID-19 pandemic: results from southern Italy. Amyotroph Lateral Scler Frontotemporal Degener 2020;21(7–8):542–8.
49. Vitacca M, Comini L, Tentorio M, et al. A pilot trial of telemedicine-assisted, integrated care for patients with advanced amyotrophic lateral sclerosis and their caregivers. J Telemed Telecare 2010;16(2):83–8.
50. Helleman J, Van Eenennaam R, Kruitwagen ET, et al. Telehealth as part of specialized ALS care: feasibility and user experiences with "ALS home-monitoring and coaching". Amyotroph Lateral Scler Frontotemporal Degener 2020;21(3–4):183–92.
51. Hobson EV, Baird WO, Partridge R, et al. The TiM system: developing a novel telehealth service to improve access to specialist care in motor neurone disease using user-centered design. Amyotroph Lateral Scler Frontotemporal Degener 2018;19(5–6):351–61.
52. van Eijk RPA, Bakers JNE, Bunte TM, et al. Accelerometry for remote monitoring of physical activity in amyotrophic lateral sclerosis: a longitudinal cohort study. J Neurol 2019;266(10):2387–95.
53. Corcia P, Pradat PF, Salachas F, et al. Causes of death in a post-mortem series of ALS patients. Amyotroph Lateral Scler 2008;9(1):59–62.
54. Vitacca M, Paneroni M, Trainini D, et al. At home and on demand mechanical cough assistance program for patients with amyotrophic lateral sclerosis. Am J Phys Med Rehabil 2010;89(5):401–6.
55. Pinto A, Almeida JP, Pinto S, et al. Home telemonitoring of non-invasive ventilation decreases healthcare utilisation in a prospective controlled trial of patients with amyotrophic lateral sclerosis. J Neurol Neurosurg Psychiatry 2010;81(11): 1238–42.
56. Ando H, Ashcroft-Kelso H, Halhead R, et al. Experience of telehealth in people with motor neurone disease using noninvasive ventilation. Disabil Rehabil Assist Technol 2019;5:1–7.
57. Pulley MT, Brittain R, Hodges W, et al. Multidisciplinary amyotrophic lateral sclerosis telemedicine care: the store and forward method. Muscle Nerve 2019; 59(1):34–9.
58. Van De Rijn M, Paganoni S, Levine-Weinberg M, et al. Experience with telemedicine in a multi-disciplinary ALS clinic. Amyotroph Lateral Scler Frontotemporal Degener 2018;19:143–8.
59. Zheng Y, Head BA, Schapmire TJ. A systematic review of telehealth in palliative care: caregiver outcomes. Telemed J E Health 2016;22(4):288–94.

60. Maese JR, Seminara D, Shah Z, et al. Perspective: what a difference a disaster makes: the telehealth revolution in the age of COVID-19 pandemic. Am J Med Qual 2020;35(5):429–31.
61. Ramsetty A, Adams C. Impact of the digital divide in the age of COVID-19. J Am Med Inform Assoc 2020;27(7):1147–8.
62. Howard IM, Kaufman MS. Telehealth applications for outpatients with neuromuscular or musculoskeletal disorders. Muscle Nerve 2018;58(4):475–85.
63. Helleman J, Kruitwagen ET, van den Berg LH, et al. The current use of telehealth in ALS care and the barriers to and facilitators of implementation: a systematic review. Amyotroph Lateral Scler Frontotemporal Degener 2020;21(3–4):167–82.
64. Govindarajan R, Berry JD, Paganoni S, et al. Optimizing telemedicine to facilitate amyotrophic lateral sclerosis clinical trials. Muscle Nerve 2020;62(3):321–6.

Telerehabilitation for Amputee Care

Joseph Webster, MD[a],*, Patricia Young, MSPT, CP[b,1], Jessica Kiecker, OTR/L[c]

KEYWORDS

- Teleamputation clinic • Virtual amputation clinic • Amputation • Rehabilitation
- Telerehabilitation

KEY POINTS

- Patients with limb loss have unique characteristics and rehabilitation needs related to the utilization of prosthetic limbs that need to be considered when services are being provided through a virtual platform.
- Rehabilitation of the person with limb loss ideally involves a collaborative interdisciplinary team; therefore, a team approach with virtual care services is recommended.
- The types of amputation rehabilitation services that can be provided virtually are numerous and vary from a full interdisciplinary team clinic to peer support visitation.
- When considering the provision of virtual amputation rehabilitation care, the benefits of enhanced access to highly specialized services, reduced patient travel burden, and improved continuity of care should all be considered.

INTRODUCTION

Advances in medical services, rehabilitation interventions, and artificial limb technologies have made management of the person with limb loss increasingly complex.[1,2] Individuals with amputation, whether from traumatic injuries or disease processes, have unique needs and require specialized management expertise in order to facilitate optimal outcomes.[3,4] These management considerations begin prior to the amputation itself and persist throughout the lifetime of the individual. These wide-ranging clinical needs are comprised of issues related to the amputation itself, issues related to other body parts impacted by the traumatic injury or disease process, and longer-term secondary health conditions.[5,6]

[a] Central Virginia Veterans Affairs Healthcare System, 1201 Broad Rock boulevard, Richmond, VA 23249, USA; [b] Amputation System of Care, Office of Connected Care, VA Central Office, Washington, DC, USA; [c] Department of PM&R, Minneapolis VA Health Care System, 1 Veterans Dr., Minneapolis, MN 55417, USA
[1] Present address: 1201 Broad Rock Blvd, PM&RS (117), Richmond, VA 23249
* Corresponding author.
E-mail address: joseph.webster@va.gov

Phys Med Rehabil Clin N Am 32 (2021) 253–262
https://doi.org/10.1016/j.pmr.2020.12.002
1047-9651/21/Published by Elsevier Inc.

Provision of amputation rehabilitation services through a virtual platform creates challenges and opportunities.[2,4,7] Care for the individual with limb loss is facilitated when services are provided by an interdisciplinary team with expertise in amputation rehabilitation. The evaluation and management of patients with an amputation require effective communication and care coordination by the clinical team. This is especially true when some or all these services are being provided by means of telerehabilitation.[2,4,7] In addition, telerehabilitation services provide the ability to connect amputation care subject matter experts with patients in more remote or underserved areas where services are not available locally. For patients with more complex amputation or artificial limb needs, telerehabilitation offers the opportunity to connect local providers with more specialized clinicians in order to maximize patient outcomes.[2,4,7]

BACKGROUND

Limb amputation has medical, functional, social, and psychological ramifications for the individual and his or her family members. Whether services are provided in person or via telehealth, these varied considerations require specialized and comprehensive management across a spectrum of health care settings and for the duration of an individual's lifespan.[1–4] Management strategies need to address issues related to the amputation itself and various underlying medical conditions or associated traumatic injuries. Clinicians must also be mindful of longer-term secondary health conditions that can develop as the person with limb loss ages. Optimal management encompasses an interdisciplinary program of services ranging from the latest practices in medical interventions to prosthetic limb technology and advanced rehabilitation strategies.[1–4]

Some amputation-related considerations are more prevalent and of greater severity in the early recovery period following amputation, whereas others develop later and have the potential for progressive worsening over time. Issues related to the amputation itself include changes in residual limb size, shape, and pressure tolerance over time, which have the potential to impact successful wearing of a prosthesis.[8] For patients with limb loss who wear a prosthesis, residual limb skin irritation or breakdown can result from pressure, shear, and skin maceration inside the socket.[8] Heterotopic ossification (HO), the formation of bone tissue outside of the normal bone structure, can also create difficulties or inability to wear a prosthesis.[9] Amputation-related pain conditions include residual limb pain and phantom limb pain. Although residual limb pain management often involves addressing the fit of the prosthesis, phantom limb pain may require a more multifaceted approach including desensitization, electrical stimulation, medication management and graded motor imagery. Telerehabilitation can play an important role in managing these conditions by helping to assure regular follow-up visits while minimizing patient travel.[10–12]

Telerehabilitation services can play a role in assisting with the psychological adjustments and continuity of care challenges that are often present following limb loss. Loss of a limb is a life-changing event involving adjustment to potential physical limitations and body image changes.[13,14] Whether provided in person or virtually, peer support services have demonstrated benefits in assisting with this adjustment process. If the amputation was the result of a traumatic injury, issues related to posttraumatic stress disorder (PTSD) and anxiety may also need to be addressed. Over the course of time, patients with limb loss may develop secondary conditions such as musculoskeletal overuse syndromes and back pain.[5,6,15,16] In association with lifestyle modifications that are required following limb loss, metabolic and cardiovascular complications can develop. In addition, living with limb loss involves dealing with the need for artificial limb repairs and replacement and an increasing dependence on other mobility aids and durable medical equipment over time.

IMPORTANCE AND PROGRAM DEVELOPMENT IN THE DEPARTMENT OF VETERANS AFFAIRS

Telehealth services have been implemented in the Department of Veterans Affairs (VA) as a means to improve access to care and the patient experience.[7] The VA's Amputation System of Care (ASoC) is an integrated, national health care delivery system that provides lifelong holistic care and care coordination for veterans who have undergone amputation.[2,4] Through close collaboration with primary care and other specialty care services, the ASoC assures that all medical, rehabilitation, and prosthetic needs of the veteran with an amputation are met. Within the ASoC, a telehealth program has been deployed to improve outcomes by providing specialized amputation clinic and rehabilitation services closer to the veteran's home.[2,4] Since 2008, there has been steady growth in VA's virtual amputation care services, and the type of services offered has expanded to provide greater services in the veteran's home and local community, with the goal to enhance the quality and consistency of amputation rehabilitation services.

TYPES OF VIRTUAL AMPUTATION CARE SERVICES

Virtual amputation care services provide people living with limb loss access to specialty clinical services regardless of their proximity to a medical center. Patients can potentially connect to their amputation care team from various locations: a local clinic site, their own home, or the office of a prosthetist located in the community. Virtual care not only improves access for individuals living in rural areas, but it also connects larger medical center sites with smaller facilities to provide care where specialized amputation care services are not available.[3,7] Virtual care can be used by all members of an amputation rehabilitation specialty team including physician, prosthetist, physical therapist, occupational therapist, RT, rehabilitation psychology, social work, and nursing to provide a full spectrum of services as needed for each individual with limb loss.[17–21]

Prior to the COVID-19 pandemic, virtual care services were primarily used to connect amputation specialty teams located at a medical facility with the recipient of care located at a satellite site or a partnering medical center. Now, with pandemic-driven precautions and advancements in the use of hand-held devices, patients can utilize application-based virtual medical rooms to remain in the comfort of their home while connecting with their treatment team or individual team members.[18,21] **Table 1** details the options available to provide virtual amputation care services.

Interdisciplinary Team Amputation Clinic

The first, and most common, clinic is the interdisciplinary (IDT) amputation clinic. This clinic includes a full amputation care team (physician, physical or occupational therapist, and prosthetist) at a medical center. If the patient is seen in his or her home using an application-based virtual platform, the individual may or may not have a family member present to assist with camera manipulation or provide assistance with safe mobility. If the patient is located either in a medical clinic or in a collaborating medical center, a telepresenter can support the patient during the visit. The telepresenter is generally a nurse or medical assistant, but a physical or occupational therapist may also assist the visit if available.[7,18,21] Services in the IDT amputation clinic include initial evaluations and follow-up visits, artificial limb and rehabilitation prescription, checkout

Table 1
Options for provision of virtual amputation care services

Clinic Type	Locations	Members of the Team	Services Provided
Interdisciplinary team	Medical center to medical center	Specialty care team (physician, therapist, and prosthetist) connects with treating team and patient	Initial patient evaluations and follow-up visits
	Medical center to satellite clinic	Specialty team connects with patient and presenter	Artificial limb and rehabilitation prescription
	Provider/team to patient home	Specialty team connects with patient (family member, if needed)	Check-out of a new prosthesis after delivery
	Provider/team to prosthetist's office	Specialty team connects with patient and prosthetist	Follow-up for comorbidities and complications
Prosthetist only	Medical center to medical center	Prosthetist connects with treating team and patient	Assist prescribing team in developing prosthesis prescription
	Provider to home	Prosthetist connects with patient (family member, if needed)	Check-out of a new prosthesis or changes in prescription
	Provider to a Prosthetist in Another Location	Prosthetist connects with patient and patient's local prosthetist	
Support group	Medical center to medical center	Support group leader (therapist, social worker, psychologist) connects with patients in multiple sites via videoconferencing	Patient are able to interact and establish peer supports
	Medical center to satellite clinic		Patients are provided counseling support and education
	Individual peer support to home		

after delivery of new prosthesis, and follow-up for amputation-related comorbidities and complications such as skin breakdown and postamputation pain conditions.

Prosthetist Support Clinic

The prosthetist support clinic incorporates a prosthetist at a medical center or other location connecting with the patient and other members of the clinical team (physician and therapist) at a collaborating medical center to complete the treatment team. The prosthetist in this clinic contributes to the prosthesis prescription, assists in completing the checkout process after delivery of a new prosthesis, and can assist in directing prosthesis prescription modifications. A prosthesis checkout appointment may occur with the individual at home or in the office of another prosthetist located in the patient's local community.[4,7]

Amputee Support Groups

Virtual amputee support groups connect people in the limb loss community providing an opportunity to interact using virtual platforms.[7] Individuals may be at home, at a medical clinic or hospital location, or even a prosthetist office or other public gathering space. The opportunity to interact provides support and often a chance for education organized by the support group leader. One-on-one virtual peer mentorship is also an option for patients looking for a more individualized, personal connection with a certi-fied peer visitor.

Virtual Amputation Care Therapy Services

A crucial component of amputation rehabilitation is the provision of therapy services to ensure optimal and safe use of a lower or upper extremity prosthetic limb. Although some aspects of amputation rehabilitation therapy services are best provided in per-son, many aspects can be provided through virtual platforms.[7,17,18,21] In order to ensure the highest level of safety, initial prosthetic gait training for patients with lower extremity amputation likely requires in-person hands-on therapy services. This is especially true for those individuals who are new to wearing a prosthesis or when impaired balance or coordination is present. In these circumstances, the primary gait training may need to be in person, but virtual visits can still be utilized for follow-up appointments as part of a continued therapy program. Therapists who are experts in providing upper extremity amputation prosthetic training are less widely available because of the lower prevalence of persons with upper extremity amputa-tion. This issue reinforces the need for virtual amputation care services for those with upper extremity amputation. Virtual care for upper extremity amputation pros-thetic training enables the patients to be connected with experts who can integrate training into their activities of daily living, instrumental activities of daily living, and vocational tasks.[20]

Although prosthetic gait training is commonly an essential aspect of amputation rehabilitation, there are many other important aspects of rehabilitation that may be able to be provided either in person or virtually. Therapy interventions for pain man-agement can be provided virtually and may include training in desensitization, training in use of a TES unit and the performance of mirror therapy. Instruction and mainte-nance of a home exercise program is also important for the person with limb loss and can often be achieved through a virtual platform. **Table 2** provides additional amputation-related therapy interventions that can potentially be provided through a virtual platform, including training in the performance of activities of daily living, the performance of a home safety evaluation, and many more interventions.[19]

BENEFITS

Virtual care access to a full amputation care clinic team or individual team members enhances the quality of the care received by the person with limb loss and brings many additional benefits along the way. These additional benefits include

- Reduced travel burden on the person with limb loss and his or her family; this is especially important for those with significant functional impairments or transpor-tation limitations
- Increased access to specialty amputation and prosthetic services including fabrication and fitting of a prosthetic limb
- The opportunity for the clinic team to conduct a visit with a patient at home allows the team to assess needs within the home and promote safety and indepen-dence in everyday tasks
- The potential for the clinic team to see the patient while the patient is visiting another provider in the community such as a prosthetist; this has the potential to enrich team collaboration and complete immediate prosthetic device modifications

Table 2
Potential virtual amputation care therapy services

Therapy Services Category	Therapy Interventions
Prosthetic gait training and gait optimization	Training on gait technique using external feedback and cueing
Activities of daily living training	Training includes donning and doffing of prosthesis during daily routine
Instrumental activities of daily living	Training in health management and maintenance (care of prosthesis, wearing schedule, sock ply management, and skin checks) meal preparation, shopping, home management, and driving/transportation
Home exercise program instruction	Performance in home setting with emphasis on safest locations in the home for exercise performance
Pain management interventions	Instruction and training in desensitization, visualization, mirror therapy, TENS unit
Management of secondary conditions	Education and training to prevent overuse syndromes such as knee arthritis on contralateral limb
DME and assistive technology evaluations	Highlighting where durable medical equipment and assistive technology devices can enhance home safety
Home safety evaluations	Highlighting safety in home through adaptive equipment use and modification recommendations in the home
Wheeled mobility evaluations	Evaluation includes wheelchair measurements and assessments to ensure wheelchair use is feasible in the home

- The accommodation of the patient's work schedule can eliminate the need for the patient to take time off from work for travel and the clinic appointment itself
- The development of innovative clinical practices that involve various medical professionals enhancing the patient's experience

CHALLENGES AND LIMITATIONS

The effectiveness of virtual amputation care services can be limited by the skill and expertise of the telepresenter assisting in the clinical evaluation at the patient location. If available, it is recommended to have a telepresenter with the patient who can assist with hands-on musculoskeletal, vascular, neurologic, and skin/wound assessments.[7] When evaluating prosthetic gait, the safety of the patient always needs to be a high priority, especially if the person has balance impairments or limited experience wearing a prosthetic limb. The space available for walking may also be a limiting factor when assessing prosthetic gait. It is vital that there is enough distance for the person to complete full strides toward and away from the camera.

The importance of residual limb management is crucial in persons with limb loss. When a person is instructed to doff the prosthesis for skin inspection of the residual limb, the person's comfort level with removing clothing in front of a camera needs to be taken into consideration. It is imperative for a provider to consider the location and camera view to promote the feeling of privacy. When evaluating skin and wounds, it is important to have extra lighting and a ruler or tape measure available that can be used to measure a wound for tracking purposes. A specialized high-resolution camera may be beneficial when a provider needs to perform a detailed wound examination.

Providing virtual care services in the patient's home may pose some of the same challenges and limitations, along with different ones, as the patient may have more limited support for the visit in his or her home. Another challenge for patients can be the lack of familiarity with the technology used for virtual care visits, especially if he or she is using a personal devices. Individuals may be used to virtually connecting with family/friends with the platform on their device, but they might not be trained with more secure platforms that are used for medical appointments. There are features within these virtual applications that are imperative for an individual to operate such as flipping the camera and the use of audio and microphone in order to have a successful visit.

Aspects of the physical examination may be challenging to complete during a virtual encounter. This can include assessment of range of motion (ROM) in the patient's lower extremity or upper extremity without the expertise of a medical professional to obtain exact measurements. If a telepresenter is not available to complete a hands-on lower extremity ROM and strength assessment, a provider may be able to observe ROM at the hip and knee during a gait/functional evaluation as the patient walks toward and away from the camera. Similar observations can be made with the upper extremity prosthetic user when he or she is performing an everyday activities of daily living task; range at the shoulder and elbow can be evaluated as he or she reaches.

Technical limitations include not having a strong enough Internet or cell tower connection. This may cause freezing or an unclear image on the screen for the virtual appointment with the provider. In this case, the provider may recommend the person attempt the virtual appointment at another location or use a different device owned by a family member/friend/caregiver. Patients who do not have a useable device may be able to qualify for a loaner devices to complete virtual appointments. These devices can be sent out to the patient, but do require familiarity with the technology.

One other challenge can be the acceptance, integration, and participation of virtual care modalities by both patients and providers.[18] Some individuals may not fully embrace virtual care and some may see this as an intrusion into their private lives if a clinician is "seeing me in my home." However, many other patients report high satisfaction with this care delivery modality. Providers, on the other hand, are typically trained in face-to-face clinical assessment and treatment and transitioning to the utilization of virtual care modalities does require additional training and taking the time to develop adequate comfort with the technology to successfully provide virtual care. In addition, the technology evolves and continuously changes with upgrades to improve the experience. Providers need to be willing to stay up to date with the evolving technology and successfully complete the training with the current platform being used for virtual care appointments.

FUTURE DIRECTIONS

Individuals with limb loss require specialized management of ongoing medical and rehabilitation needs. Utilizing virtual care modalities can provide interaction and support from the vast array of necessary rehabilitation providers to patients in their local and/or home environments. Implementation of virtual care into every rehabilitation provider's standard of practice is an opportunity to provide the same level of specialized care and full spectrum of services to all patients with limb loss, whether they live close to a medical facility or in more rural, remote areas.

There has been tremendous growth in the use and effectiveness of virtual amputation care services, and it is anticipated that these opportunities will continue to expand in the future. Developments enabling the utilization of computer, tablet, and smartphone applications for patients to be able to send the provider videos of their gait in different settings or pictures of their wounds could enhance care. The use of Bluetooth sensors on prosthetic limbs to automatically analyze gait and transmit activity level information to providers could contribute to the providers' overall evaluation in addition to enabling the use of outcomes-based measurements. The collection of outcomes will assist in measuring and identifying the effectiveness of various treatments offered to those with limb loss through virtual care. It is anticipated that these technology advances and comfort with virtual care platforms will continue to enhance care and improve the patient experience in the future.

CLINICS CARE POINTS

- When amputation care services are being provided through a virtual platform, maintaining a team approach is highly recommended.
- Persons with amputation have unique rehabilitation needs related to the utilization of prosthetic limbs that add to the complexity of providing virtual amputation services.
- Special precautions may be required when performing virtual gait training for individuals who are new to wearing a prosthesis or when impaired balance or coordination is present in order to ensure the highest level of patient safety.
- There are many important aspects of amputation rehabilitation that may be able to be provided virtually. Potential virtual services include prosthetic gait training, ADL training, home exercise program instruction, pain management interventions, assistive technology evaluations, and home safety evaluations.
- There are many ways in which virtual amputation services may be provided to best accommodate the patient and to maximize the expertise of the treating team: into the home for home assessments, into the prosthetist's office for follow-up modifications and alignment changes, or into the clinic from another clinic or medical center location for the sharing of teams with expertise in a certain area of amputation care.

DISCLOSURE

The authors have nothing to disclose. The authors have no commercial or financial conflicts of interest.

REFERENCES

1. Resnik L, Meucci MR, Lieberman-Klinger S, et al. Advanced upper limb prosthetic devices: implications for upper limb prosthetic rehabilitation. Arch Phys Med Rehabil 2012;93(4):710–7.
2. Webster JB, Poorman CE, Cifu DX. Guest editorial: Department of Veterans Affairs Amputations System of Care: 5 years of accomplishments and outcomes. J Rehabil Res Dev 2014;51(4):vii–xvi.

3. VA/DoD Clinical Practice Guideline for Rehabilitation of Individuals with Lower Limb Amputation. 2017. Available at: https://www.healthquality.va.gov/guidelines/rehab/amp/index.asp. Accessed September 18, 2020.

4. Webster JB, Scholten J, Young P, et al. Ten-year outcomes of a systems-based approach to longitudinal amputation care in the US Department of Veteran Affairs. Fed Pract 2020;37(8):360–7.

5. Farrokhi S, Mazzone B, Eskridge S, et al. Incidence of overuse musculoskeletal injuries in military service members with traumatic lower limb amputation. Arch Phys Med Rehabil 2018;99(2):348–54.e1.

6. Butowicz CM, Dearth CL, Hendershot BD. Impact of traumatic lower extremity injuries beyond acute care: movement-based considerations for resultant longer-term secondary health conditions. Adv Wound Care (New Rochelle) 2017;6(8): 269–78.

7. Scholten J, Poorman C, Culver L, et al. Department of Veterans Affairs polytrauma telerehabilitation: twenty-first century care. Phys Med Rehabil Clin N Am 2019; 30(1):207–15.

8. Highsmith MJ, Kahle JT, Klenow TD, et al. Interventions to manage residual limb ulceration due to prosthetic use in individuals with lower extremity amputation: a systematic review of the literature. Technol Innov 2016;18(2–3):115–23.

9. Edwards DS, Kuhn KM, Potter BK, et al. Heterotopic ossification: a review of current understanding, treatment, and future. J Orthop Trauma 2016;30(Suppl 3): S27–30.

10. Rothgangel AS, Braun S, Schulz RJ, et al. The PACT trial: Patient Centered Telerehabilitation: effectiveness of software-supported and traditional mirror therapy in patients with phantom limb pain following lower limb amputation: protocol of a multicentre randomized controlled trial. J Physiother 2015;61(1):42 [discussion: 42].

11. Rothgangel A, Braun S, Winkens B, et al. Traditional and augmented reality mirror therapy for patients with chronic phantom limb pain (PACT study): results of a three-group, multicentre single-blind randomized controlled trial. Clin Rehabil 2018;32(12):1591–608.

12. Rothgangel A, Braun S, Smeets R, et al. Design and development of a telerehabilitation platform for patients with phantom limb pain: a user-centered approach. JMIR Rehabil Assist Technol 2017;4(1):e2.

13. Bhatnagar V, Richard E, Melcer T, et al. Lower-limb amputation and effect of post-traumatic stress disorder on Department of Veterans Affairs outpatient cost trends. J Rehabil Res Dev 2015;52(7):827–38.

14. Talbot LA, Brede E, Metter EJ. Psychological and physical health in military amputees during rehabilitation: secondary analysis of a randomized controlled trial. Mil Med 2017;182(5):e1619–24.

15. Norvell DC, Czerniecki JM, Reiber GE, et al. The prevalence of knee pain and symptomatic knee osteoarthritic among veteran traumatic amputees and non-amputees. Arch Phys Med Rehabil 2005;86:487–93.

16. Miller MJ, Stevens-Lapsley J, Fields TT, et al. Physical activity behavior change for older veterans after dysvascular amputation. Contemp Clin Trials 2017; 55:10–5.

17. Agostini M, Moja L, Banzi R, et al. Telerehabilitation and recovery of motor function: a systematic review and meta-analysis. J Telemed Telecare 2015;21(4): 202–13.

18. Elnitsky C, Latlief G, Gavin-Dreschnack D, et al. Lessons learned in pilot testing specialty consultations to benefit individuals with lower limb loss. Int J Telerehabil 2012;4(2):3–10.
19. Cason J. Telehealth opportunities in occupational therapy through the Affordable Care Act. Am J Occup Ther 2012;66:131–6.
20. Schmeler M, Schein R, McCue M, et al. Telerehabilitation clinical and vocational applications for assistive technology:research, opportunities, and challenges. Int J Telerehabil 2009;1(1):59–72.
21. Cason J. Telehealth: a rapidly developing service delivery model for occupational therapy. Int J Telerehabil 2014;6(1):29–35.

Cardiopulmonary Telerehabilitation

Dixie Aragaki, MD[a,b,]*, Jerry Luo, MD[c], Elizabeth Weiner, MD[c], Grace Zhang, MD[c], Babak Darvish, MD[d]

KEYWORDS

- Telehealth • Telerehabilitation • Cardiac rehabilitation • Pulmonary rehabilitation
- Home-based rehabilitation

KEY POINTS

- Comprehensive cardiopulmonary telerehabilitation programs can include remote monitoring, health coaching, virtual education tools, and social networking to enhance interest and motivation.
- Cardiac and pulmonary telerehabilitation programs have been shown to be safe and effective alternatives to center-based rehabilitation programs.
- The optimization of various telemedicine platforms and tools (for remote cardiorespiratory monitoring and therapy interventions) continues to grow and enhance care.
- A thoughtful team-oriented patient-centered approach can ensure higher-risk patients are triaged to the most appropriate care setting.

INTRODUCTION

Chronic heart failure (CHF) and chronic obstructive pulmonary disease (COPD) frequently coexist in older frail adults because of common risk factors. These conditions are associated with frequent exacerbations leading to vicious cycles of dyspnea, reduced activity, impaired function, and social isolation, and are ultimately leading causes of mortality.[1] The prevalence of CHF in patients with COPD is more than 20% and that of COPD in patients with CHF ranges from 10% to 40%.[2] More urgent

[a] Department of Medicine, Division of Physical Medicine and Rehabilitation, David Geffen School of Medicine at UCLA, Los Angeles, CA USA; [b] Physical Medicine and Rehabilitation Service, VA Greater Los Angeles Healthcare System, 11301 Wilshire Boulevard (117), Los Angeles, CA 90073, USA; [c] Physical Medicine and Rehabilitation Residency (PGY-2), Greater Los Angeles VA Healthcare System, West Los Angeles VA Medical Center, 11301 Wilshire Boulevard (117), Los Angeles, CA 90073, USA; [d] Cardiopulmonary Telehealth Service, Physical Medicine and Rehabilitation Service, Greater Los Angeles Healthcare System, West Los Angeles VA Medical Center, 11301 Wilshire Boulevard (117), Los Angeles, CA 90073, USA
* Corresponding author. Physical Medicine and Rehabilitation Service, VA Greater Los Angeles Healthcare System, 11301 Wilshire Boulevard (117), Los Angeles, CA 90073, USA
E-mail address: Dixie.aragaki@va.gov

Phys Med Rehabil Clin N Am 32 (2021) 263–276
https://doi.org/10.1016/j.pmr.2021.01.004
1047-9651/21/Published by Elsevier Inc.

than ever is the call to help patients with cardiovascular and pulmonary disease safely and effectively access comprehensive rehabilitative programs that can improve quality of life.

Telerehabilitation enables virtual care by facilitating remote interactions between patients and providers using information and communication technology. It can use videoconferencing, telephone, email, secure messaging, smartphones, personal computers, wearable sensors, and other electronic gadgetry to engage participants of various levels of technological proficiency. Despite the virtual nature, cardiopulmonary telerehabilitation programs deliver real results for patients, families, caregivers, and an allied health care team.

Cardiac rehabilitation (CR) is a class IA recommendation for secondary prevention of cardiovascular disease (CVD)[3] yet remains poorly used, with studies reporting enrollment rates of only 25% to 30% of eligible patients in the United States.[4,5] Contributing factors to low participation include clinical provider awareness and referral patterns; facility or community resources; logistic impediments (eg, transportation, distance, schedule conflicts, caregiver responsibilities); and patient-dependent factors, such as motivation and health status. Telerehabilitation programs offer the advantage of reducing some logistical barriers while achieving comparable safety and efficacy to center-based care models for low-to-moderate-risk patients.[5–7] However, virtual CR faces separate challenges including a paucity of specific recommended protocols for patients with high complexity and cardiovascular risk. Although the Centers for Medicare and Medicaid Services expanded reimbursement for telehealth during the SARS-CoV-2 (COVID-19) pandemic to facilitate the path for clinicians to reach patients sequestered in their homes, no similar reimbursement allowance was arranged for home-based CR as of 2020.[8] In the setting of the COVID-19 global pandemic with public health recommendations emphasizing social distancing and imposing periodic or partial closures of outpatient services and gyms, virtual CR programs have emerged as necessary alternatives to facility-based care. Home-based cardiac telerehabilitation programs can help select appropriate patients, avoid delays in treatment, improve participation in secondary prevention programs, preserve delivery of care in a cost-effective and convenient manner, and mitigate risk of infections and preventable hospitalizations.[8]

Before the COVID-19 pandemic, concerns about limited access to hospital- or community-based pulmonary rehabilitation (PR) programs were expressed worldwide. For instance, only 0.5% to 2.0% of eligible patients in Portugal were reported to have access to a PR program.[9] Despite the well-supported benefits of PR, including improvement in functional capacity, limb muscle function, dyspnea, and psychosocial outcome measures, such as quality of life and self-efficacy, it is troubling that overall use of PR programs has been low.[10,11] One analysis revealed that only 3% of Medicare beneficiaries with COPD participate in traditional PR programs in the United States.[12] Given the recent rise in public acceptance of telehealth care options, there is likely an even lower use of pulmonary telerehabilitation programs. Insufficient funding, resources, reimbursement, awareness, and additional patient-related barriers to enrollment are cited as contributors to the gap in delivery of PR programs to patients who could benefit.[11,13]

Since the COVID-19 global outbreak, stakeholders have been pressed to expand access to the proven physiologic and psychosocial benefits of PR for patients with preexisting chronic pulmonary disease and newly acquired infectious respiratory illness. The closures of many community gyms and outpatient clinics have prompted technological solutions to overcome hindrances imposed by social distancing and lack of physical treatment spaces. The multidisciplinary nature of traditional PR programs involves a team of skilled providers to provide key components of medical clearance, exercise training, health coaching, and behavior modification to optimize respiratory fitness. However, lack of official endorsement for a standardized virtual care version of a multidisciplinary PR approach by leading professional organizations, such as the American Thoracic Society or the European Respiratory Society, leaves challenges in telehealth care planning, coordination, and implementation. Despite these challenges, studies have demonstrated effectiveness of home-based programs comparable with facility-based programs, including decreased acute COPD exacerbations and hospitalizations with superior reduction in emergency department visits.[14]

Cardiac and pulmonary telerehabilitation programs should be considered safe and effective components of a sustainable solution to meet the needs of patients with acute or chronic, preexisting or newly acquired, cardiopulmonary diseases. This review highlights clinical considerations, current evidence, global context, potential barriers, advantages, recommendations, and future directions of cardiopulmonary telerehabilitation.

NATURE OF THE PROBLEM/CONSIDERATIONS

Given the poor referral patterns, enrollment levels, and completion rates for traditional center-based CR programs, society has needed alternative strategies to deliver care in a convenient flexible manner.[7] With the emergence of the COVID-19 pandemic in early 2020, the global ability to offer care was further challenged. Home-based CR has increasingly been proposed because patients of all age groups show a growing ability to use information and communication technology to connect with their care providers.[15] A Pew Research Center survey in 2016 revealed that 80% of US adults ages 65 and older owned a cellphone and 42% had smartphones (up from 18% in 2013). Access to the Internet, tablets, computers, and social media is correlated with age, household income, and educational level.[16] It is important to take these patient-centered factors into consideration when trying to implement virtual CR programs. Additional challenges include limited facility and staff resources, paucity of standardized virtual CR protocols, lack of reimbursement, and underdeveloped virtual care infrastructure to meet privacy policy and documentation standards.

Part of the solution requires bridging the digital divide so people of broader ages, socioeconomic backgrounds, and technological familiarity can use communication technology. The Veterans Affairs system offers a good example of meeting this need through its recent creation of a national "digital divide" consultation that offers technical assistance and loaner tablets or smartphones to facilitate telehealth (eg, VA Video Connect, "my HealtheVet").

Another consideration is how to reach eligible patients in a fluctuating period of care-delivery restrictions and physical distancing recommendations. Changes in staffing, referral practices, early discharge emphasis, and intermittent closures of outpatient services can result in losing touch with patients in need of continuity of care. The Italian Association of Clinical Cardiology published a position paper describing frequently observed clinical scenarios. Delayed presentation and treatment were common themes in the postsurgery and postacute coronary syndrome patient population for fear of nosocomial infections. Observed direct effects of COVID-19 infection include acute cardiac injury presenting as elevated cardiac troponins, cardiomyopathy, and heart failure.[17] Indirect effects include quarantine-induced stress with restricted physical activities, reduced adherence to prescribed therapy, limited access to follow-up visits, social isolation, depression, behavioral addictive disorders, weight gain, and a cascade of sequelae from unsuccessful implementation of secondary prevention strategies.[17]

Patients with preexisting CVD are at increased risk of severe illness and worse outcome from COVID-19 infection given profound impacts on the pulmonary system and association with multiorgan failure, acute hypoxic myocardial injury, myocarditis, and arterial and venous thromboembolism.[18] Vascular complications, such as pulmonary embolism, deep vein thrombosis, disseminated intravascular coagulation, acute coronary syndrome, ischemic stroke, and arterial and capillary embolism, have been reported in approximately 20% of patients with COVID-19.[19] Therefore, residual impacts, such as deconditioning, focal neurologic deficits, risks of extended anticoagulation therapy, and possible development of post-phlebitic syndrome are contextual factors to consider because therapeutic and educational programs should be tailored to meet specific needs.

To maximize success, virtual cardiopulmonary rehabilitation programs should prioritize basic, safe, and timely care options over comprehensive or complex approaches.[5] Considering the status in resources and limitations of the health care recipients and providers is crucial to bridging the digital divide and implementing feasible solutions.

CURRENT EVIDENCE

There exists strong evidence for health benefits of PR, yet implementation is low with only 3% to 16% of appropriate patients with COPD being referred to PR and only 1% to 2% gaining access.[20] Transportation has been reported as the most common barrier to PR participation.[21] Therefore, pulmonary telerehabilitation has gained support. Health counseling via telephone was reported by patients with moderate to severe COPD to result in behavioral changes (eg, increased physical activity, smoking cessation) and increased motivation to maintain a healthier lifestyle.[22] There is moderate evidence that virtual PR can increase quality of life, reduce hospital admissions and emergency department visits, and reduce health care costs in patients with chronic pulmonary disease.[23]

In support of sustained PR outcomes, a 2-year pilot study showed full completion rate and improvement in 6-minute-walk distance with maintained physical performance, health status, and quality of life.[24] Most telehealth PR programs use regular telephone calls (eg, weekly calls for 8 weeks followed by transition to monthly telephone calls for up to a year) with reinforcement, feedback, and support provided via Web sites, mobile phone text messages, or live video-calls. A meta-analysis investigating effects of telehealth in patients with COPD found improvements in physical activity level,[25] which is importantly the strongest predictor for mortality in patients with COPD.[26]

In a study of elderly patients with combined COPD and CHF, a 4-month telerehabilitation program was deemed feasible, safe, and effective demonstrating improvements in walking distance, quality of life, dyspnea, physical activity profile, disability, and time-to-event (defined as hospitalization or death) compared with a control group[1] receiving standard care. The intervention group patients were followed via structured telephone calls with individualized exercise programs using mini-ergometer, callisthenic exercises, and pedometer-based walking and monitoring was done with pulse oximeter, portable one-lead electrocardiograph, and use of the Borg Rating of Perceived Exertion scale.[1]

Similar to PR, CR also suffers from low enrollment rates.[27] Multiple randomized controlled trials and meta-analyses have found cardiac telerehabilitation to be as effective as traditional center-based rehabilitation for patients with history of coronary atherosclerotic disease, myocardial infarction, revascularization, or heart failure.[28–30] Patients are remotely monitored using devices (eg, video, pulse oximeters, pedometers) to collect health data, such as daily physical activity and heart rate, to provide feedback.[31] Benefits of cardiac telerehabilitation include cost, convenience, increased participation, decreased transport needs, and empowerment of patients engaged in their rehabilitation experience through education by professionals and self-monitoring at home.[32,33]

In a randomized controlled study consisting of patients with documented coronary artery disease or previous myocardial infarction completing a 12-week CR program, peak oxygen uptake significantly increased in home-based and center-based groups, but the center-based group reported more sedentary time (quantified as <1.5 metabolic equivalent tasks [METs]).[31] Another randomized controlled trial supported these findings in heart failure patients. Their results showed no significant difference between home-based telerehabilitation and traditional center-based programs in gains in 6-minute-walk distance.[34]

In a systematic review and meta-analysis of 17 randomized trials by Buckingham and colleagues,[35] there was no difference in adverse events or all-cause mortality noted at 1-year follow-up, nor was any difference observed in the number of cardiac events, including coronary revascularization, recurrent myocardial infarctions, or heart failure–related admissions between home- and center-based groups. In one 6-year follow-up study,[36] general hospitalizations were greater for the center-based group compared with the home-based group and home-based programs seemed to confer higher adherence. Ultimately, there was no significant difference in secondary outcomes, including exercise capacity, modifiable risk factors, quality of life, and cardiac events when comparing home-based with center-based rehabilitation, suggesting that home-based programs are an adequate alternative to center-based programs.[35]

Cost of telerehabilitation programs is another important factor to consider with far-reaching consequences on access to care and future policies. Currently, the best conducted cost-analysis studies of cardiac telerehabilitation are based in Europe and New Zealand. The Telerehab III trial, conducted in Belgium, was a multicenter randomized controlled trial originally designed to assess the long-term efficacy of cardiac telerehabilitation compared with usual care. Frederix and colleagues[37] collected data from this study and performed a cost analysis, primarily focusing on incremental cost-effectiveness and number of lost workdays. Within the 1-year follow-up period, there was a statistically significant lower incremental cost per patient and significantly fewer days lost because of cardiovascular rehospitalizations compared with the control group.[37] A long-term follow-up study to the Telerehab III trial was conducted to gauge the cost impact of an additional 6-month cardiac telerehabilitation regimen at 2-year follow-up and still showed cost-savings and overall efficacy in the Internet-based therapy group.[38]

In a more recent New Zealand study,[33] similar cost reductions were found for virtual CR involving a 12-week smartphone and chest-worn wearable sensor-based platform compared with a supervised control group. Delivery of the telerehabilitation protocol was found to be substantially less expensive. Similarly, a Netherlands comparison trial found evidence that telerehabilitation had a 75% to 95% probability of being more cost-effective.[39]

The cost and efficiency at which cardiac telerehabilitation can be delivered help determine if it is a suitable option. Although further studies need to be conducted within the United States to conclusively determine the cost-effectiveness of cardiopulmonary telerehabilitation, current evidence is optimistic.

CLINICAL RELEVANCE

CR can have life-saving benefits, because just a 1-MET improvement in functional capacity bestows a 17% to 30% reduction in all-cause mortality.[40] One study examining a large pool of Medicare beneficiaries with coronary artery disease found a 21% to 34% lower mortality rate in those who completed CR compared with those who did not.[41] It also seems that reductions in mortality rates are dose-dependent. A study of greater than 30,000 Medicare beneficiaries participating in CR showed reduction in morbidity at 4 years was better if patients attended greater than 11 sessions out of a full 36 sessions offered. When mortality risk of those who attended all 36 sessions was compared with the risk of patients who attended fewer sessions, they observed that each additional six sessions was associated with a 6% reduction in mortality.[42] This underscores the importance of encouraging patients to not only initiate a CR program but to also choose a program they are most likely to complete in full.

Benefits of CR reach beyond those with typical CVD. Cancer survivors have a 1.3- to 3.6-fold increase in mortality risk and a 1.7- to 18.5-fold increase in incidence of CVD risk factors compared with people without a cancer history.[43] A comprehensive CR program focused on nutrition, physical activity, and appropriate management of cardiotoxic oncologic therapies is useful. Exercise has been shown to improve cardiorespiratory fitness after completion of cancer treatment, indicating lower mortality, less symptom burden, and lower treatment-related toxicities in this population. The connection between CVD risk factors and outcomes among cancer survivors clearly identifies a need for accessibility and feasibility of rehabilitation.[43] Patients undergoing treatment of cancer or recovering from illness are also particularly vulnerable to COVID-19, and careful consideration must be taken when determining if a face-to-face evaluation is justifiable. This presents another opportunity for telerehabilitation to protect frailer patients from potential exposure to a public health threat.

Not only does the presence of CVD increase COVID-19 fatality rates up to 10-fold, the pandemic-strained health care system has delayed routine care for many patients with CVD, leading to a greater risk of future cardiovascular events and death.[44] Many beneficial, but elective, interventions, such as coronary angiograms, pacemaker, or implantable cardioverter defibrillator device placement, and cardiac surgeries have been postponed. Even patients who experience an acute coronary event fear going to the hospital, and admissions to cardiac intensive care units have been reduced and follow-up care appointments are fewer than usual because of concerns of COVID-19 exposure.[45] This can result in a cycle of patients being untreated or undertreated for existing cardiovascular conditions and potentially suffering adverse outcomes.

Cardiac telerehabilitation will become more important following the resolution of the COVID-19 pandemic. Some long-term sequelae for those recovering from the virus include cardiac injury, coagulation disorders, stroke, and critical illness myopathy and polyneuropathy.[46] Home-based rehabilitation allows for initiation of therapy and education while keeping these patients safely isolated from others early in the recovery phase.

APPLICATION

Center-based CR has a class IA recommendation by the American Heart Association, the American College of Cardiology, and the European Society of Cardiology for secondary prevention after an acute coronary syndrome, coronary revascularization, or in the setting of stable angina or symptomatic peripheral arterial disease. CR is also recommended after heart valve surgery, cardiac transplantation, and CHF with reduced ejection fraction.[7,15]

During the COVID-19 global pandemic, some inpatient CR units have been closed or converted to emergency COVID units and the medical staff detailed to fulfill other hospital operation duties. Phase I inpatient CR programs noted reduced referrals for patients with nonemergent cardiothoracic surgeries and procedures that were deferred because of fear of nosocomial infections.[45] Because of the higher COVID-19 mortality rates of elderly patients with preexisting cardiopulmonary disease,[47] health care systems have emphasized the importance of reducing unnecessary hospital visits. Traditional phase II outpatient CR programs have largely been postponed but core elements are effectively delivered through telemedicine.[5]

Fig. 1 presents the generally accepted three-phase model of CR programs with additional components of telehealth to augment the outpatient phase II and longer-term maintenance phase III after completion of the inpatient phase I. The major components of an outpatient cardiopulmonary telerehabilitation program are shown in **Fig. 2**.

COMPLICATIONS/CONCERNS

During a global health crisis, such as the COVID-19 pandemic, providers face the challenge of performing a risk-benefit analysis to triage patients to either in-person evaluation or virtual care. It can feel like a high-stakes gamble where the risks of offering a virtual CR program without the typical face-to-face clearance evaluation must be balanced with the benefits of initiating valuable elements of CR while preventing unnecessary infectious disease exposure.

Leading organizations consider a symptom-limited graded exercise test (GXT) to be the gold standard for exercise prescription formulation and risk stratification. However, because of the predominant droplet and probable airborne mode of SARS-CoV-2 virus transmission, face-to-face encounters and nonemergent aerosol-generating

Phases of Cardiac Rehabilitation + Telehealth

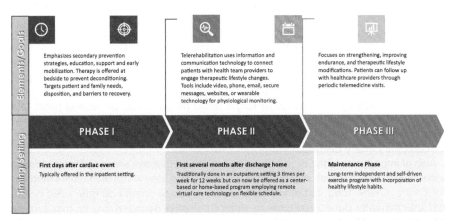

Fig. 1. Scheme of the three-phase model of cardiac rehabilitation with additional telehealth components to augment the outpatient intervention period (phases II and III) after completion of the traditional early inpatient treatment period (phase I).

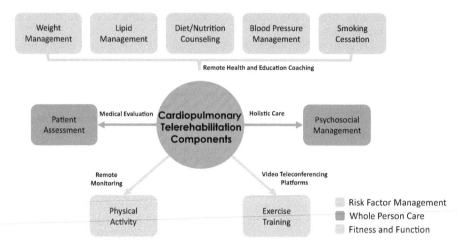

Fig. 2. Key components of cardiopulmonary rehabilitation are vital to center-based and home-based programs. These secondary prevention strategies incorporate elements from risk factor management to whole person care to fitness and function. These interventions are achieved remotely through use of information and communication technology.

procedures, such as a GXT, have been largely discouraged.[47] Nonetheless, a GXT should be performed under safest conditions possible (eg, preprocedure COVID-19 testing and proper personal protective equipment) if clinically indicated for particularly higher risk patients (eg, active cardiopulmonary symptoms, exercise-related arrhythmias, or significantly reduced ejection fraction). If a GXT is not available or deemed necessary, a careful decision-making process can permit alternative methods of assessing functional capacity (eg, Duke Activity Status Index, self-administered 6-minute-walk test). Home-based exercise prescriptions should be conservative, slowly titrated, and monitored via wearable heart-rate monitors/sensors or exertion level estimates (eg, the "talk test" or Borg Rating of Perceived Exertion).[5] Before the COVID-19 pandemic, surveys done by US[48] and Dutch clinics[49] reported that up to 70% of CR programs did not perform a baseline GXT before initiating CR and used other methods to create exercise prescriptions.[40] Therefore, a cautious prescription for physical activity is arguably better than the alternative of withholding CR completely.

Moderate-intensity exercise programs are guided by parameters, such as the Karvonen formula (eg, 40%–60% of the heart rate reserve plus resting heart rate), 55% to 70% peak heart rate, 4 to 6 METs, or the "speech rule" (ie, respiratory rate allows conversation).[50] In the absence of a baseline GXT, commonly used techniques for prescribing exercise include using the Borg rating of perceived exertion in a range of 11 to 14 or creating a conservative target pulse range based on resting heart rate plus 20 to 30 beats per minute.[40] The rating of perceived exertion is closely related to physiologic responses to exercise, such as lactate threshold, even in patients with coronary artery disease.[51]

Also of importance is the blood pressure and blood glucose response to exercise in patients with hypertension and diabetes mellitus, especially when on multiple medications with variable food and fluid intake. Blood pressure should be measured before and intermittently during exercise to detect possible hypertensive or hypotensive response to exercise. A systolic blood pressure greater than 200 mm Hg or a diastolic blood pressure greater than 100 mm Hg is used as a relative indication to terminate exercise.[50] A decrease in systolic blood pressure greater than 10 mm Hg less than baseline while exercising is also a reason for holding activity and seeking evaluation for cardiac ischemia before continuing a telerehabilitation program. For patients with diabetes, initial exercise workload should be cautious to prevent hypoglycemic events possibly triggered by skeletal muscle consumption in proportion to exercise intensity. Patients should be advised to check their blood glucose levels before and after the first few exercise sessions if they do not have a recent history of being physically active. A small snack (with ~15 g of carbohydrate) is given if blood sugar levels are low (<70 mg/dL) and repeated if still low on a recheck 15 minutes later. Exercise progression are gradually and safely achieved through routine remote telerehabilitation program participation.

Patients with CHF are considered to be at higher risk for an exercise-related event and warrant telehealth screening for warning signs, such as active cardiopulmonary symptoms, vital sign abnormalities, weight trends (eg, sudden increase can signal fluid retention), and absence or even reversal of expected progress. If a CR team member suspects worsening exercise intolerance or significant ischemia at low work rates (<2 METs), exercise should be terminated, and the patient directed for appropriate reassessment.[52]

Serious adverse CVD events are estimated to occur in about 1 per every 50,000 patient-hours during center-based CR, but the incidence of adverse events experienced during cardiac telerehabilitation is not well established.[4] Cardiopulmonary arrests, arrhythmias, angina, syncope, and ST-segment changes on electrocardiogram are typically categorized as true adverse events.[53] The incidence of such events during cardiac telerehabilitation should ideally occur at comparable or lower rates than traditional center-based CR to be suitable. Fortunately, there are some promising studies in support of telerehabilitation safety.

There have been several reviews demonstrating optimistic findings in favor of telerehabilitation. A European multinational randomized clinical trial demonstrated that there was no significant increase in adverse events between participation in cardiac telerehabilitation compared with no rehabilitation at all. Snoek and colleagues[54] concluded that based on these findings, telerehabilitation may safely offer improved physical fitness and activity to elderly patients that decline traditional center-based CR. Frederix and colleagues reviewed 37 publications using a variety of telemedicine formats including telephone, Internet-based, and videoconferencing interventions. Seven of these 37 publications evaluated safety and after pooled analysis, the telerehabilitation format was found to be favored in terms of adverse events and rehospitalizations because of cardiovascular reasons (odds ratio, 1.30; 95% confidence interval, 1.13–1.50).[55] Two additional systematic reviews corroborated these findings, reporting a negligible difference in adverse events attributed to participation in telerehabilitation.[28,56] Although many prior studies have been statistically underpowered and conducted in a non-US population, cardiac telerehabilitation seems to be a suitable alternative to center-based rehabilitation provided patients are adequately risk-stratified (low-to-moderate-risk cardiac patients) before engaging in therapies.[4]

FUTURE DIRECTIONS/SUMMARY

Further studies investigating the safety and efficacy of cardiopulmonary telerehabilitation will help set standardized guidelines, especially in light of the recent pandemic, which has left many COVID-19 survivors in need of care.[57] In fact, among patients that required intensive care unit hospitalization, many develop long-lasting cardiac consequences, including venous thromboembolisms, myocarditis, or myocardial ischemic injury.[57] In a study performed in Switzerland among COVID-19 survivors,

Table 1	
Seven tips for starting a cardiopulmonary telerehabilitation program	
Make it simple	Use existing staff and resources with the mantra, "Use what works and work with what you got." A telephone is effective if your patient or team does not have secure videoconferencing or smartphone technology available.
Make it timely	Do not delay care if you can start even just a hybrid model or partial aspect of the multidisciplinary program safely.
Make it focused	Target your dedicated telehealth virtual sessions on core elements, such as medical advice, physical therapeutic activities, psychological counseling, dietary education, smoking cessation, and other topics.
Make it practical	Consider helpful tools that are easy to use and may be available at your facility, such as blood pressure cuffs, pedometers, pulse oximeters, pedal exercise machines, loaner tablets or smartphones, and illustrated exercise pamphlet materials.
Make it social	To reduce feelings of social isolation, introduce patient group sessions for dietician, psychologist, physiologist, and other multidisciplinary team members.
Make it better	Keep assessing and seeking ways to improve the program based on feedback from patients, providers, and other stakeholders. Provide updates to colleagues, department and facility leadership, and funding resources when positive outcomes and milestones are achieved to share success stories.
Make it last	Strengthen and reinforce your team and resources. Even after COVID-19 or another public health threat, plan for cardiopulmonary telerehabilitation programs to continue offering a safe and effective alternative to center-based care.

some of whom required mechanical ventilation, 2 to 4 weeks of acute inpatient cardiopulmonary rehabilitation improved exercise capacity measured by the 6-minute-walk test.[57] A need for an alternative to acute inpatient rehabilitation for those who cannot feasibly access these health services has arisen. Furthermore, those who pose a high risk for reinfection may find it safer to participate in rehabilitation in a socially distanced manner. When remotely guided physical exercise and multidisciplinary secondary prevention measures are used in conjunction, these interventions have been shown to reduce future adverse events and help patients manage risk factors.[44]

Moving forward, cardiopulmonary telerehabilitation should be made widely accessible and incorporate new lessons learned from the COVID-19 pandemic and harness the power of information and communication technology to provide evidence-based patient-centered care. **Table 1** lists recommendations to facilities or health care groups seeking to develop a cardiopulmonary telerehabilitation program.

CLINICS CARE POINTS

- Cardiac and pulmonary telerehabilitation are safe, convenient, and cost-effective alternatives to traditional center-based rehabilitation programs and facilitate patient participation by reducing logistical and financial barriers.
- Comprehensive telerehabilitation programs can include remote monitoring, health coaching, virtual education tools, and social networking to enhance interest and motivation.
- Potential limitations of cardiopulmonary telerehabilitation include willingness and ability of enrolled patients to engage in telehealth technologies in addition to limitations on resources, reimbursement, and policies within health care organizations.

- Because of the increased health risks faced by patients with cardiopulmonary disease, telemedicine offers the benefit of a remote visit type during an ongoing pandemic (especially when the infectious disease impacts cardiac and respiratory systems).

DISCLOSURE

The authors have nothing to disclose.

REFERENCES

1. Bernocchi P, Vitacca M, La Rovere MT, et al. Home-based telerehabilitation in older patients with chronic obstructive pulmonary disease and heart failure: a randomised controlled trial. Age Ageing 2018;47(1):82–8.
2. Hawkins NM, Virani S, Ceconi C. Heart failure and chronic obstructive pulmonary disease: the challenges facing physicians and health services. Eur J Heart Fail 2013;34:2795–803.
3. Piepoli MF, Corrà U, Adamopoulos S, et al. Secondary prevention in the clinical management of patients with cardiovascular diseases. Core components, standards and outcome measures for referral and delivery: a policy statement from the cardiac rehabilitation section of the European Association for Cardiovascular Prevention & Rehabilitation. Endorsed by the Committee for Practice Guidelines of the European Society of Cardiology. Eur J Prev Cardiol 2014;21(6):664–81.
4. Thomas RJ, Beatty AL, Beckie TM. Home-based cardiac rehabilitation: a scientific statement from the American Association of Cardiovascular and Pulmonary Rehabilitation, the American Heart Association, and the American College of Cardiology. J Am Coll Cardiol 2019;74:133–53.
5. Moulson N, Bewick D, Selway T, et al. Cardiac rehabilitation during the COVID-19 era: guidance on implementing virtual care. Can J Cardiol 2020;36(8):1317–21.
6. Scherrenberg M, Wilhelm M, Hansen D, et al. The future is now: a call for action for cardiac telerehabilitation in the COVID-19 pandemic from the secondary prevention and rehabilitation section of the European Association of Preventive Cardiology. Eur J Prev Cardiol 2020. https://doi.org/10.1177/2047487320939671. 2047487320939671.
7. Kumar KR, Pina IL. Cardiac rehabilitation in older adults: new options. Clin Cardiol 2020;43(2):163–70.
8. Drwal KR, Forman DE, Wakefield BJ, et al. Cardiac rehabilitation during COVID-19 pandemic: highlighting the value of home-based programs. Telemed J E Health 2020;26(11):1322–4.
9. Jacome C, Marques A, Oliveira A, et al. Letter to the editor pulmonary telerehabilitation: an international call for action. Pulmonol 2020;26(6):335–7.
10. Spruit MA, Singh SJ, Garvey C, et al. An official American Thoracic Society/European Respiratory Society statement: key concepts and advances in pulmonary rehabilitation. Am J Respir Crit Care Med 2013;188:e13–64.
11. Rochester CI, Vogiatzis I, Holland AE, et al. An official American Thoracic Society/European Respiratory Society policy statement: enhancing implementation, use, and delivery of pulmonary rehabilitation. Am J Respir Crit Care Med 2015;192:1373–86.
12. Nishi SP, Zhang W, Kuo YF, et al. Pulmonary rehabilitation utilization in older adults with chronic obstructive pulmonary disease, 2003 to 2012. J Cardiopulm Rehabil Prev 2016;36:375–82.

13. Garvey C, Novitch RS, Porte P, et al. Editorial healing pulmonary rehabilitation in the United States: a call to action for ATS members. Am J Respir Crit Care Med 2019;8:944–6.

14. Vasilopoulou M, Pappaioannou AI, Kaltsakas G, et al. Home-based maintenance telerehabilitation reduces the risk for acute exacerbations of COPD, hospitalisations, and emergency department visits. Eur Respir J 2017;49:1602129.

15. Beckie TM. Utility of home-based cardiac rehabilitation for older adults. Clin Geriatr Med 2019;35(4):499–516.

16. Anderson M, Perrin A. Tech adoption climbs among older adults. In: Pew Research Center Internet & Technology. 2017. Available at: https://www.pewresearch.org/internet/2017/05/17/technology-use-among-seniors/. Accessed December 13, 2020.

17. Mureddu GF, Ambrosetti M, Venturini E, et al. Cardiac rehabilitation activities during the COVID-19 pandemic in Italy. Position Paper of the AICPR (Italian Association of Clinical Cardiology, Prevention and Rehabilitation). Monaldi Arch Chest Dis 2020;90(2). https://doi.org/10.4081/monaldi.2020.1439.

18. Huang C, Wang Y, Li X, et al. Clinical features of patients infected with 2019 novel coronavirus in Wuhan, China. Lancet 2020;395:497–506.

19. Zhai Z, Li C, Chen Y, et al. Prevention and treatment of venous thromboembolism associated with coronavirus disease 2019 infection: a consensus statement before guidelines. Thromb Haemost 2020;120(6):937–48.

20. Johnston K, Grimmer-Somers K. Pulmonary rehabilitation: overwhelming evidence but lost in translation? Physiother Can 2010;62:368–73.

21. Thorpe O, Johnston K, Kumar S. Barriers and enablers to physical activity participation in patients with COPD: a systematic review. J Cardiopulm Rehabil Prev 2012;32:359–69.

22. Walters JA, Cameron-Tucker H, Courtney-Pratt H, et al. Supporting health behavior change in chronic obstructive pulmonary disease with telephone health-monitoring: insights from a qualitative study. BMC Fam Pract 2012;13:55.

23. McLean S, Nurmatov U, Liu JL, et al. Telehealthcare for chronic obstructive pulmonary disease. Cochrane Review and meta-analysis. Br J Gen Pract 2012;62(604):e739–49.

24. Zanaboni P, Hoaas H, Lien LA, et al. Long-term exercise maintenance in COPD via telerehabilitation: a two-year pilot study. J Telemed Telecare 2016;23(1):74–82.

25. Lundell S, Holmner Å, Rehn B. Telehealthcare in COPD: a systematic review and meta-analysis on physical outcomes and dyspnea. Respir Med 2015;109(1):11–26.

26. Waschki B, Kirsten A, Holz O, et al. Physical activity is the strongest predictor of all-cause mortality in patients with COPD: a prospective cohort study. Chest 2011;140:331–42.

27. Chan C, Yamabayashi C, Syed N, et al. Exercise telemonitoring and telerehabilitation compared with traditional cardiac and pulmonary rehabilitation: a systematic review and meta-analysis. Physiother Can 2016;68(3):242–51.

28. Huang K, Liu W, He D, et al. Telehealth interventions versus center-based cardiac rehabilitation of coronary artery disease: a systematic review and meta-analysis. Eur J Prev Cardiol 2015;22(8):959–71.

29. Anderson L, Sharp GA, Norton RJ, et al. Home-based versus centre-based cardiac rehabilitation. Cochrane Database Syst Rev 2017;6(6):CD007130.

30. Batalik L, Filakova K, Batalikova K, et al. Remotely monitored telerehabilitation for cardiac patients: a review of the current situation. World J Clin Cases 2020;8(10): 1818–31.

31. Avila A, Claes J, Goetschalckx K, et al. Home-based rehabilitation with telemonitoring guidance for patients with coronary artery disease (short-term results of the TRiCH Study): randomized controlled trial. J Med Internet Res 2018;20(6):e225.

32. Brouwers RWM, van Exel HJ, van Hal JMC, et al. Cardiac telerehabilitation as an alternative to centre-based cardiac rehabilitation. Neth Heart J 2020;28(9): 443–51.

33. Maddison R, Rawstorn JC, Stewart RAH, et al. Effects and costs of real-time cardiac telerehabilitation: randomised controlled non-inferiority trial. Heart 2019; 105(2):122–9.

34. Hwang R, Bruning J, Morris NR, et al. Home-based telerehabilitation is not inferior to a centre-based program in patients with chronic heart failure: a randomised trial. J Physiother 2017;63(2):101–7.

35. Buckingham SA, Taylor RS, Jolly K, et al. Home-based versus centre-based cardiac rehabilitation: abridged Cochrane systematic review and meta-analysis. Open Heart 2016;3(2):e000463.

36. Arthur HM, Smith KM, Kodis J, et al. A controlled trial of hospital versus home-based exercise in cardiac patients. Med Sci Sports Exerc 2002;34:1544–50.

37. Frederix I, Hansen D, Coninx K, et al. Effect of comprehensive cardiac telerehabilitation on one-year cardiovascular rehospitalization rate, medical costs and quality of life: a cost-effectiveness analysis. Eur J Prev Cardiol 2016;23(7): 674–82.

38. Frederix I, Solmi F, Piepoli MF, et al. Cardiac telerehabilitation: a novel cost-efficient care delivery strategy that can induce long-term health benefits. Eur J Prev Cardiol 2017;24(16):1708–17.

39. Kraal JJ, Van den Akker-Van Marle ME, Abu-Hanna A, et al. Clinical and cost-effectiveness of home-based cardiac rehabilitation compared to conventional, centre-based cardiac rehabilitation: Results of the FIT@Home study. Eur J Prev Cardiol 2017;24(12):1260–73.

40. Mytinger M, Nelson RK, Zuhl M. Exercise prescription guidelines for cardiovascular disease patients in the absence of a baseline stress test. J Cardiovasc Dev Dis 2020;7(2):15.

41. Suaya JA, Stason WB, Ades PA, et al. Cardiac rehabilitation and survival in older coronary patients. J Am Coll Cardiol 2009;54:25–33.

42. Hammill BG, Curtis LH, Schulman KA, et al. Relationship between cardiac rehabilitation and long-term risks of death and myocardial infarction among elderly Medicare beneficiaries. Circulation 2010;121:63–70.

43. Gilchrist SC, Barac A, Ades PA, et al. Cardio-oncology rehabilitation to manage cardiovascular outcomes in cancer patients and survivors. a scientific statement from the American Heart Association. Circulation 2019;138:e997–1012.

44. Nicholls SJ, Nelson M, Astley C, et al. Optimising secondary prevention and cardiac rehabilitation for atherosclerotic cardiovascular disease during the COVID-19 pandemic: a position statement from the Cardiac Society of Australia and New Zealand (CSANZ). Heart Lung Circ 2020;29(7):e99–104.

45. Vigorito C, Faggiano P, Mureddu GF. COVID-19 pandemic: what consequences for cardiac rehabilitation? Monaldi Arch Chest Dis 2020;90(1). https://doi.org/10.4081/monaldi.2020.1315.

46. Sheehy LM. Considerations for postacute rehabilitation for survivors of COVID-19. JMIR Public Health Surveill 2020;6(2):e19462.

47. CDC Coronavirus Disease 2019 (COVID-19) overview and infection prevention and control priorities in non-US healthcare settings. Available at: https://www.cdc.gov/coronavirus/2019-ncov/hcp/non-us-settings/overview/index.html#transmission. Accessed November 29, 2020.

48. O'Neil S, Thomas A, Pettit-Mee R, et al. Exercise prescription techniques in cardiac rehabilitation centers in midwest states. J Clin Physiol 2018;7:8–14.

49. Vromen T, Spee R, Kraal J, et al. Exercise training programs in Dutch cardiac rehabilitation centres. Neth Heart J 2013;21:138–43.

50. Ambrosetti M, Abreu A, Corrà U, et al. Secondary prevention through comprehensive cardiovascular rehabilitation: from knowledge to implementation. 2020 update. A position paper from the Secondary Prevention and Rehabilitation Section of the European Association of Preventive Cardiology. Eur J Prev Cardiol 2020. https://doi.org/10.1177/2047487320913379. 2047487320913379.

51. Scherr J, Wolfarth B, Christle JW, et al. Associations between Borg's rating of perceived exertion and physiological measures of exercise intensity. Eur J Appl Physiol 2013;113:147–55.

52. Myers J. Principles of exercise prescription for patients with chronic heart failure. Heart Fail Rev 2008;13:61–8.

53. Gibbons RJ, Balady GJ, Bricker JT, et al. ACC/AHA 2002 guideline update for exercise testing: summary article. A report of the American College of Cardiology/American Heart Association Task Force on Practice Guidelines (Committee to Update the 1997 Exercise Testing Guidelines) [published correction appears in J Am Coll Cardiol. 2006 Oct 17;48(8):1731]. J Am Coll Cardiol 2002;40(8):1531–40.

54. Snoek JA, Prescott EI, van der Velde AE, et al. Effectiveness of home-based mobile guided cardiac rehabilitation as alternative strategy for nonparticipation in clinic-based cardiac rehabilitation among elderly patients in Europe: a randomized clinical trial. JAMA Cardiol 2020;e205218. https://doi.org/10.1001/jamacardio.2020.5218.

55. Frederix I, Vanhees L, Dendale P, et al. A review of telerehabilitation for cardiac patients. J Telemed Telecare 2015;21(1):45–53.

56. Hwang R, Bruning J, Morris N, et al. A systematic review of the effects of telerehabilitation in patients with cardiopulmonary diseases. J Cardiopulm Rehabil Prev 2015;35(6):380–9.

57. Hermann M, Pekacka-Egli A-M, Witassek F, et al. Feasibility and efficacy of cardiopulmonary rehabilitation after COVID-19. Am J Phys Med Rehabil 2020; 99(10):865–9.

Cancer Telerehabilitation

Philip Chang, DO[a],*, Arash Asher, MD[b]

KEYWORDS

- Telerehabilitation • Cancer rehabilitation • Telemedicine • Oncology rehabilitation

KEY POINTS

- Patients with cancer are at increased risk for severe illness from coronavirus disease 2019 (COVID-19).
- Telemedicine is an important tool in providing cancer rehabilitation medicine services and has the potential to reach more remote populations.
- Telemedicine can be an adequate substitute for in-person visits in many situations.
- Preparation and triaging of patients to the appropriate encounter type (in person or virtual) is critical to a successful visit.

INTRODUCTION
Background

The pandemic caused by the novel coronavirus disease 2019 (COVID-19) has expedited the transition to telemedicine across the spectrum of medical care. Several health systems have increased the proportion of patients seen via telemedicine, with some reporting 6-fold increases in telemedicine encounters.[1] Not only has this growth occurred in specialties ranging from urology[2] to allergy and immunology[3] but there has also been a concordant increase in interest from the general population.[4] The benefits of telemedicine during a pandemic are both clear and lifesaving as has been observed with the preservation of limited medical supplies, namely personal protective equipment, and the promotion of social distancing.

It is now well established that COVID-19 does not affect everyone equally, and older adults and those with certain medical conditions are at increased risk for severe illness.[5] The Centers for Disease Control and Prevention (CDC) recognizes that patients of any age with comorbidities of obesity, chronic kidney disease, COPD, serious heart disease, type 2 diabetes mellitus, sickle cell disease, immunocompromised state, and cancer are all at increased risk for severe illness.[5] There is strong and

[a] Department of Physical Medicine and Rehabilitation, Cedars-Sinai Samuel Oschin Comprehensive Cancer Institute, 8700 Beverly Boulevard, NT Lower Level, AC 1050, Los Angeles, CA 90048, USA; [b] Wellness, Resilience and Survivorship, Department of Physical Medicine and Rehabilitation, Cedars-Sinai Samuel Oschin Comprehensive Cancer Institute, 8700 Beverly Boulevard, NT Lower Level, AC 1109, Los Angeles, CA 90048, USA
* Corresponding author.
E-mail address: Philip.chang@cshs.org

Phys Med Rehabil Clin N Am 32 (2021) 277–289
https://doi.org/10.1016/j.pmr.2020.12.001
1047-9651/21/© 2020 Elsevier Inc. All rights reserved.

consistent evidence for cancer in particular as being an important risk factor. One of the initial studies from China showed that patients with cancer had a higher mortality at 5.6% compared with 2.3% in the general population.[6] A larger international retrospective study with 928 patients with cancer showed that 40% of patients were hospitalized, 13% were intubated, and there was a case fatality rate of 13%.[7] Similarly, a prospective cohort study in 800 patients reported an overall mortality of 23%.[8] These and several other studies[9–11] indicate that COVID-19 disproportionately affects patients with cancer with increased rates of intubation and death.[12]

Apart from the serious risks associated with the novel coronavirus and other communicable diseases, patients with cancer face additional barriers to receiving traditional in-person care. It has been estimated that less than 15% of patients receive their cancer care at tertiary care centers.[13] Although there has been rapid growth in the last 10 years, cancer rehabilitation remains an emerging field, and most specialized providers are concentrated in these tertiary care centers, which are not widely accessible to the population at large. It is common for patients to live very far from the facilities where they receive cancer treatment, with 1 study indicating that 24% of Medicare beneficiaries drive more than an hour to reach their care sites.[14] These additional cost and travel burdens are often compounded by the significant physical ailments that accompany malignancies, including pain, fatigue, and often physical disability.

As such, it is vital that telemedicine becomes an essential component of comprehensive cancer rehabilitation care, because it has the capacity not only to keep patients safer but also to reduce significant travel burdens and reach currently unreached communities. The remainder of this article discusses the advantages and disadvantages of telemedicine as well as the various factors to be considered when providing telemedicine rehabilitation services to patients with cancer.

DISCUSSION
Advantages of Telemedicine

As outlined earlier, there are several advantages to telemedicine for patients with cancer (**Box 1**), perhaps foremost of which is the ability to keep the patient in a safer and more isolated environment. In addition to surgery, the 2 primary treatment modalities for cancer are radiation therapy and systemic therapy, which often includes chemotherapy. Both of these therapies put patients at increased risk for neutropenia, which is commonly defined as an absolute neutrophil count (ANC) of less than 1500 cells/μL in an adult. The severity and duration of neutropenia have been shown to pose a greater risk for life-threatening infection, with 10% risk in patients with ANC less

---

Box 1
Telemedicine advantages and disadvantages

Advantages
  Decreased travel time and costs
  Improved isolation and social distancing
  Increased convenience for patients
  Reaching more remote communities

Disadvantages
  Increased social isolation
  Limitations in physical examination
  Technical difficulties
  Unable to provide interventions

than 1000/μL for 1 week and 50% infection risk if ANC is less than 1000/μL for 4 weeks.[15] Patients are at risk not only for contracting and developing serious complications secondary to COVID-19 but also from other common opportunistic infections, including methicillin-resistant *Staphylococcus aureus* (MRSA) and viridans group streptococci.[16] These risks are further amplified in patients who have received allogeneic bone marrow transplants, who are frequently on immunosuppressants. Keeping patients out of clinics, waiting rooms, and hospital settings may in some circumstances be lifesaving.

In addition to increased infection risk, patients with cancer also have increased risk for developing thrombosis. Some reports have stated that cancer-associated thrombosis accounts for 20% of all incidents of thrombosis worldwide[17] and that it is the second leading cause of death in patients with cancer.[18] Venous stasis, a key component of the Virchow triad in the development of venous thrombosis, may occur with prolonged periods of immobility, such as extended car travel. For those patients who do travel long distances to reach their cancer centers, telemedicine may be a good method to help mitigate such risks.

Aside from the physical risks of travel, patients and their caregivers often note the difficulties and increased stress of having to travel for frequent clinic visits. For some patients, travel distances can be significant and parking costs and gas fees can quickly add up. It is common for patients with cancer to have a large care team consisting of a surgeon, radiation oncologist, medical oncologist, primary care provider, and multiple members of a supportive care team. Although many cancer centers try to coordinate and consolidate care to reduce the number of trips taken, often this is not feasible. Patients with cancer also frequently have the added burden of reduced functional ability compounding travel difficulties. Problems with gait and balance are common among older individuals, but adjusted prevalence rates are even higher among patients with cancer, including prostate, breast, lung, and non-Hodgkin lymphoma.[19] A study on 244 patients receiving outpatient cancer treatment showed that 17.8% of patients reported difficulties with balance and 22% reported problems with gait.[20] Cancer-related fatigue is even more common, with reports of almost universal prevalence throughout the course of a disease, affecting virtually all patients while on chemotherapy and up to 30% of patients who have finished treatment.[21] Such functional deficits increase the difficulty of transferring in and out of cars, walking from distant parking lots, and navigating complex hospital corridors. Telemedicine can significantly alleviate these burdens, as 1 study in a vascular surgery practice showed significant decreases in travel time, travel distance, and cost for patients.[22]

Disadvantages of Telemedicine

Although telemedicine has shown itself to be an important and likely essential tool in the care of patients with cancer, it is not a perfect substitute for in-person visits. In the realm of a neuromusculoskeletal centric specialty, perhaps the most striking difficulty comes from the limitations in performing a physical examination. Although guidelines for conducting a musculoskeletal physical examination have recently become available[23] in which providers instruct patients and able helpers through physical examination maneuvers, specificities and sensitivities of these new techniques are not yet available. In addition, physicians may be apprehensive about making a diagnosis when they have not been able to physically examine patients the way they were trained to do. Some physicians may practice differently under such circumstances, whether it be ordering a more intensive work-up or being more hesitant when ordering interventional procedures such as nerve blocks or epidural injections. Much remains unknown on this front and future studies are needed.

Although technology has undoubtedly made extraordinary progress in the last 20 years, it is still common to run into technical difficulties. Because an unprecedented number of meetings have now been shifted to online platforms, virtually everyone has experienced a dropped call, a frozen screen, loss of audio/video, or some other malfunction, which can be irritating, to say the least. When technical difficulties do occur, they may lead to frustrations on the sides of both patients and health care providers, adding stress to an already stressful situation and undermining the purpose of the encounter. These challenges may disproportionately affect those with poorer technologic literacy, and they may have increased difficulty troubleshooting problems. It is hoped that, as technology continues to advance, such issues can be minimized, but for now they remain as a continuing challenge.

Reimbursement for services could be an issue for a subset of patients, limiting the scope of telemedicine. As of this writing, there are 71 National Cancer Institute (NCI)–designated cancer centers operating in 36 states.[24] It is common for patients to travel significant distances to receive care at an NCI-designated cancer center as they perform many of the ongoing clinical trials, and a 2015 study showed superior survival rates compared with non–NCI-designated centers.[25] As such, cancer centers close to state borders may have patients seeking out-of-state care, and some payers may not cover out-of-state telemedicine visits. As of 2019, there are 9 states that issue special licenses or certificates allowing providers to render telemedicine services in states where they are not located.[26] It should be noted that state laws and regulations regarding reimbursement for telehealth services are frequently evolving because of the COVID-19 pandemic.[26]

Another area of concern is the potential for creating greater gaps in health care disparity. A survey study seeking to understand barriers to telemedicine use in rural emergency departments found that 46% of the emergency departments surveyed did not use telemedicine, and cost was the most commonly cited barrier to adoption.[27] Care should be taken moving forward to ensure more equitable distribution of health care resources.

Finally, the negative impacts of social isolation, which may lead to loneliness, cannot be overstated. Cancer is already known to be potentially isolating because cancer and its treatment may contribute to individuals feeling cut off from their normal social networks. One sample of 94 patients with gynecologic cancer found that 44% of women had moderate levels of loneliness and a further 8.5% had moderately high or high levels of loneliness.[28] Other groups, such as those with head and neck cancer, are also known to be more socially isolated because of issues related to eating, drinking, and body image changes.[29] Given the recognition among many patients with cancer of the higher risks of COVID-19 complications, many feel even more lonely and isolated given current pandemic circumstances. Chronic loneliness is associated with worse cancer outcomes; higher rates of pain, depression, and fatigue; as well as higher hazard ratios among breast cancer survivors.[30,31] The personal, face-to-face engagement with the health care team, which may include nurses, parking attendants, check-in clerks, and of course physicians, is absent with telemedicine and may have quality-of-life and health risks of its own.

Approach to Care: Preparing for a Telemedicine Visit

Before conducting a telemedicine visit, it is necessary to review the policies and practices of the individual institution. Policies on which telemedicine platforms are acceptable for use vary from institution to institution, and clinicians should be aware of which platforms can be used and on what specific devices in order to maintain compliance with the Health Insurance Portability and Accountability Act (HIPAA) guidelines.

Regulations were relaxed during the onset of the pandemic with the use of popular video chatting applications, including Facetime (Apple Inc, Cupertino, CA), Google Hangouts (Google LLC, Mountain View, CA), and Skype (Skype Technologies, Palo Alto, CA), permitted without risk of penalty for noncompliance of HIPAA rules.[32] However, these allowances should be assumed to be temporary, and clearance from an individual institution's administration should be obtained.

Likewise, institutions may have requirements for documentation to maintain compliance with state and federal regulations. In addition to the standard documentation requirements per evaluation and management guidelines, additional documentation of the patient's consent to the telemedicine visit, visit start time, visit end time, location of the patient, location of the provider, and participants in the encounter may be required. Premade templates or so-called smart phrases in an institution's electronic medical record may be available and can be tested before the encounter.

Institutional procedures for patient intake for telemedicine visits should be reviewed. During typical in-person clinic visits, patients are seen by a nurse or medical assistant who may take vitals, do a medication reconciliation, provide instruction on the completion of intake forms, and possibly take a brief history and review of systems. Except for vitals, it is possible for these other aspects of intake to be streamlined into the telemedicine encounter, and discussions with the clinic team should take place.

Before the encounter, patients may benefit from receiving specific instructions on how to set up the visit. If it is a phone visit, specifications can be made as to who will be calling who and at which phone number. If it is a video visit, instructions can be given as to what tasks should be completed beforehand (ie, medication reconciliation, intake forms) and then how to open the visit. Instructions on how to proceed if technical difficulties such as loss of connection occur can also be given. For patients with functional deficits presenting to a rehabilitation specialist, considerations should be given to ensure a thorough and safe examination. Patients may be instructed to wear comfortable clothing that allows for direct visualization of relevant musculoskeletal structures and to have a family member or friend available for assistance with examination maneuvers. Laskowski and colleagues[23] recently published instructions on performing a telemedicine musculoskeletal examination, which may serve as a helpful reference. Patients should be advised to make sure they are in an area with enough space to move around comfortably and to walk around for proper gait analysis. In addition, providers should also make sure they are creating a setting with appearance and environment to match the professionalism of an in-patient visit.[33] Further tips on conducting telemedicine rehabilitation visits can be found in a recently published article from Verduzco-Gutierrez and colleagues.[33]

Approach to Care: Triaging a Telemedicine Visit

Although it is important to take all the measures discussed earlier into account, perhaps most important is triaging each patient to the appropriate visit type. Because telemedicine is likely to continue as an integral part of medical and rehabilitation care moving forward, further research will be needed in determining which patients should present for phone visits, video visits, and for in-person encounters. Because data are currently unavailable for this in the area of cancer rehabilitation medicine, the authors make the following suggestions based on their experiences. We understand that, in the constantly evolving and heterogeneous setting of a global pandemic, situations are different and will change from location to location, and so the following should only be considered when possible and practical.

Considering telemedicine as the default visit type

As has previously been outlined, patients with cancer differ significantly from other rehabilitation patient populations because they are often immunocompromised, especially patients on active chemotherapy and/or radiation therapy, putting them at increased risk for communicable disease, including severe illness and increased mortality from COVID-19.[6–12] As of this writing, the COVID-19 pandemic continues. Although the roll out of vaccinations has started, the duration of efficacy and the effects on transmission of the virus have not been established. As a state of unprecedented increased risk continues, it may be prudent to use telemedicine visits as the default visit type when indicated (**Box 2**) and possible not only to protect vulnerable patients with cancer but to continue to promote quarantine and social distancing as a medical community.

Telemedicine for follow-up visits

Telemedicine is well suited for follow-up visits, particularly if patients have had their initial evaluations in person with a complete physical examination. A useful paradigm may be to categorize follow-up patients as having stable/improving problems, worsening problems, or new problems. Patients with problems that are likely to be stable or improving can adequately be serviced through telemedicine visits. For example, a well-known patient with cancer-related cognitive impairment on methylphenidate for reduced attention can be seen through a video or phone visit. Likewise, a patient who had recently received a corticosteroid injection for de Quervain tenosynovitis secondary to aromatase inhibitor–associated musculoskeletal symptoms can also be followed up through video or phone. Follow-up visits in patients with worsening problems in certain situations may also adequately be serviced through telemedicine. Patients requiring medication titrations such as a gabapentinoid for chemotherapy-induced peripheral neuropathy or a trial of a different muscle relaxant for spasms secondary to radiation fibrosis syndrome can be accommodated through telemedicine. In contrast, certain situations, such as worsening back pain in a patient with metastatic breast cancer where there may be a concern for new or worsening spinal metastasis, are best evaluated in person. If appropriate, a telemedicine encounter may be used to do an initial evaluation to triage the patient for an urgent in-person evaluation or a higher level of care. Follow-up visits for patients with new problems may be triaged based on the nature of the new problem and, in that regard, can be treated as new patients.

Box 2
Suggested indications for telemedicine visits

Cancer-related fatigue

Follow-up after a procedure

Follow-up for a stable problem

Lifestyle counseling

Medication rotation

Medication titration

Preoperative counseling

Cancer-related cognitive impairment

Telemedicine for new patients

It is in the opinion of the authors that new patients with cancer or known patients with cancer with new problems relating to the neuromusculoskeletal system should be evaluated in person whenever possible. However, there are clinical scenarios in which a video visit may be entirely appropriate. For example, new patients with osteosarcomas who are presenting for preamputation counseling can be fully accommodated through a video visit. Likewise, patients presenting for exercise, dietary, or lifestyle counseling may do well with telemedicine. Patients presenting for pure cognitive complaints may also be sufficiently evaluated through video. Situations in which a new diagnosis must be made or where an interventional procedure will likely be indicated would best be triaged for an in-person encounter, because a significant proportion of the diagnoses cancer physiatrists make are clinically based on a comprehensive physical examination. Furthermore, establishing a baseline sense of a patient's neurologic function is essential to detect future changes in function. Because significant knowledge of a patient's chief complaint is required for triage beforehand, careful chart review and clarification from referring providers may be needed. Providers can then relay to scheduling teams about which visit type is preferred for an individual patient. The authors acknowledge that, as telemedicine physical examination skills evolve and improve over time, the utility of telemedicine in new patient encounters may expand.

Provider and patient comfort level

Ultimately, it is up to individual providers and patients to determine what they think about conducting visits through telemedicine or in person. Many patients are understandably reluctant about entering into hospital or clinic settings where people with COVID-19 are receiving care. In such situations, reassurance and education on precautions that are used should be given to alleviate concerns if an in-person evaluation is indicated. However, there are risks and factors (eg, living with other elderly or vulnerable populations) that providers may be unaware of, so the decision should ultimately be left up to the patient. Similarly, some providers may themselves be at increased risk for severe illness or have circumstances in which isolation may be favored. There may also be providers less comfortable managing patient problems through telemedicine with greater preference for in-person evaluations. There are many unique situations and each should be taken on a case-by-case basis.

Complications/Concerns

In triaging patients for a particular visit type, it is essential to consider the unique complications that patients with cancer face. Missing increased weakness or a cranial nerve deficit may translate to missing an area of new metastasis or disease recurrence with the potential for significant and irreversible loss of function. When there is concern for any of the following, the authors recommend an in-person evaluation for an in-depth physical examination if possible (**Box 3**).

Acute pain in the setting of lytic lesions

Bone is the third most common location for metastases after the liver and lungs, with an estimated 250,000 patients developing osseous metastases.[34] Lesions from breast, lung, prostate, kidney, and thyroid make up 80% of osseous metastases, and the most common cause of cancer pain is from bony lesions.[35] As an extremely common source of pain and potential morbidity, it is important to catch because there are effective treatments, the most commonly used of which is radiation therapy. Evaluating patients in person may help to distinguish possible bone pain from other sources (eg, visceral, myofascial, neuropathic) in addition to helping to evaluate for

---

Box 3
Suggested indications for in-person visits

Administration of interventional procedure

Concern for pathologic fracture

New musculoskeletal complaint

New or worsening back pain

Worsening or new neurologic deficit

---

functional pain. Functional pain is an important characteristic because it is a criterion in measuring risk of pathologic fracture and indication for prophylactic fixation.[36]

Spinal pain

Back pain is one of the most common patient complaints, with an estimated lifetime prevalence up to 85%.[37] There are myriad causes of back pain, and most of it is self-limiting. However, in patients with cancer, it may be a harbinger of serious complications, with spinal metastasis and associated nerve root and spinal cord compression occurring in 5% to 10% of patients with systemic disease.[38] These patients are best evaluated with a comprehensive in-person musculoskeletal and neurologic physical examination to rule out malignant causes of pain. There should be a low threshold for ordering spinal MRI, because urgent referral to neurosurgery and/or radiation oncology is needed in select cases. In addition, many patients with cancer have increased risk for vertebral compression fractures, especially in the setting of lytic lesions, corticosteroid use, or previous radiation therapy.[39,40] Patients may present with acute functional pain and are best evaluated in person to rule out cord compression.

Chemotherapy-induced peripheral neuropathy affecting gait

Several chemotherapeutic agents associated with distal symmetric polyneuropathy cause primarily sensory symptoms. However, a few agents, including the taxanes, vinca alkaloids, and bortezomib, occasionally cause weakness. It is essential to know whether weakness is occurring in addition to reduced proprioception because both significantly alter ambulatory ability and place the patient at increased fall risk. If these complications are occurring to a significant degree, care should be coordinated with the medical oncologist to consider dose reduction or therapy rotation, because this can blunt or reduce neuropathic symptoms.[41]

Peripheral neuropathies

Aside from the more common chemotherapy-induced neuropathies, more focal neuropathies at the level of the root, plexus, or nerve secondary to compression from primary or metastatic lesions can also occur. In these patients, as with all the other patients discussed so far presenting with neurologic deficits, it is important to examine the patient in person if possible to establish a baseline level of function and monitor for future decline. Depending on the site, extent of injury, and overall clinical picture, it may be possible to decompress the affected nerve with radiation or surgery, so early detection is key. Neuropathies associated with lymphoproliferative disorders[41] or, to a lesser extent, paraneoplastic syndromes[42] may also be present. In such cases, a thorough physical examination to characterize the neuropathy is essential in pinpointing an accurate diagnosis.

Delivering Care

Physical therapy, occupational therapy, speech therapy, and neuropsychology are all essential components of rehabilitation care. Many of these services are also now available through telemedicine (called telerehabilitation) in varying degrees. Some therapy centers, including ReVital (Select Medical, Mechanicsburg, PA), which offers therapy services specifically for cancer survivors, offer telemedicine therapy services starting with the initial evaluation. Other centers may require an initial in-person visit followed by subsequent telemedicine visits. A recent survey study by Tenforde and colleagues[43] showed that patients had overall high satisfaction with these types of services in outpatient practices. Similarly, a survey study in an outpatient rehabilitation musculoskeletal practice also showed high patient satisfaction.[44] Additional resources, including survivorship programs, have also had some success moving to telemedicine platforms.

Survivorship and Wellness Programs

Many cancer programs around the country now support several wellness and survivorship programs, given the increased recognition of this type of programming on the overall quality of life of patients with cancer and even possibly cancer biology.[45] Because these programs are generally considered as not being critical, they are almost unequivocally put on hold with the current pandemic. However, like some other cancer programs, our institution was able to pivot and adapt the following programs to a virtual format:

- Gentle Yoga for Wellness
- Art Therapy
- Cancer Exercise Recovery Program
- Emerging from the Haze[46]
- Growing Resilience and Courage (GRACE) with cancer
- Nutrition in Your Kitchen (cancer survivorship cooking demonstration/education program)
- How to Address Stress – Yoga

Given the psychoeducational nature of these programs, these types of wellness interventions provide an opportunity for virtual adaptation given that they do not require in-person physical examinations or procedures. Other programs, such as support groups and mindfulness-based stress-reduction programs, which have also shown evidence-based benefits for cancer survivors,[47] can also easily be adapted to a virtual program. Based on the authors' experience thus far, attendance and satisfaction with these virtual programs have been high, with many participants reporting that these types of supportive programs have provided a reprieve from the stressors related to cancer and the pandemic in a convenient environment. Our group is also in the midst of a clinical pilot study to assess the impact of a virtual adaptation of Emerging from the Haze (our cognitive rehabilitation program for cancer-related cognitive impairment) on patient-reported outcomes. Clearly, much more work is needed to assess the impact of these types of wellness and survivorship programs as they are modified to the virtual format.

GOALS

The medical community's ability to adapt to telemedicine platforms over the course of the last year has been impressive, but there is still much to do. If telemedicine continues to make up a significant proportion of patient encounters, which seems likely for the time being, then establishing the accuracy of our physical examination techniques will be important. Developing an evidence-based consensus as to which patient problems are best addressed by phone and video visits, and what situations require an in-person encounter to guide triaging practices, would also be helpful. Questions that need to be answered include whether providers will be comfortable ordering an interventional procedure such as an ultrasonography-guided botulinum toxin injection or an epidural steroid injection based on a telemedicine encounter. In addition, monitoring the care clinicians give and looking out for complications or possible misses caused by lack of in-person care will need to be ongoing.

SUMMARY

Telemedicine looks as though it will remain a fixture of comprehensive cancer rehabilitation care for the clear benefits it can offer to a vulnerable patient population. By allowing patients to stay at home, it promotes social distancing, reduces the risk of contracting communicable disease, and is likely to be an essential tool in providing currently sequestered services to more remote communities. With adequate preparation, cancer rehabilitation telemedicine can serve as a suitable substitute for in-person encounters in several situations. Still, there are limits with technologic deficits, reimbursement questions, and the inability to conduct hands-on physical examinations. Therefore, it will be important to appropriately triage patients to the most suitable visit type, whether telemedicine or in person, with aims of reducing unnecessary risks, monitoring for potential complications, and having productive encounters.

CLINICS CARE POINTS

- Telemedicine is an invaluable tool in continuing cancer rehabilitation medicine services while keeping patients with cancer who are vulnerable to severe illness from COVID-19 safe.
- Barriers to an effective telemedicine practice may include technical difficulties, which should be anticipated and prepared for.
- It is important to review institutional policies regarding permitted telemedicine platforms and required documentation.
- Because of the increased health risks faced by patients with cancer, consider telemedicine as a default visit type in the setting of an ongoing pandemic.
- Chart review and a clear understanding of the patient's reason for referral are key to triaging future visits for either phone, video, or in-person.
- Patients with cancer with acute pain complaints, spinal pain, or any type of progressive neurologic deficit should be seen in person if safe and practical.

DISCLOSURE

The authors have nothing to disclose.

REFERENCES

1. Wosik J, Fudim M, Cameron B, et al. Telehealth transformation: COVID-19 and the rise of virtual care. J Am Med Inform Assoc 2020;27(6):957–62.
2. Novara G, Checcucci E, Crestani A, et al. Telehealth in urology: a systematic review of the literature. How much can telemedicine be useful during and after the COVID-19 pandemic? Eur Urol 2020;18. https://doi.org/10.1016/j.eururo.2020.06.025.

3. Mustafa SS, Yang L, Mortezavi M, et al. Patient satisfaction with telemedicine encounters in an allergy and immunology practice during the coronavirus disease 2019 pandemic. Ann Allergy Asthma Immunol 2020;125(4):478–9.

4. Hong Y-R, Lawrence J, Williams D, et al. Population-level interest and telehealth capacity of US hospitals in response to COVID-19: cross-sectional analysis of google search and national hospital survey data. JMIR Public Health Surveill 2020;6(2):e18961.

5. CDC. Coronavirus disease 2019 (COVID-19). Centers for disease control and prevention. Published February 11, 2020. Available at: https://www.cdc.gov/coronavirus/2019-ncov/index.html. Accessed October 26, 2020.

6. Wu Z, McGoogan JM. Characteristics of and important lessons from the coronavirus disease 2019 (COVID-19) outbreak in China: summary of a report of 72 314 cases from the Chinese center for disease control and prevention. JAMA 2020; 323(13):1239–42.

7. Kuderer NM, Choueiri TK, Shah DP, et al. Clinical impact of COVID-19 on patients with cancer (CCC19): a cohort study. Lancet 2020;395(10241):1907–18.

8. Lee LY, Cazier J-B, Angelis V, et al. COVID-19 mortality in patients with cancer on chemotherapy or other anticancer treatments: a prospective cohort study. Lancet 2020;395(10241):1919–26.

9. Dai M, Liu D, Liu M, et al. Patients with cancer appear more vulnerable to SARS-CoV-2: a multicenter study during the COVID-19 outbreak. Cancer Discov 2020; 10(6):783–91.

10. Yang F, Shi S, Zhu J, et al. Clinical characteristics and outcomes of cancer patients with COVID-19. J Med Virol 2020. https://doi.org/10.1002/jmv.25972.

11. Tian J, Yuan X, Xiao J, et al. Clinical characteristics and risk factors associated with COVID-19 disease severity in patients with cancer in Wuhan, China: a multicentre, retrospective, cohort study. Lancet Oncol 2020;21(7):893–903.

12. Fung M, Babik JM. COVID-19 in immunocompromised hosts: What we know so far. Clin Infect Dis 2020;27. https://doi.org/10.1093/cid/ciaa863.

13. Cheville AL, Mustian K, Winters-Stone K, et al. cancer rehabilitation: an overview of current need, delivery models, and levels of care. Phys Med Rehabil Clin N Am 2017;28(1):1–17.

14. Rocque GB, Williams CP, Miller HD, et al. Impact of travel time on health care costs and resource use by phase of care for older patients with cancer. J Clin Oncol 2019;37(22):1935–45.

15. Crawford J, Dale DC, Lyman GH. Chemotherapy-induced neutropenia: risks, consequences, and new directions for its management. Cancer 2004;100(2): 228–37.

16. Ng A, Oo T. Hematologic and thromboembolic complications of cancer and their treatment. In: cancer rehabilitation. 2nd edition. Springer Publishing Company; 2019. p. 482–93.

17. Heit JA, O'Fallon WM, Petterson TM, et al. Relative impact of risk factors for deep vein thrombosis and pulmonary embolism: a population-based study. Arch Intern Med 2002;162(11):1245–8.

18. Khorana AA, Francis CW, Culakova E, et al. Thromboembolism is a leading cause of death in cancer patients receiving outpatient chemotherapy. J Thromb Haemost 2007;5(3):632–4.

19. Huang MH, Blackwood J, Godoshian M, et al. Prevalence of self-reported falls, balance or walking problems in older cancer survivors from surveillance, epidemiology and end results-medicare health outcomes survey. J Geriatr Oncol 2017; 8(4):255–61.

20. Cheville AL, Beck LA, Petersen TL, et al. The detection and treatment of cancer-related functional problems in an outpatient setting. Support Care Cancer 2009; 17(1):61–7.
21. Gerber LH, Weinstein AA. Evaluation and management of cancer-related fatigue. In: cancer rehabilitation. 2nd edition. Springer Publishing Company; 2019. p. 960–71.
22. Paquette S, Lin JC. Outpatient telemedicine program in vascular surgery reduces patient travel time, cost, and environmental pollutant emissions. Ann Vasc Surg 2019;59:167–72.
23. Laskowski ER, Johnson SE, Shelerud RA, et al. The Telemedicine Musculoskeletal Examination. Mayo Clin Proc 2020;95(8):1715–31.
24. NCI-Designated Cancer Centers - National Cancer Institute. Published April 5, 2012. Available at: https://www.cancer.gov/research/infrastructure/cancer-centers. Accessed October 26, 2020.
25. Wolfson JA, Sun C-L, Wyatt LP, et al. Impact of care at comprehensive cancer centers on outcome: Results from a population-based study. Cancer 2015; 121(21):3885–93.
26. Current state laws and reimbursement policies | CCHP Website. Available at: https://www.cchpca.org/telehealth-policy/current-state-laws-and-reimbursement-policies#. Accessed October 26, 2020.
27. Zachrison KS, Boggs KM, Hayden EM, et al. Understanding barriers to telemedicine implementation in rural emergency departments. Ann Emerg Med 2020; 75(3):392–9.
28. Sevil U, Ertem G, Kavlak O, et al. The loneliness level of patients with gynecological cancer. Int J Gynecol Cancer 2006;16(Suppl 1):472–7.
29. Rozniatowski O, Reich M, Mallet Y, et al. Psychosocial factors involved in delayed consultation by patients with head and neck cancer. Head Neck 2005;27(4): 274–80.
30. Holt-Lunstad J, Smith TB, Baker M, et al. Loneliness and social isolation as risk factors for mortality: a meta-analytic review. Perspect Psychol Sci 2015;10(2): 227–37.
31. Kroenke CH, Michael YL, Poole EM, et al. Postdiagnosis social networks and breast cancer mortality in the after breast cancer pooling project. Cancer 2017; 123(7):1228–37.
32. COVID-19 frequently asked questions (FAQs) on medicare fee-for-service (FFS) billing. Available at: https://www.cms.gov/files/document/03092020-covid-19-faqs-508.pdf. Accessed October 26, 2020.
33. Verduzco-Gutierrez M, Bean AC, Tenforde AS, et al. How to conduct an outpatient telemedicine rehabilitation or prehabilitation visit. PM R 2020;12(7):714–20.
34. Morris J, Belzarena A, Boland P. Bone metastases. In: cancer rehabilitation. 2nd edition. Springer Publishing Company; 2019. p. 780–6.
35. Buckwalter JA, Brandser EA. Metastatic disease of the skeleton. Am Fam Physician 1997;55(5):1761–8.
36. Mirels H. Metastatic disease in long bones. A proposed scoring system for diagnosing impending pathologic fractures. Clin Orthop 1989;249:256–64.
37. Money S, Smith S. Spine disorders in cancer. In: cancer rehabilitation. 2nd edition. Springer Publishing Company; 2019. p. 729–36.
38. Plotkin SR, Wen PY. Neurologic complications of cancer therapy. Neurol Clin 2003;21(1):279–318, x.
39. Deyo RA, Rainville J, Kent DL. What can the history and physical examination tell us about low back pain? JAMA 1992;268(6):760–5.

40. Sahgal A, Atenafu EG, Chao S, et al. Vertebral compression fracture after spine stereotactic body radiotherapy: a multi-institutional analysis with a focus on radiation dose and the spinal instability neoplastic score. J Clin Oncol 2013;31(27): 3426–31.

41. Weimer L, Brannagan T. Peripheral neuropathy in cancer. In: cancer rehabilitation. 2nd edition. Springer Publishing Company; 2019. p. 658–76.

42. Antoine J-C, Camdessanché J-P. Paraneoplastic neuropathies. Curr Opin Neurol 2017;30(5):513–20.

43. Tenforde AS, Borgstrom H, Polich G, et al. Outpatient physical, occupational, and speech therapy synchronous telemedicine: a survey study of patient satisfaction with virtual visits during the COVID-19 pandemic. Am J Phys Med Rehabil 2020; 99(11):977–81.

44. Tenforde AS, Iaccarino MA, Borgstrom H, et al. Telemedicine during COVID-19 for outpatient sports and musculoskeletal medicine physicians. PM R 2020; 12(9):926–32.

45. Andersen BL, Goyal NG, Weiss DM, et al. Cells, cytokines, chemokines, and cancer stress: a biobehavioral study of patients with chronic lymphocytic leukemia. Cancer 2018;124(15):3240–8.

46. Myers JS, Cook-Wiens G, Baynes R, et al. Emerging from the haze: a multicenter, controlled pilot study of a multidimensional, psychoeducation-based cognitive rehabilitation intervention for breast cancer survivors delivered with telehealth conferencing. Arch Phys Med Rehabil 2020;101(6):948–59.

47. Xunlin NG, Lau Y, Klainin-Yobas P. The effectiveness of mindfulness-based interventions among cancer patients and survivors: a systematic review and meta-analysis. Support Care Cancer 2020;28(4):1563–78.

Telerehabilitation for Geriatrics

Mooyeon Oh-Park, MD, MS[a],*, Henry L. Lew, MD, PhD[b,c], Preeti Raghavan, MD[d]

KEYWORDS

• Telehealth • Social isolation • Quality of life • Patient and caregiver centeredness

KEY POINTS

- Telehealth use was accelerated by the coronavirus disease 2019 pandemic and became an essential part of the rehabilitation service.
- Telehealth has a great potential in alleviating social isolation as well as addressing the medical needs of older individuals.
- Challenges to effective and efficient implementation include willingness to adapt to the technology by older adults, reliable Internet connections, identifying the area where telehealth is most effective, and evaluating the patients and administrative outcomes of telehealth interventions.

INTRODUCTION

Advancements in medical science and technology, along with global increases in life expectancy, are changing the way health care services are delivered to the aging society.[1] Telerehabilitation is a specific area of telehealth that refers to clinical rehabilitation services involving evaluation, diagnosis, and treatment.[2] It is an attractive option for older adults who may have multiple comorbidities and challenges in commuting to clinicians' offices. The coronavirus disease 2019 (Covid-19) pandemic required clinicians to modify the way rehabilitation care is delivered to patients, particularly to the geriatric population, because of their increased risk of developing serious illness. Limited access to in-person services and the concern about potential exposure to severe acute respiratory syndrome coronavirus-2 (SARS-CoV-2) also accelerated the acceptance of telerehabilitation by many patients. In addition, recent changes in rules,

[a] Department of Rehabilitation Medicine, Albert Einstein College of Medicine, Montefiore Health System, Burke Rehabilitation Hospital, 785 Mamaroneck Avenue, White Plains, NY 10605, USA; [b] Department of Communication Sciences and Disorders, University of Hawai'i at Mānoa, John A. Burns School of Medicine, 677 Ala Moana Boulevard, Suite 625, Honolulu, HI 96813, USA; [c] Department of Physical Medicine and Rehabilitation, Virginia Commonwealth University School of Medicine, Richmond, Virginia, USA; [d] Department of Physical Medicine and Rehabilitation and Neurology, Johns Hopkins University School of Medicine, 600 North Wolfe Street, Baltimore, MD 21287, USA
* Corresponding author.
E-mail address: MOhPark@Burke.org

Phys Med Rehabil Clin N Am 32 (2021) 291–305
https://doi.org/10.1016/j.pmr.2021.01.003

regulation, and insurance reimbursement allowed clinicians to use telerehabilitation more broadly than it has ever been used before.

The convergence of medicine and informatics will inevitably lead to the development of new interdisciplinary research models and products for the care of older adults. The widespread use of telerehabilitation provides an opportunity for clinical researchers to examine its outcomes and efficacy.[2] This article reviews the scope, need, and implementation of telehealth and telerehabilitation in the aging population from the perspective of both clinicians, patients, and caregivers.

AGING POPULATION IN THE UNITED STATES

According to the US Census Bureau, the population of individuals aged 65 years and older is expected to double from 43.1 million in 2012 to 83.7 million in 2050.[3] The proportion of older adults has been steadily increasing from 9.8% in 1970 to 13% in 2010 and is estimated to be more than 20% of the US population by 2030. The proportion of the oldest-old (aged $\geq$85 years) is also expected to increase dramatically, from 1.9% of the US population in 2012 to 4.5% in 2050.[3] The potential burden of the dependent older population on the working-age population is measured by the old-age dependency ratio [(population aged $\geq$65 years /population 18–64 years) $\times$ 100].[3] The old-age dependency ratio is projected to increase from 21 in 2010 to more than 30 by 2030. Although older women are projected to continue to outlive men, life expectancy is expected to increase more for men than for women. This changing sex ratio has implications for the types of care that are available to the older population. Both men and women are expected to survive to older ages, spouses may be able to care for one another longer, and there could be an increased demand for assisted-care settings for couples. The older population in the United States will also become more racially and ethnically diverse because the proportion of minority individuals is projected to increase from 20.7% in 2010 to 39.1% in 2050. From a global perspective, although the percentage of older individuals in the United States is not the highest, it has the largest number of people aged 65 years and older among the developed countries.[3] The projected growth of the older population in the United States poses major challenges to policy makers and programs (eg, Medicare) and will affect families, businesses, and health care providers.

POTENTIAL ROLE OF TELEHEALTH AND TELEREHABILITATION FOR OLDER ADULTS

One of the main challenges in the aging population is a high prevalence of chronic diseases and need for medical care.[3] Telehealth facilitates a broad scope of practice, which includes monitoring and assessment of patients and delivery of many interventions remotely (**Box 1**). Patients in the United States spend an average of 2 hours, including travel and wait time, for a 20-minute in-person office visit.[4,5] Telehealth leads to improved quality of health care by facilitating compliance with home programs,[6] with patient outcomes compatible with face-to-face service.[7] Telehealth can be beneficial to both patients and caregivers, especially during transitions between different health care settings. Care transition is a high-risk period for care quality and patient safety, specifically for older adults with complex medical needs who often undergo multiple transitions.[8] Transitions are plagued with discontinuity and a lack of coordination.[9] Gaps in communication and timely delivery of information are known barriers for interprofessional teams working along the continuum of care.[8] Strategies to improve transition of care can include telehealth to enhance communication and education of the patient and family caregivers[10] to ensure that there are no gaps in information sharing and understanding.[8]

Box 1
Potential role of telehealth and telerehabilitation for older adults

Use of telehealth in older adults
- Remote monitoring of chronic conditions (eg, vital signs, weight, blood glucose)
- Receiving laboratory results and medical reports
- Accessing personal health records
- Physician visits via videoconferencing

Use of telerehabilitation in older adults
- Facilitating transition of care between different health care settings (eg, acute hospitals, rehabilitation hospitals, nursing homes, home care)
- Fall prevention and reducing functional decline
- Cognitive rehabilitation
- Rehabilitation therapy for specific conditions (eg, cardiac disease, osteoarthritis)
- Combating loneliness and social isolation
- Home safety monitoring

Preventive home visitation programs are effective for older adults in preventing further functional decline and reducing the risk of nursing home admissions when multiple follow-up home visits are provided and the individuals have a lower risk for death.[11] The limitations of home rehabilitation programs include the cost of travel, and the absence of health care personnel with detailed medical knowledge of the patient's complex medical conditions. Several studies have shown the effectiveness of telerehabilitation in older adult populations in optimizing the management of chronic diseases or transition of care at home after being discharged from the hospital.[12–14]

Telerehabilitation is an area in which the focus of care is on rehabilitation of individuals with cognitive, psychosocial, and/or physical impairments. Telerehabilitation has number of advantages, including reduced travel and the time and costs associated with it, longer consultation duration, and a potential increase in the pool of specialists who are available for consultation.[15]

Although recent advances in technology have been rapidly adopted by health care to enable telerehabilitation, there is still a need to define what is delivered, how it is delivered, to whom, by whom, and how effective it is.[2] The technology must facilitate accessibility and compliance, and also be adaptable and engaging to optimize use.[16] In addition, without proactive efforts to ensure equity, current implementation of telehealth and telerehabilitation may increase disparities in health care access for vulnerable older populations with limited technology literacy or access.[17]

CONSIDERATIONS IN IMPLEMENTING TELEHEALTH AND TELEREHABILITATION IN OLDER ADULTS

Potential advantages and disadvantages of telehealth are summarized in **Box 2**. Despite the advantages of telehealth mentioned earlier, older adults are especially challenged in using and adopting telehealth technology widely.[18] A large-scale study of 1.1 million patients who completed 2.2 million care visits was conducted to identify the characteristics of individuals who chose telehealth versus in-person visits.[19] Patients aged 65 years and older were 2.4 times less likely to choose a video visit rather than an in-person office visit compared with young adults.[19]

One of the greatest challenges in using telerehabilitation for older adults is limited digital literacy. Only 55% to 60% of Americans aged 65 years or older own a smartphone or have home Internet access.[20] Only 60% of this population is able to send an email or search a Web site.[20,21] Virtual health visits can be especially challenging for older patients with cognitive impairment, language barriers, or lack of access to

---

Box 2
Potential advantages and disadvantages of telerehabilitation in geriatric population

Potential advantages of telerehabilitation in geriatric populations
- Enhanced accessibility in older adults with limited transportation
- Avoid potential exposure to SARS-CoV-2 virus
- Avoid the hassle, time, and cost associated with transportation

Potential disadvantages of telerehabilitation in geriatric populations
- Requires a certain degree of technology literacy
- Individuals with hearing loss, visual impairment, or cognitive impairment may need caregiver assistance
- Increases patient responsibility to report health status and self-examination
- Patient safety issues
- Human connection may not be established and patient engagement can be challenging

---

technology. Guidance is also needed in converting a designated area at home into a distraction-free examination room for appointments or a therapy gym.

Several factors relate to the acceptance of telehealth in older adults. Performance expectancy, effort expectancy, and perceived privacy and security are direct predictors of their intention to use videoconferencing. Self-efficacy plays a role in their intention to use, as well as their actual use, of technology. Both self-efficacy and digital literacy play a major role in older adults' capacity to use digital technology.[22] In another study about perceptions regarding telehealth, older adults expressed concern about access to their personal health data by unauthorized persons and their need to be able to control authorization for third-party access and by close family members.[23] Family caregivers are the primary source of help for older adults in using telehealth platforms. Older adults' reluctance to allow family members to access their health records combined with their suboptimal ability to use the technology were found to be the main contributors to their anxiety about using telehealth services. This information underscores the importance of technical support to facilitate telehealth.[23]

Key actions recommended for clinicians and health systems to ensure equitable access to telehealth include (1) identify potential disparities in access, (2) mitigate digital literacy and resource barriers by education and training to acquire a digital skill set and information about low-cost broadband Internet in their area, and (3) health system leadership buy-in and advocacy for policies and infrastructure to facilitate equitable telehealth access.[17]

Frontline Clinicians' Perception of Telehealth and Telerehabilitation

It has been shown that the perception of clinicians on telehealth greatly influences the belief of patients in the value of telehealth.[19] A recent study surveyed physical therapists on telerehabilitation care of individuals with osteoarthritis, and suggested that telerehabilitation can (1) protect patient privacy (>75% agreed/strongly agreed), (2) save patients' time (76% agreed/strongly agreed), and (3) increase convenience for patients (80% agreed/strongly agreed).[24] The survey also revealed that lack of physical contact, low confidence in using Internet video technologies, and inexperience with telerehabilitation were barriers. These factors were significantly associated with reduced interest in delivering telephone and/or video-based services.[24] Providers often struggle with platform connectivity, provider-directed patient self-examination, and establishing an emotional connection with patients.[25] Because hands-on techniques cannot be implemented, clinicians should reevaluate their practice patterns and reallocate their time, resources, and focus.[26] Only 54% of physical therapists provided care based on the recommendations.[27] It is important to emphasize that clinicians should provide care that is best practice for the patient's conditions, regardless of the method of delivery. Well-designed telerehabilitation for specific populations with established protocols (eg, after total knee arthroplasty) showed high clinician satisfaction.[28] Defining the patient population appropriate for telerehabilitation, and establishing best practices for what to deliver, and how to deliver it through an iterative processes will clarify future use of telerehabilitation by clinicians and patients.[2]

Engagement and Communication with Patient and Family Caregiver

Patient engagement is a key driver of high-quality health care outcomes. Virtual health care places greater responsibility on patients to prepare for the visit, to examine themselves, and to report their health.[29] This responsibility can be motivating for some older adults, but it can be challenging for many. Family caregivers are often involved in multiple aspects of clinical care of older adults, including making appointments and setting up telerehabilitation visits. Telerehabilitation can promote care that is centered on the patient and caregivers by placing emphasis on communication, education, and self-management.[26] Best-practice guidelines are available for telepresence communication.[29,30] The Academy of Communication in Healthcare (ACH) has published useful tips on their Web site.[30,31] Key pointers include preparation with intention, listening intently and completely, agreement on what matters most, connecting with the patient's story, and exploring emotional cues.[29] **Box 3** summarizes useful tips for clinicians for telehealth visits. It is important to educate therapists that telerehabilitation is an adjunct to in-person interventions, and to train them formally to maximize the benefits of telerehabilitation to facilitate self-management. In addition, physical examination tools for clinicians can be built into telerehabilitation software platforms (eg, goniometers and tape measures to assess range of motion or edema) to facilitate the sessions.[32] Education sessions and a digital library for home exercise programs may also support clinicians' ability to train and educate patients.

OUTCOMES OF TELEREHABILITATION

The effectiveness of telerehabilitation has been studied in older patients with diverse diagnoses to examine functional outcomes and satisfaction, although several studies had small sample sizes and no control group. Patient outcomes are reported to be satisfactory with telerehabilitation in those with humeral fractures,[33] total knee arthroplasty,[28] and heart failure.[34] In terms of the cost analysis of telerehabilitation, the evidence is conflicting.[35] Health care expenditure of telerehabilitation was comparable with in-person rehabilitation after total knee arthroplasty.[36] Cost-utility analysis of cardiac telerehabilitation shows that it is effective and can increase participation, but

---

Box 3
Useful tips for clinicians providing telerehabilitation for older adults

- Coaching model for patients to increase patients' accountability for each session
- Relationship-centered communication skills
- Teach-back techniques to ensure that the proper understanding of instructions and training is provided to the patients
- Listening to both content and emotions of patients

cost-utility analysis depends on the cost of the technology used.[37,38] Hybrid approaches combining in-person interventions and telerehabilitation (eg, telephone calls, home visits, telerehabilitation visits) have shown improved patient outcomes in terms of function and depression, and reduced caregiver stress in the stroke population[39] and those with total knee arthroplasty.[40] Randomized controlled trials have recently been initiated to examine the effectiveness of telerehabilitation in patients with osteoarthritis[41] and in those with chronic stroke.[42]

EXAMPLE OF TELEREHABILITATION USE
Hip Fracture Rehabilitation in Older Adults

Hip fractures occur predominantly in the geriatric population, with a lifetime risk of 9% for women and 4% for men.[43] Hip fractures are a major public health issue in terms of morbidity, mortality, health care costs, and societal burden.[44,45] Up to 20% of individuals die within a year following hip fractures.[46] Thirty-five percent of older adults are not able to walk independently and approximately 30% do not regain their prefracture levels of activities of daily living (ADL) after sustaining hip fractures.[47] After a hip fracture, older adults may develop delirium, weight loss, depression, pain, pressure injuries, falls, and urinary incontinence, which can increase the need for health care services. One-third of older adults with hip fracture are readmitted to the hospital within 30 days of their discharge home. These individuals typically have multiple risk factors for falls, including chronic medical conditions that require long-term follow-up care.

Telehealth has been recognized as a promising alternative to in-person care, especially during the Covid-19 pandemic. Home rehabilitation has generally been successful in facilitating recovery of ADL function and ambulation.[48,49] Randomized controlled trials of the effectiveness of a telerehabilitation intervention compared with face-to-face home visits and usual care of community-dwelling older adults after hip fracture are ongoing.[50] Older adults with hip fracture also have gait and balance disturbances that need to be addressed during telerehabilitation. The next part of this article also applies to older adults after hip fracture.

Rehabilitation for Older Adults with Balance and Gait Impairment

Telerehabilitation starts with proper assessment of gait and balance in older patients. Clinicians should be familiar with pathologic gait patterns and relate them to the history and physical examination findings.[51] Gait needs to be examined both qualitatively and quantitatively. Key components of a fall prevention program include strengthening, increasing endurance, and balance training, which need to take place in a safe manner during telerehabilitation. Traditional testing may need to be modified because of space limitations at home. For example, the 10-m walk test to measure gait speed can be replaced by a 4-m walk test.[52] Evaluation of proximal lower limb muscle strength can be tested by a 5-times chair rise test. Balance can be tested with a functional reach test.

In terms of telerehabilitation for balance training, a home exercise program with reported feasibility and effectiveness is generally recommended.[32] Telerehabilitation using tai chi exercise has been studied for its compliance and effectiveness, as well as for balance outcomes and fall reduction, and was found to be more effective than a home-based video and as effective as in-person programs.[53,54] Wu and colleagues[53] reported that tai chi performed 3 times a week for 15 weeks in a televideoconferencing program showed 78% compliance and willingness to continue the tele-exercise program. This study also reported improvement in single-leg stance time by 43%, timed up-and-go test by 21%, and reduced body sway during quiet stance by 8%. Other investigators have shown that Web-based tele-exercise using elastic resistance bands and balance exercises for 20 to 40 minutes, 3 times a week, for 12 weeks improves performance on the chair sit-to-stand test and Berg Balance Scale, and reduces fear of falling.[55] A home exercise program delivered by telerehabilitation to 283 older adults discharged from the hospital reduced risk of falls by 40%.[56] These studies suggest that balance training is feasible and effective through telerehabilitation.

Older Adults with Sarcopenia

Sarcopenia is age-associated decline in muscle mass, strength, and quality, which contributes to falls, disability, and mortality in older adults.[57] The prevalence of sarcopenia ranges from 9.9% to 40% in community-dwelling older adults, depending on the definitions.[58] Sarcopenia is not simply a gradual loss of muscle mass; it is exacerbated by periods of inactivity (eg, hospitalization). Patients with acute loss of muscle mass and function often do not recover fully to the level before the inactive period.[59]

The Covid-19 pandemic is an unprecedented health crisis that necessitated the implementation of travel restrictions, quarantine, and social distancing. These restrictions are particularly stringent for older adults because of the risk of serious illness in cases of Covid-19 infection. The restrictions have had a profound effect on reduction in physical activity and changes in dietary habits that could potentially lead to loss of muscle mass and function (**Box 4**).[60] A recent study that investigated physical activity levels during the Covid-19 lockdown showed that participants had lower heart rate, longer sleeping hours, and increased phone usage.[61] In addition, reduced physical activity may reduce the effectiveness of feedback systems for body mass regulation and affect appetite, resulting in potential weight gain.[60] The skeletal muscles serve as an endocrine organ and produce myokines in response to physical activity, which regulates the immune system.[60,62] Social isolation also may have significant implications on mental health and well-being in addition to reduced physical activities.

Exercise is the primary intervention to remedy the progression of sarcopenia. A recent qualitative survey study reported decreased participation of seniors attending group physical activity even before the implementation of quarantine measures.[63] These seniors expressed the need for physical activity during the pandemic, indicating support for home exercise programs.[63]

The first step in starting a home-based exercise training program is initial evaluation of physical performance.[64] One home-based training strategy implemented during the Covid-19 pandemic recommends a structure that includes warm-up, main exercise, and cool-down activity.[64] For each exercise, there are 3 levels of difficulty (easy, medium, and difficult), which are prescribed based on the functional level of the individual

---

Box 4
Potential impact of the Covid-19 pandemic on older adults

- Reduced physical activity and associated loss of muscle mass, increasing risk of falls
- Poor appetite control (potential overconsumption of ultraprocessed food, risk of poor nutrition, weight gain or loss)
- Reduced exposure to sun and vitamin D
- Impaired sleep and immunity
- Poor glucose control for patients with diabetes mellitus
- Social isolation affecting mental health and well-being, potentially affecting cognitive function

at the initial assessment. Ensuring the safety of the patient is essential for a tele-exercise program. Ming and colleagues[65] created an exercise video for Japanese older adults consisting of 10 minutes of functional training performed 3 times a day, 7 days a week, with the goal of 150 minutes of physical activity per week. Setting goals and celebrating progress is no different from that needed for in-person training. In terms of equipment, simple and inexpensive tools are preferable. Resistance bands can be an excellent alternative to free weights or machines for strength training. In home settings, older adults may use exercise regimens that are of lower intensity, but at higher repetitions until momentary muscle failure is achieved to induce muscle hypertrophy.[66] Hong and colleagues[67] reported that a resistive exercise program delivered via telerehabilitation resulted in improved lower limb muscle mass, appendicular lean soft tissue, and total muscle mass.

Older adults may have misperceptions of increased risk of heart attack or stroke by participating in resistive exercise and it is important to answer any questions and concerns.[68] Clinicians should also keep older adults motivated to increase adherence by involving participants in exercise selection and program design, seeking feedback for intensity of exercise, providing positive feedback, and being transparent about the future training sessions.[60]

Home Safety Assessment

Home safety assessment and modifications recommended by occupational therapists have been shown to be effective in preventing falls. There is increasing demand for home modification services in the aging population, and the focus has shifted toward providing community-based services to enable people to live at home instead of in a nursing home. Gitlin and colleagues[69] found that, after a home visit, 80% of patients needed adjustments to assistive devices, 45% of them needed additional equipment, and 65% of them reported they were not using the recommended equipment because of safety issues or poorly fitting equipment. However, older adults may not receive home safety assessments because of service delivery costs, lack of available therapists, or because of an expansive geographic area.[70] A pilot study reported that a telehealth occupational therapy home modification intervention was not only feasible but was also highly satisfactory to older adults.[70] The intervention was delivered using participant-owned smart phones, tablets, or computers. Participants and caregiver assistants were provided a Web site with resources including educational handouts and instructional videos on how to record the problems related to the home and activity, and possible funding sources. The caregiver communicated with the occupational therapist in real time, and also sent video recordings of the problems related to the home and the activity before the session. During the intervention, the occupational therapist and the patient collaboratively generated a list of client-centered occupational problems to be addressed through home modification. The telerehabilitation intervention led to improvement in patients' perceptions of performance in multiple areas, including in the shower, for mobility, transfers, carrying items, and cutting food, and also improved home safety scores. The challenges for tele–home safety assessment interventions are slow video processing speed and poor image quality. However, with increasing high-speed Internet connections, there is great potential for the use of tele–home safety evaluation and modification.

Cognitive Telerehabilitation for Older Adults with Cognitive Impairment

Dementia affects 46.8 million people worldwide and is an increasing burden on families and on society. In addition, cognitive disorders are common in many neurologic conditions (eg, stroke, traumatic brain injury). The Cognitive Rehabilitation Task Force of the American Congress of Rehabilitation Medicine recently published a systematic review focusing on the recommendations for evidence-based practice of cognitive rehabilitation for attention deficits after brain injury or stroke, compensatory strategies for mild memory deficits, metacognitive strategy training for deficits in executive functioning, and comprehensive holistic neuropsychological rehabilitation to reduce cognitive and functional disability after brain injury or stroke.[71] With limited success of pharmacologic agents, cognitive rehabilitation therapy has been an attractive adjunct intervention. Cognitive rehabilitation therapy is defined as functionally oriented therapeutic cognitive activities directed to achieve functional improvement. Cognitive rehabilitation programs are most effective when they are delivered intensively over a prolonged period of time. In the current pandemic situation with reduced access to care, cognitive telerehabilitation is a promising alternative to in-person programs. A recent systematic review of 5 publications showed that cognitive telerehabilitation interventions had effects comparable with conventional face-to-face rehabilitation in patients with mild cognitive impairment, Alzheimer disease, and frontotemporal dementia.[72] Cognitive telerehabilitation uses several methods and technologies. In addition to delivering conventional cognitive rehabilitation using information and communication by the therapist, virtual reality, augmented reality, and games can also be used (**Table 1**). Virtual reality allows the user to be immersed in a computer-generated environment in a naturalistic way.[73] Serious games (SGs) are digital applications specialized for purposes other than entertainment, such as training and educating, informing, communicating, or enhancing the user's cognitive and/or physical function.[74] Programs using SGs can offer challenging, rewarding, motivating, and interactive experiences that can be shared with other players. This method can provide constructive home-based learning opportunities at low cost.[73] Programs using

Table 1
Advantages and disadvantages of technologies used in cognitive rehabilitation

Technology Used in Cognitive Telerehabilitation	Advantages	Disadvantages
VR	• Allow transfer skills by using diverse environment compared with repetitive training in a fixed conventional rehabilitation setting • Adaptable to the individual's skill level with immediate feedback • Higher compliance than conventional rehabilitation • Can be performed by the supervision of caregivers • May aim to improve both physical and cognitive function	• VR systems can be cumbersome and expensive • Lack of specific VR features (eg, immersion or sense of presence) may result in limited effectiveness
SGs	• Allows adaptation to the level of participants • Highly engaging, can play with others • Low cost and available at home • Performance analysis in real time	• Lack of theoretic models behind development in many products • Lack of regulation for development, marketing, and use of SG with vulnerable population for safety and respecting ethical principles

Abbreviations: SG, serious games; VR, virtual reality.

such technology can be tailored to focus on discernment, short-term memory, problem solving, attention, and spatial orientation for patients with early stages of cognitive impairment.[75] The programs tend to focus on object recognition, communication, reaction time, and memory for patients with moderate cognitive impairment.[75] Further studies with long-term follow-up are needed to evaluate the effectiveness of SGs in cognitive rehabilitation.

Remote Monitoring of Older Adults

Several technologies allow individuals to be monitored without requiring caregivers to operate the devices. Home telemonitoring is intended to detect early deterioration to prevent medical emergencies and reduce hospital readmission. Ultimately, these technologies aim not only to increase older adults' independence but also to reduce the burden and caregiving time of family caregivers and improve quality of life for both older adults and caregivers.[1] Remote monitoring uses cameras, bed sensors, wearable sensors, and/or automatic lights to monitor the individual's behavior.[76] Alerts are sent to the caregiver if any unusual activity patterns are noted. A recent systematic review showed that remote monitoring reduced 6-month mortality but not readmission rates or 1-year mortality in patients with heart failure.[77] A recent review on technology use in fall prevention showed that the effectiveness of these technologies needs further examination in real-world settings.[78]

Reduction of Caregiver Burden

According to the report of the National Alliance for Caregiving (NAC) and the American Association of Retired Persons (AARP), more than 1 in 5 Americans (21.3%) are now caregivers, having provided care to an adult or child with special needs in the past 12 months.[79] The number of caregivers in the United States is currently estimated at 53 million adults, up from the estimated 43.5 million caregivers in 2015. The increase of more than 8 million caregivers is primarily driven by the significant increase in those who care for adults aged 50 years or older (79% of all caregivers).[79] The physical and emotional toll on caregivers has been documented and includes high incidence of chronic diseases and impaired psychological function. Caregivers also report that they spend more than 10% of their annual income on caregiving expenses, including transportation and travel and accommodating their work schedules using vacation and sick time. From this perspective, telehealth is an attractive alternative to conventional in-person care for many caregivers. Several telehealth programs have targeted support for family caregivers of older adults with dementia.[76] The Veterans Health Administration's Telehealth Education Program is designed to enhance the knowledge, skills, and feelings of support for the spouse caregivers of veterans with dementia through a teleconference once a week for 10 weeks. This intervention saved $2768 per patient at 6 months.[80] Tindall and colleagues[81] reported that telerehabilitation of 16 speech therapy sessions for patients with Parkinson disease saved 48 hours of time, more than 92 hours of work time, and $1024 for each caregiver.

SUMMARY AND FUTURE DIRECTIONS

The acceptance and implementation of telerehabilitation has been rapidly accelerated by the COVID-19 pandemic,[81,82] and telehealth is expected to serve a greater role in the delivery of health care in the future. Clinicians should keep in mind that, regardless of the delivery method of care, they must provide care that aligns with clinical practice guidelines and recommendations with conscious effort to engage both the patient and caregiver. Future research on telerehabilitation should examine the impact of recent regulatory changes on the delivery of rehabilitation, and further define the population that can most benefit from telerehabilitation. The future of rehabilitation will likely involve a balance of in-person and virtual care, with strategic use of various technologies.[16] Supporting older adults with user-friendly technology with equity in mind and training of clinicians for patient engagement skills will be instrumental to the success of telerehabilitation in improving outcomes of older adults.

CLINICS CARE POINTS

- The older population is expected to double from 43.1 million in 2012 to 83.7 million in 2050. Prevalence of chronic diseases and need for medical care are expected to increase accordingly.

- Telehealth and telerehabilitation are increasingly used for monitoring, assessments, and intervention purposes in geriatric populations with diverse diagnoses.

- The role of telehealth and telerehabilitation during the Covid-19 pandemic has been expanded more than ever.

- Digital literacy in the geriatric population and proper training of clinicians based on best practice of virtual care are instrumental in the success of telehealth and telerehabilitation implementation.

DISCLOSURE

The authors have nothing to disclose.

REFERENCES

1. Sapci AH, Sapci HA. Innovative assisted living tools, remote monitoring technologies, artificial intelligence-driven solutions, and robotic systems for aging societies: systematic review. JMIR Aging 2019;2(2):e15429.
2. Prvu Bettger J, Resnik LJ. Telerehabilitation in the age of COVID-19: an opportunity for learning health system research. Phys Ther 2020;100(11):1913–6.
3. Ortman JM, Velkoff VA. Census 2014. An Aging Nation: the older population in the United States; 2014, p. 25-1140.
4. Daschle T, Dorsey ER. The return of the house call. Ann Intern Med 2015;162(8): 587–8.
5. Ray KN, Chari AV, Engberg J, et al. Disparities in time spent seeking medical care in the United States. JAMA Intern Med 2015;175(12):1983–6.
6. Emmerson KB, Harding KE, Taylor NF. Providing exercise instructions using multimedia may improve adherence but not patient outcomes: a systematic review and meta-analysis. Clin Rehabil 2019;33(4):607–18.
7. Speyer R, Denman D, Wilkes-Gillan S, et al. Effects of telehealth by allied health professionals and nurses in rural and remote areas: a systematic review and meta-analysis. J Rehabil Med 2018;50(3):225–35.
8. Sims-Gould J, Byrne K, Hicks E, et al. Examining "success" in post-hip fracture care transitions: a strengths-based approach. J Interprof Care 2012;26(3): 205–11.
9. McLeod J, Stolee P, Walker J, et al. Measuring care transition quality for older patients with musculoskeletal disorders. Musculoskeletal Care 2014;12(1):13–21.
10. Popejoy LL, Dorman Marek K, Scott-Cawiezell J. Patterns and problems associated with transitions after hip fracture in older adults. J Gerontol Nurs 2013;39(9): 43–52.

11. Stuck AE, Egger M, Hammer A, et al. Home visits to prevent nursing home admission and functional decline in elderly people: systematic review and meta-regression analysis. JAMA 2002;287(8):1022–8.

12. Sanford JA, Griffiths PC, Richardson P, et al. The effects of in-home rehabilitation on task self-efficacy in mobility-impaired adults: a randomized clinical trial. J Am Geriatr Soc 2006;54(11):1641–8.

13. Tousignant M, Boissy P, Corriveau H, et al. In home telerehabilitation for older adults after discharge from an acute hospital or rehabilitation unit: A proof-of-concept study and costs estimation. Disabil Rehabil Assist Technol 2006;1(4): 209–16.

14. Gaikwad R, Warren J. The role of home-based information and communications technology interventions in chronic disease management: a systematic literature review. Health Informatics J 2009;15(2):122–46.

15. Cason J. Telehealth: a rapidly developing service delivery model for occupational therapy. Int J Telerehabil 2014;6(1):29–35.

16. Jayasree-Krishnan V, Ghosh S, Palumbo A, et al. Developing a framework for designing and deploying technology-assisted rehabilitation post stroke: a qualitative study. Am J Phys Med Rehabil 2020. https://doi.org/10.1097/PHM. 0000000000001634.

17. Nouri S, Khoong EC, Lyles CR, et al. Addressing equity in telemedicine for chronic disease management during the Covid-19 pandemic. NEJM Catal Innov Care Deliv 2020.

18. Foster MV, Sethares KA. Facilitators and barriers to the adoption of telehealth in older adults: an integrative review. Comput Inform Nurs 2014;32(11):523–33, quiz 534–25.

19. Reed ME, Huang J, Graetz I, et al. Patient characteristics associated with choosing a telemedicine visit vs office visit with the same primary care clinicians. JAMA Netw Open 2020;3(6):e205873.

20. Demographics of internet and home broadband usage in the United States. Available at: http://www.pewinternet.org/fact-sheet/internet-broadband/. Accessed November 03, 2020.

21. San Francisco digital equity. Digital Equity. San Francisco mayor's office of housing and community development. City and county of San Francisco. 2018. Available at: https://sfmohcd.org/digital-equity. Accessed November 03, 2020.

22. van Houwelingen CT, Ettema RG, Antonietti MG, et al. Understanding older people's readiness for receiving telehealth: mixed-method study. J Med Internet Res 2018;20(4):e123.

23. Cimperman M, Brencic MM, Trkman P, et al. Older adults' perceptions of home telehealth services. Telemed J E Health 2013;19(10):786–90.

24. Lawford BJ, Bennell KL, Kasza J, et al. Physical therapists' perceptions of telephone- and internet video-mediated service models for exercise management of people with osteoarthritis. Arthritis Care Res 2018;70(3):398–408.

25. Srinivasan M, Asch S, Vilendrer S, et al. Qualitative assessment of rapid system transformation to primary care video visits at an academic medical center. Ann Intern Med 2020;173(7):527–35.

26. Pugliese M, Wolff A. The value of communication, education, and self-management in providing guideline-based care: lessons learned from musculoskeletal telerehabilitation during the COVID-19 crisis. HSS J 2020;16(Suppl 1):1–4.

27. Zadro J, O'Keeffe M, Maher C. Do physical therapists follow evidence-based guidelines when managing musculoskeletal conditions? Systematic review. BMJ Open 2019;9(10):e032329.
28. Tousignant M, Boissy P, Moffet H, et al. Patients' satisfaction of healthcare services and perception with in-home telerehabilitation and physiotherapists' satisfaction toward technology for post-knee arthroplasty: an embedded study in a randomized trial. Telemed J E Health 2011;17(5):376–82.
29. Srinivasan M, Phadke AJ, Zulman D, et al. Enhancing patient engagement during virtual care: a conceptual model and rapid implementation at an academic medical center. NEJM Catal Innov Care Deliv 2020.
30. Cooley L. Fostering human connection in the Covid-19 virtual health care realm. NEJM Catal Innov Care Deliv 2020.
31. Academy of Communication in Healthcare. Covid-19 communication resources. Available at: https://achonline.org/COVID-19#resources. Accessed November 20, 2020.
32. Hayes D. Telerehabilitation for older adults. Top Geriatr Rehabil 2020;36(4): 205–2011.
33. Tousignant M, Giguere AM, Morin M, et al. In-home telerehabilitation for proximal humerus fractures: a pilot study. Int J Telerehabil 2014;6(2):31–7.
34. Tousignant M, Mampuya WM, Bissonnette J, et al. Telerehabilitation with live-feed biomedical sensor signals for patients with heart failure: a pilot study. Cardiovasc Diagn Ther 2019;9(4):319–27.
35. Kairy D, Lehoux P, Vincent C, et al. A systematic review of clinical outcomes, clinical process, healthcare utilization and costs associated with telerehabilitation. Disabil Rehabil 2009;31(6):427–47.
36. Tousignant M, Moffet H, Nadeau S, et al. Cost analysis of in-home telerehabilitation for post-knee arthroplasty. J Med Internet Res 2015;17(3):e83.
37. Hwang R, Morris NR, Mandrusiak A, et al. Cost-utility analysis of home-based telerehabilitation compared with centre-based rehabilitation in patients with heart failure. Heart Lung Circ 2019;28(12):1795–803.
38. Kidholm K, Rasmussen MK, Andreasen JJ, et al. Cost-utility analysis of a cardiac telerehabilitation program: the teledialog project. Telemed J E Health 2016;22(7): 553–63.
39. Bernocchi P, Vanoglio F, Baratti D, et al. Home-based telesurveillance and rehabilitation after stroke: a real-life study. Top Stroke Rehabil 2016;23(2):106–15.
40. Fusco F, Turchetti G. Telerehabilitation after total knee replacement in Italy: cost-effectiveness and cost-utility analysis of a mixed telerehabilitation-standard rehabilitation programme compared with usual care. BMJ Open 2016;6(5):e009964.
41. Bennell KL, Keating C, Lawford BJ, et al. Better Knee, Better Me: effectiveness of two scalable health care interventions supporting self-management for knee osteoarthritis - protocol for a randomized controlled trial. BMC Musculoskelet Disord 2020;21(1):160.
42. Allegue DR, Kairy D, Higgins J, et al. Optimization of upper extremity rehabilitation by combining telerehabilitation with an exergame in people with chronic stroke: protocol for a mixed methods study. JMIR Res Protoc 2020;9(5):e14629.
43. Nguyen ND, Ahlborg HG, Center JR, et al. Residual lifetime risk of fractures in women and men. J Bone Miner Res 2007;22(6):781–8.
44. Caeiro JR, Bartra A, Mesa-Ramos M, et al. Burden of first osteoporotic hip fracture in Spain: a prospective, 12-month, observational study. Calcif Tissue Int 2017;100(1):29–39.

45. Leal J, Gray AM, Prieto-Alhambra D, et al. Impact of hip fracture on hospital care costs: a population-based study. Osteoporos Int 2016;27(2):549–58.
46. Kanis JA, Oden A, Johnell O, et al. The components of excess mortality after hip fracture. Bone 2003;32(5):468–73.
47. Bertram M, Norman R, Kemp L, et al. Review of the long-term disability associated with hip fractures. Inj Prev 2011;17(6):365–70.
48. Edgren J, Salpakoski A, Sihvonen SE, et al. Effects of a home-based physical rehabilitation program on physical disability after hip fracture: a randomized controlled trial. J Am Med Directors Assoc 2015;16(4):350 e351–357.
49. Ziden L, Kreuter M, Frandin K. Long-term effects of home rehabilitation after hip fracture - 1-year follow-up of functioning, balance confidence, and health-related quality of life in elderly people. Disabil Rehabil 2010;32(1):18–32.
50. Gilboa Y, Maeir T, Karni S, et al. Effectiveness of a tele-rehabilitation intervention to improve performance and reduce morbidity for people post hip fracture - study protocol for a randomized controlled trial. BMC Geriatr 2019;19(1):135.
51. Pirker W, Katzenschlager R. Gait disorders in adults and the elderly : a clinical guide. Wien Klin Wochenschr 2017;129(3–4):81–95.
52. Briggs BC, Jain C, Morey MC, et al. Providing rural veterans with access to exercise through gerofit. Fed Pract 2018;35(11):16–23.
53. Wu G, Keyes LM. Group tele-exercise for improving balance in elders. Telemed J E Health 2006;12(5):561–70.
54. Wu G, Keyes L, Callas P, et al. Comparison of telecommunication, community, and home-based Tai Chi exercise programs on compliance and effectiveness in elders at risk for falls. Arch Phys Med Rehabil 2010;91(6):849–56.
55. Hong J, Kong HJ, Yoon HJ. Web-based telepresence exercise program for community-dwelling elderly women with a high risk of falling: randomized controlled trial. JMIR MHealth UHealth 2018;6(5):e132.
56. Bernocchi P, Giordano A, Pintavalle G, et al. Feasibility and clinical efficacy of a multidisciplinary home-telehealth program to prevent falls in older adults: a randomized controlled trial. J Am Med Directors Assoc 2019;20(3):340–6.
57. Cruz-Jentoft AJ, Bahat G, Bauer J, et al. Sarcopenia: revised European consensus on definition and diagnosis. Age Ageing 2019;48(4):601.
58. Mayhew AJ, Amog K, Phillips S, et al. The prevalence of sarcopenia in community-dwelling older adults, an exploration of differences between studies and within definitions: a systematic review and meta-analyses. Age Ageing 2019;48(1):48–56.
59. English KL, Paddon-Jones D. Protecting muscle mass and function in older adults during bed rest. Curr Opin Clin Nutr Metab Care 2010;13(1):34–9.
60. Kirwan R, McCullough D, Butler T, et al. Sarcopenia during COVID-19 lockdown restrictions: long-term health effects of short-term muscle loss. GeroScience 2020;42(6):1547–78.
61. Sun S, Folarin AA, Ranjan Y, et al. Using smartphones and wearable devices to monitor behavioral changes during COVID-19. J Med Internet Res 2020;22(9):e19992.
62. Pedersen BK, Febbraio MA. Muscles, exercise and obesity: skeletal muscle as a secretory organ. Nat Rev Endocrinol 2012;8(8):457–65.
63. Goethals L, Barth N, Guyot J, et al. Impact of home quarantine on physical activity among older adults living at home during the COVID-19 pandemic: qualitative interview study. JMIR Aging 2020;3(1):e19007.

64. Guadalupe-Grau A, Lopez-Torres O, Martos-Bermudez A, et al. Home-based training strategy to maintain muscle function in older adults with diabetes during COVID-19 confinement. J Diabetes 2020;12(9):701–2.

65. Aung MN, Yuasa M, Koyanagi Y, et al. Sustainable health promotion for the seniors during COVID-19 outbreak: a lesson from Tokyo. J Infect Dev Ctries 2020;14(4):328–31.

66. Van Roie E, Delecluse C, Coudyzer W, et al. Strength training at high versus low external resistance in older adults: effects on muscle volume, muscle strength, and force-velocity characteristics. Exp Gerontol 2013;48(11):1351–61.

67. Hong J, Kim J, Kim SW, et al. Effects of home-based tele-exercise on sarcopenia among community-dwelling elderly adults: body composition and functional fitness. Exp Gerontol 2017;87(Pt A):33–9.

68. Burton E, Farrier K, Lewin G, et al. Motivators and barriers for older people participating in resistance training: a systematic review. J Aging Phys Act 2017;25(2): 311–24.

69. Gitlin LN, Miller KS, Boyce A. Bathroom modifications for frail elderly renters: outcomes of a community based program. Technol Disabil 1999;10:141–9.

70. Renda M, Lape JE. Feasibility and effectiveness of telehealth occupational therapy home modification interventions. Int J Telerehabil 2018;10(1):3–14.

71. Cicerone KD, Goldin Y, Ganci K, et al. Evidence-based cognitive rehabilitation: systematic review of the literature from 2009 through 2014. Arch Phys Med Rehabil 2019;100(8):1515–33.

72. Cotelli M, Manenti R, Brambilla M, et al. Cognitive telerehabilitation in mild cognitive impairment, Alzheimer's disease and frontotemporal dementia: a systematic review. J Telemed Telecare 2019;25(2):67–79.

73. Mantovani E, Zucchella C, Bottiroli S, et al. Telemedicine and virtual reality for cognitive rehabilitation: a roadmap for the COVID-19 pandemic. Front Neurol 2020;11:926.

74. Robert PH, Konig A, Amieva H, et al. Recommendations for the use of Serious games in people with alzheimer's disease, related disorders and frailty. Front Aging Neurosci 2014;6:54.

75. Ning H, Li R, Ye X, et al. A review on serious games for dementia care in ageing societies. IEEE J Transl Eng Health Med 2020;8:1400411.

76. Quinn WV, O'Brien E, Springan G. Using Telehealth to improve home-based care for older adults and family caregivers. May 2018. AARP Public Policy Institute.

77. Pekmezaris R, Tortez L, Williams M, et al. Home telemonitoring in heart failure: a systematic review and meta-analysis. Health Aff 2018;37(12):1983–9.

78. Oh-Park M, Doan T, Dohle C, et al. Technology utilization in fall prevention. Am J Phys Med Rehabil 2020. https://doi.org/10.1097/PHM.0000000000001554.

79. The National Alliance for Caregiving (NAC) and AARP. Caregiving in the U.S. 2020: Executive summary. 2020.

80. Wray LO, Shulan MD, Toseland RW, et al. The effect of telephone support groups on costs of care for veterans with dementia. Gerontologist 2010;50(5):623–31.

81. Tindall LR, Huebner RA. The impact of an application of telerehabilitation technology on caregiver burden. Int J Telerehabil 2009;1(1):3–8.

82. Lew HL, Oh-Park M, Cifu DX. The War on COVID-19 Pandemic: Role of Rehabilitation Professionals and Hospitals. Am J Phys Med Rehabil 2020;99(7):571–2.

Telehealth in Pediatric Rehabilitation

Nancy Hsu, PsyD, LCP[a], Eugenio Monasterio, MD[b], Olivier Rolin, MD, PhD[b],*

KEYWORDS

• Pediatric rehabilitation • Telehealth • Telerehabilitation • Physiatry

KEY POINTS

- Telerehabilitation increases access to high-quality pediatric rehabilitation care for people in rural and remote areas.
- Distancing the therapist from the patient helps to maintain the fidelity of therapists to a role as a coach for caregivers to support enrichment of activities where children live, learn, and play.
- The use of telehealth visits can greatly enhance the connectivity of the interdisciplinary rehabilitation team and bring a group of specialists to a patient and his or her family at 1 time.
- Although many studies report equivalent outcomes between in-person care and telerehabilitation, these results may not be generalized to the real-world experience where practitioners are not trained and patients are not actively volunteering to receive telerehabilitation.

INTRODUCTION

Pediatric rehabilitation focuses on optimizing function and quality of life of children through a holistic and transdisciplinary patient-centered team approach. Pediatric rehabilitation is unique in that the team must adapt to the evolving needs of patients throughout the developmental process. While care of infants focuses on acquisition of motor, cognitive, communication, self-care, and language skills, older children may be more focused on integration into school and community pursuits and eventually transitioning to vocational endeavors. Pediatric rehabilitation is also broad in its scope of diagnoses, which include neurodevelopmental disorders, concussion and traumatic brain injury, spinal cord injury and spina bifida, myopathies, peripheral polyneuropathies, connective tissue disorders, pain, and musculoskeletal injuries. Lastly,

There are no conflicts of interest to disclose.
[a] Department of Physical Medicine and Rehabilitation, Virginia Commonwealth University Health Sciences, 1223 E Marshall Street, Richmond, VA 23298, USA; [b] Department of Physical Medicine and Rehabilitation, Virginia Commonwealth University Health Sciences, Children's Hospital of Richmond at VCU, Children's Pavilion, 1000 E Broad Street, Richmond, VA 23219, USA
* Corresponding author.
E-mail address: olivier.rolin@vcuhealth.org

pediatric rehabilitation practitioners cannot focus solely on the child being treated but must also educate and empower the child's parents or caretakers to support the execution of a plan of care in daily life. Relative to other rehabilitation disciplines, pediatrics has a significant shortage of providers, and rural and remote areas often have no specialized pediatric rehabilitation providers at all. Studies have shown successful utilization of videoconference-mediated telehealth across a variety of clinical settings, including primary care, neurology, psychology, psychiatry, and radiology.[1] Telerehabilitation can provide the necessary gateway to increasing access to high-quality pediatric rehabilitation. In 2015, the Pew Research Center Internet, Science, and Tech Report revealed that approximately 68% of the US population had smartphones, and 45% had tablet computers.[2] Furthermore, 88% of American teens ages 13 to 17 had or had access to a mobile phone, and most teens (73%) had smartphones.

As with general rehabilitation, pediatric rehabilitation care involves collaboration of physical medicine and rehabilitation (PM&R) physicians with physical therapists (PTs), occupational therapists (OTs), speech and language pathologists (SLPs), neuropsychologists (NPs), orthoptists, prosthetists, and specialists in durable medical equipment. It is beyond the scope of this article to review all specific applications of telerehabilitation for each specific discipline, patient condition, and intervention. This article will provide an overview of the growing application of telerehabilitation to enhance patient access to services and highlight particular instances where telerehabilitation may be equivalent or superior to in-person care. This article will also discuss examples of how teleconference can improve the collaboration between members of the rehabilitation team.

Where possible, this article will refer to peer-reviewed literature; however, telerehabilitation practice remains relatively new, and prior to the COVID-19 pandemic, represented a small percentage of rehabilitation care. In 2016, only 15% of all pediatric clinicians had used telehealth at least once in the prior year,[3] with payment and billing being the most cited cause for reluctance to incorporate telehealth into their practice. Since the COVID-19 pandemic, provider and patient comfort with telerehabilitation care has evolved rapidly by necessity, and practitioners of telerehabilitation are proceeding with minimal training. Within the authors' institution, practitioners across all rehabilitation disciplines have generally appreciated the opportunity to integrate telehealth into their practices and expressed a desire to continue using telehealth in their practices. However, the need for tactile assessment and feedback remains essential to evaluation and treatment of certain conditions, and individual differences in personality and preferred method of learning can affect preference for in-person versus virtual interaction.

PHYSICAL AND OCCUPATIONAL THERAPIES

Early intervention (EI) practitioners have been among the early adopters of telerehabilitation. The Individuals with Disabilities Education Act Part C urges prompt delivery of rehabilitation services to be provided to every infant and toddler at risk for disability in the settings where they live, learn, and play.[4] The mandate to provide services to families in their homes prompted the integration of telerehabilitation into EI services in order to expand accessibility of care to remote and rural areas.[5]

EI therapy prioritizes supporting the parent-child interaction, with the goal to elicit consistent high-quality interactions beginning in early infancy. Although skilled EI physical and occupational therapists may be experts in optimally handling children to facilitate movement and motor learning, the sustained value of their work derives from coaching parents. EI therapists must help parents master the provision of warm, sensitive, and responsive interactions and to create opportunities for motor development that are embedded in the child's daily life activities and play time.[6] Responsive caregiving in early infancy is central to not only achievement of motor milestones, but also cognitive development and social-emotional processing that is crucial for cultivating exploratory behavior that begets learning throughout development.[7]

By physically distancing the rehabilitation specialist from the parent-child dyad, telehealth delivery of therapy depends on and facilitates use of family coaching strategies. In a study assessing practitioner behavior during a telehealth EI treatment for children with hearing impairments, practitioners demonstrated increased use of family-centered behaviors during telehealth sessions, compared with historic norms reported for in-person intervention. Key provider behaviors included observation, parent practice with feedback, and child behavior with provider feedback.[8] In a group of infants with delayed developmental milestones receiving EI, family social outcomes such as infant positive behavior, parent positive behavior, and maternal postpartum depression improved equally in a telehealth intervention compared with in-person intervention.[9] In addition to social and behavioral outcomes, telehealth was successfully used to deliver a highly protocolled constraint-induced movement therapy program to improve upper extremity function in infants with asymmetric CP. Reported parent fidelity throughout a 4-week program was greater than 93%; there was no loss to follow-up, and a significant improvement was found in a primary motor outcome measure of unimanual fine motor control of the impaired extremity.[10]

Although these studies represent a small sampling of EI therapies and diagnoses, they demonstrate that EI telehealth can: improve provider fidelity to the role as coach, yield equivalent outcomes for social and behavioral outcomes, and deliver effective treatment for motor impairments. These findings are highly encouraging given that lack of interpersonal warmth and the absence of tactile facilitation of movement are perceived limitations of telehealth intervention.[11] Subjective benefits cited by recipients of telehealth EI intervention include flexibility, accessibility, and versatility. For example, telehealth practitioners could facilitate visits during nontraditional times such as important daily routines like dressing and bathing and meal times, to provide relevant situational coaching.[5]

There was comparatively less reporting on PT and OT outcomes for school-aged children. One pilot program included children ages 6 to 11 years with impaired fine motor and/or visual motor skills impacting their handwriting, with most reporting high satisfaction.[12] In a virtual reality telehealth trial, 3 adolescents with hemiplegia participated in remotely monitored videogame gaming with a sensor glove fitted to the hemiplegic hand and attached to a console installed in their home. All 3 participants improved the ability of their hemiplegic hand to lift objects, improved finger range of motion based on remote measurements, and showed expanded spatial in brain motor circuitry on fMRI during a grip task.[13] Another study assessed a 6-week telehealth intervention for sensory processing in 4 children with autism. Three of the children improved, or made no changes, in their sensory processing, while a forth demonstrated worsened processing outcomes.[14] Regarding patient and family satisfaction, a recent survey performed in Massachusetts reported a high satisfaction rating (93.7%–99%) with telerehabilitation services, with 86% of participants placing high value in future telehealth visits.[11] Parents and patient care advocates reported that telerehabilitation was useful in establishing a new routine, and provided structure that was highly necessary for children with behavioral problems. Other parents reported that telerehabilitation had enhanced their ability to provide care and to create play and learning opportunities outside of therapy sessions and were able to repurpose material already present in the home for therapeutic activity. Most caregivers reported a desire to continue to use telerehabilitation services even if physical distancing practices were no longer restricting the use of clinic space. Reported limitations included lack of tactile feedback, inability to provide skilled soft tissue manipulation, and absence of the healing touch. There was variability in the child's engagement with telehealth, with some being equally engaged to levels exhibited during in-person therapy, while others demonstrated limited attention. Device positioning and video quality also limited successful delivery of some therapy sessions.[11]

Prior to 2020, therapists working at rehabilitation clinics affiliated with the Children's Hospital of Richmond (CHoR) had no experience with using telehealth services. The perceived value of the telehealth therapy sessions depended greatly on the environment the patient was in, the attention span of the patient, and the ability of patients and caregivers to follow instruction. Therapists rated exercise teaching to be well suited for remote instruction. Facilitation of activities for children with developmental disorders and autism was challenging but could be successful with highly engaged caregivers who would obtain the necessary equipment and tools to enable specific tasks and be present throughout sessions in order to promote the child's engagement in therapies. Many CHoR therapists reported they would like to continue to deliver some of their care by telehealth even after restrictions on physical distancing were lifted, but that it would not be universally optimal for all patients.

SPEECH AND LANGUAGE PATHOLOGY

As SLP interventions require fewer tactile interactions than physicians or physical and occupational therapists, their mostly auditory, verbal, and visual interactions translate naturally to video conference interventions. Research on telehealth SLP interventions have been ongoing for over a decade, with findings largely demonstrating telehealth SLP interventions are equivalent to in-person interventions.

The development of language and communication skills facilitates social integration and achievement of functional independence in developing children. Speech and language impairments put children at risk for bullying, poor academic performance, and subsequent vocational and social inequality in adulthood. SLP interventions are generally recommended for children with impairments of receptive and expressive language, phonation, and articulation. SLP practitioners also provide care to facilitate swallowing and feeding for children who have challenges with oral nutrition. Disorders of language, communication, and feeding may be present in some children who are otherwise typically developing and are common in children with neurodevelopmental disorders such as cerebral palsy, autism, and other genetic disorders.[15–18] SLP therapists also treat children with disorders of attention and memory that commonly can lead to deteriorating academic performance after concussions or more significant brain injuries.[19]

Studies comparing telehealth SLP intervention with in-person service found equivalent response to therapy for multiple diagnoses and diverse outcome measures. An intervention targeting speech sounds, receptive and expressive language, pragmatics, and phonological awareness in a group of children aged 3 to 12 years found that 68% of participants achieved at or above expected levels and that 79% of participants met at least 1 therapeutic goal.[20] In a study involving 200 school children in Ohio, participants were children referred for school-based SLP intervention for any reason with therapeutic aims spanning the 12 key areas of functional communication, speech sound production, spoken language comprehension, spoken language production, intelligibility, fluency, pragmatics, voice, written composition, emergent literacy, reading comprehension, word recognition, and writing accuracy. Seventy percent of participants progressed on at least 1 level of functional communication measures (FCMs). In general, performance with telehealth compared favorably with data from the National Outcomes Measurement System (NOMS) database, with the exception of language comprehension and production, where telehealth recipients had fewer gains than historically reported in the NOMS database.[21] In a small N randomized control trial, school aged children were assigned to a telehealth group or an in-person group for a speech sound intervention. Participants received twice-weekly intervention sessions during a 5-week summer program. Children receiving telehealth and in-person services both demonstrated significant improvement on the Goldman Fristoe Test of Articulation – Second Edition, and there were no between-group differences in outcome.[22] In all, most participants were satisfied with the intervention itself and the progress achieved.[20,23] Limiting factors were reduced attention for some children[23] and suboptimal connectivity and audio output.[20]

For children with autism spectrum disorder (ASD), positive impacts on communication after telehealth therapy included improved initiation and responses as measured by formal and observation measures.[24] Telehealth therapy also supported improved use of transition words compared with baseline measures and more consistent performance. Telehealth participants with ASD improved on the Vinland Adaptive Behavior Scales-2.[25] Another study measured achievement of students with 3 goals in the domains of social, communication, and independence skills individually selected for intervention for each child. Forty-nine teacher-child dyads supported by telehealth or in-person SLP coaching demonstrated no difference in outcomes.[26] Children receiving functional analysis for behavior and functional communication training reported greater than 90% reduction in problem behaviors, with similar improvements whether children receive home-based in-person or telehealth services.[27] Compared with a waitlist group, child-parent dyads receiving SLP telehealth services had significantly reduced scores on the Screen for Anxiety and Related Emotional Disorders in Children compared with wait list controls.[28]

There is minimal literature on the use of telehealth for feeding therapy. Some patients may be well-suited for remote services; a primary in-person visit is recommended to assess intensity of behavior problems, the parent's level of comfort and engagement, the effect of setting on behavior, and the distance from the clinic. After the initial assessment session, care may be conducted by teleconference. The observations target meals in the individual's natural environment, while limiting reactivity of an observer that tends to occur in contrived clinic observations. Parents or caregivers implement the behavioral feeding intervention under the therapist's direction. Performance feedback is provided to the interventionist. If the caregiver does not respond to the behavior skills training to implement the feeding treatment, services can transition to clinic, where modeling with the client can augment the experience of the behavioral therapy. This method of telehealth feeding therapy was successful, with most beneficiaries being between 4 and 10 years old, with diagnoses such as ASD, developmental disability, or intellectual disability. Patients treated via telehealth have made demonstrated progress on individualized treatment goals, including reduced disruptive behavior during mealtimes, increased consumption of fruits and vegetables, and a greater variety of foods consumed.[29]

NEUROPSYCHOLOGY

Neuropsychology is an essential component of the pediatric rehabilitation team. Clinical neuropsychological assessment evaluates cognitive functioning, characterizes cognitive strengths and weaknesses, assists with differential diagnosis, and guides recommendations based on test results. A pediatric neuropsychologist also evaluates emotional, behavioral, and academic functioning to better inform treatment planning. Traditional neuropsychological assessment involves pencil-and-paper tests, as well as some hands-on manipulatives that are administered face to face. Although computer technology has been utilized to replace certain test administration to improve accuracy, most clinicians continue to rely heavily on the paper-and-pencil administration. In addition, the standardized norms are based on the paper-and-pencil administration. Post-COVID, given the restrictions put in place to ensure safety of the providers and patients, the practice was forced to transition to telehealth neuropsychology (teleNP).

TeleNP can offer consultative services, including educating parents/caregivers on managing their child's impulsive or aggressive behaviors following a brain injury. Aspects of neuropsychological assessment are fluidly amenable to videoconferencing, such as clinical interview, behavioral observation, and self- or parent-report measures. The teleNP interview can be used at the initial intake and evaluation to collect information to triage testing cases, determine appropriateness for teleNP, and begin the process of helping with differential diagnosis. Valuable information is also gathered through behaviors displayed by the child and interactions observed between the parents and the child.

The validity of remote computer-based neuropsychological test results has not been established. Numerous variables may influence that validity. A child's and/or parents' ability to navigate the technology and distractions in the environment can greatly influence test performance. The child could be distracted by noise in the household, particularly as more adults are working from home and school-aged children are learning virtually from home. Another consideration in pediatric teleNP is the involvement of caregivers in testing. The child may need assistance from his or her parents to prepare for testing. For children with behavioral dysregulation that might impact engagement, parents would need to encourage their child to participate.

Ransom and colleagues[30] collected a dataset consisting of the largest teleNP pediatric sample to date (N = 129). They found teleNP to be feasible with the early childhood to early adulthood populations who present with a broad range of clinical concerns. These children were evaluated for a variety of cognitive, emotional, and behavioral needs stemming from complex medical conditions, including history of traumatic brain injury, epilepsy, systemic lupus erythematosus (SLE), and pediatric cancer. Eighty-three percent of the referred children scheduled for face-to-face assessment before COVID-19 were determined by providers to be appropriate for a teleNP evaluation. However, despite the positive result of teleNP, most patients in their sample still required an in-person follow-up. Therefore, the authors recommended that pediatric teleNP be used as a screening service to determine appropriate recommendations for intervention or further assessment.

ORTHOTICS AND PROSTHETICS

Orthotics and prosthetics (O&P) are indispensable for many children with physical impairments. There was no literature found describing telehealth interventions for pediatric O&P. However, PM&R physicians, PTs, and OTs at CHoR began using teleconferencing in the spring of 2020 in order to conduct collaborative evaluations with O&P practitioners in the community. For O&P, there is no substitute for in-person visits for casting and measurement and adjustment of braces and prosthetic components to optimize fit and function. The O&P practitioners, however, do not work in isolation but rather operate as part of a team in order to provide the tools that therapists and physicians recommend for helping patients with functional goals. By comparison with clinics and therapy centers, O&P offices tend to have significantly less traffic and are often in small standalone stores amenable to physical distancing. Many patients who were anxious about visiting the PM&R clinic were comfortable with the O&P office setting. Video conferencing allowed physicians and therapists to see their patient in a location with reliable high-speed Internet and quality video. Together with the orthoptist, they could conduct clinical evaluations or observe the result of a prescribed device at the time of delivery. This way clinicians could assess the efficacy of the recommended device and sometimes make recommendations about additional components that should be added. O&P practitioners facilitating the visit are also experienced and competent at performing range of motion measurements, which are valuable to the clinical team. The collaborative visits were greatly appreciated by patients and their families whose lives so frequently revolve around visits to health care professionals and were glad to be spared an additional evaluation at another time and location. They also were generally pleased to know that their providers were communicating directly and working as a team.

PHYSICIAN SERVICES

A hybrid model of telerehabilitation in person care can greatly enhance the overall efficiency and efficacy of PM&R physician care. Here gait analysis is provided as an example of care that can be enhanced with incorporation of telehealth. Gait analysis is often used in the assessment of ambulatory children with disabilities to refine clinical decision making.[31,32] The visual assessment of walking may be augmented by video-taping with the use of slow-motion and split screens to view the child's gait simultaneously from the front, back, and side. In many centers, patients also undergo 3-dimensional gait assessment in a motion laboratory. The amount of total data stored previously made transmission of the raw data impermissible. The advancement of video and data transmission improvements have opened up the ability to transmit gait and movement analysis information for review. Where previously the large files necessitated storage on media for delayed playback, current infrastructure makes it possible to view live video with accompanying force measures, for review by an experienced team of caregivers, which will help in therapeutic and surgical outcomes.[33] The in-person physical examination of an ambulatory child with cerebral palsy remains necessary as the assessment of hypertonia, joint range of motion, muscle strength, skeletal alignment, and sensory function provides insight on of the structural and functional causes underlying the gait impairment.

Despite the importance of a quality hands-on assessment, telehealth has been a helpful adjunct in order to provide timely and convenient follow-up once an intervention has been recommended. For example, a physiatrist may determine that spasticity is limiting functional movement and prescribe a spasmolytic agent such as baclofen. Although quantitative assessment of spasticity with physical examination is necessary to make that diagnosis and treatment recommendation, assessment of benefit and medication adverse effects can be made by teleconference, observing the child functioning in his or her natural environment and receiving verbal feedback from caregivers. Based on telehealth follow-up, the physician can make decisions on whether to continue therapy, adjust a dose or switch to another medication because of intolerable effects.

Perhaps the greatest strength of telehealth beyond the convenience and the ability to expand access to care to remote and rural areas is the ability to connect a patient's care team in a unified conversation. PM&R physicians work in close collaboration with team of medical and allied health professionals without whom a treatment plan for children with complex care needs could not be effectively executed.[34] Although the PM&R physician may prescribe an intervention, therapists and O&P providers are supporting the execution of that intervention. Physicians see high volumes of patients and may have intervals of several months between visits, whereas therapists will have a smaller case load of patients with whom they have extended visits, often on a weekly basis. Therapists therefore often have detailed insights into a child's progress and functional goals. For a PM&R physician, to be able to remote in via telehealth with a child attending a therapy session makes for a high-quality visit where therapist feedback can help determine whether an intervention was helpful and help to trouble shoot alternative solutions if an intervention was not successful. Therapists are also highly skilled in physical examination and can execute advanced diagnostic examination maneuvers that may help the physician assess a problem. This model of collaborative visits has been used intermittently at CHoR and regarded as highly valuable by the therapists, physicians, and patients alike. In the authors' limited experience conducting such visits, the chief drawback has been the coordination of schedules so that all parties are available promptly at a predetermined time.

FUTURE DIRECTIONS

The use of remote assessment in pediatric rehabilitation has changed over time as technology has advanced. Access to trained caregivers, particularly in hard-to-reach and underserved communities involved members of a team, a physician, nurse or therapist to physically be present with the patient and then transmit video of the examination to the specialty team. This hybrid system of remote access can still be used, but the improvement in data and video distribution will make it more feasible for general practice rather than an infrequent event. The ability to remotely evaluate a patient by multiple caregivers at different sites opens up the idea of multidisciplinary clinics and care. Once a risk or problem has been identified, systems need to be in place to provide appropriate referral for children identified as high risk for disability, monitoring of growth and screening for physical disorders, comprehensive surveillance of development and health, and health promotion activities and targeted interventions.[35]

Prior to 2020, telehealth was used minimally by early adopters seeking to use teleconference technology to expand access to care. The widespread incorporation of telehealth in 2020 will hopefully accelerate physicians' ability to reach every child in need of rehabilitation care. Research on telehealth interventions generally reports positive outcomes, often equivalent when compared with in-person care for a broad diversity of interventions and pediatric diagnoses. Despite the apparent success of telehealth in the literature thus far, the results of these studies, which involve training of research staff, selection of motivated participants, and protocolled interventions, may not be generalizable to the experience of practitioners who had to shift to delivering telehealth without any preparation. As telehealth becomes a more sustained part of practice, clinicians will benefit from training in specifically how to direct telehealth interactions.

Although telehealth will not eliminate all in-person visits and may not be suitable for all individuals or diagnoses, it can be a highly useful adjunct to improve patient access to care at a reduced cost without compromising the effectiveness of care. Families of children with severe disabilities are regularly having to attend therapy sessions and see physicians. A great burden will be lifted from caregivers if they can be spared additional hours commuting to clinics for equally effective care that can be received at home. Furthermore, the ability of telehealth to bring a collaborating team of health providers into a single, direct conversation with the patient and family can not only consolidate the number of visits but also enable physicians, therapists, O&P specialists, and other allied health providers to share ideas and create goals that are clearly shared between the child, his or her family members, and the care team caring.

CLINICS CARE POINTS

- An in person evaluation is usually recommended prior to shifting treatment to the telerehabilitation setting.
- Physicians, therapists, neuropsychologists, orthoptists, prosthetists and durable medical equipment specialists should make use of telerehabilitation to enhance communication between members of a patient care team and reduce the number of clinical visits a patient needs.
- Training on how to use videoconferencing to deliver effective rehabilitation interventions should integrate pregraduate and post graduate curriculum for physicians and allied health providers.

REFERENCES

1. Hewitt KC, Rodgin S, Loring DW, et al. Transitioning to telehealth neuropsychology service: Considerations across adult and pediatric care settings. Clin Neuropsychol 2020;34(7–8):1335–51.
2. Myers K, Nelson E-L, Rabinowitz T, et al. American telemedicine association practice guidelines for telemental health with children and adolescents. Telemed J E Health 2017;23(10):779–804.
3. Sisk B, Alexander J, Bodnar C, et al. Pediatrician attitudes toward and experiences with telehealth use: results from a national survey. Acad Pediatr 2020; 20(5):628–35.
4. ECTA Center. Part C of IDEA. Available at: https://ectacenter.org/partc/partc.asp. Accessed November 15, 2020.
5. Cole B, Pickard K, Stredler-Brown A. Report on the use of telehealth in early intervention in colorado: strengths and challenges with telehealth as a service delivery method. Int J Telerehabil 2019;11(1):33–40.
6. Harbourne RT, Dusing SC, Lobo MA, et al. Sitting together and reaching to play (START-Play): protocol for a multisite randomized controlled efficacy trial on intervention for infants with neuromotor disorders. Phys Ther 2018;98(6):494–502.
7. Rush DD, Shelden ML. The early childhood coaching Handbook. Brookes Publishing Company; 2011.
8. Stredler-Brown Arlene. Examination of coaching behaviors used by providers when delivering early intervention via telehealth to families of children who are deaf or hard of hearing. Perspect ASHA Spec Interest Groups 2017;2(9):25–42.
9. Baggett KM, Davis B, Feil EG, et al. Technologies for expanding the reach of evidence-based interventions: preliminary results for promoting social-emotional development in early childhood. Top Early Child Spec Educ 2010; 29(4):226–38.
10. Pietruszewski L, Burkhardt S, Yoder PJ, et al. Protocol and feasibility-randomized trial of telehealth delivery for a multicomponent upper extremity intervention in infants with asymmetric cerebral palsy. Child Neurol Open 2020;7. https://doi.org/10.1177/2329048X20946214.
11. Tenforde AS, Borgstrom H, Polich G, et al. Outpatient physical, occupational, and speech therapy synchronous telemedicine: a survey study of patient satisfaction

with virtual visits during the COVID-19 pandemic. Am J Phys Med Rehabil 2020. https://doi.org/10.1097/PHM.0000000000001571.

12. Criss MJ. School-based telerehabilitation in occupational therapy: using telerehabilitation technologies to promote improvements in student performance. Int J Telerehabil 2013;5(1):39–46.

13. Golomb MR, McDonald BC, Warden SJ, et al. In-home virtual reality videogame telerehabilitation in adolescents with hemiplegic cerebral palsy. Arch Phys Med Rehabil 2010;91(1):1–8.e1.

14. Gibbs V, Toth-Cohen S. Family-centered occupational therapy and telerehabilitation for children with autism spectrum disorders. Occup Ther Health Care 2011; 25(4):298–314.

15. Guro A, Mjøen Tone R, Torstein V. Prevalence of speech problems and the use of augmentative and alternative communication in children with cerebral palsy: a registry-based study in Norway. Perspect Augment Altern Commun 2010;19(1): 12–20.

16. Tager-Flusberg H, Caronna E. Language disorders: autism and other pervasive developmental disorders. Pediatr Clin North Am 2007;54(3):469–81.

17. Reilly S, Skuse D, Poblete X. Prevalence of feeding problems and oral motor dysfunction in children with cerebral palsy: a community survey. J Pediatr 1996;129(6):877–82.

18. Levin DS, Volkert VM, Piazza CC. A multi-component treatment to reduce packing in children with feeding and autism spectrum disorders. Behav Modif 2014;38(6): 940–63.

19. Williams-Butler MA, Cantu RC. Concussion practice patterns among speech-language pathologists. Health (N Y) 2019;11(7):880–95.

20. Fairweather GC, Lincoln MA, Ramsden R. Speech-language pathology teletherapy in rural and remote educational settings: Decreasing service inequities. Int J Speech Lang Pathol 2016;18(6):592–602.

21. Gabel R, Grogan-Johnson S, Alvares R, et al. A field study of telepractice for school intervention using the ASHA NOMS K-12 Database. Commun Disord Q 2013;35(1):44–53.

22. Grogan-Johnson S, Schmidt AM, Schenker J, et al. A comparison of speech sound intervention delivered by telepractice and side-by-side service delivery models. Commun Disord Q 2013;34(4):210–20.

23. Isaki E, Fangman Farrell C. Provision of speech-language pathology telepractice services using apple iPads. Telemed J E Health 2015;21(7):538–49.

24. Baharav E, Reiser C. Using telepractice in parent training in early autism. Telemed J E Health 2010;16(6):727–31.

25. Ingersoll B, Wainer AL, Berger NI, et al. Comparison of a self-directed and therapist-assisted telehealth parent-mediated intervention for children with ASD: A Pilot RCT. J Autism Dev Disord 2016;46(7):2275–84.

26. Ruble LA, McGrew JH, Toland MD, et al. A randomized controlled trial of COMPASS web-based and face-to-face teacher coaching in autism. J Consult Clin Psychol 2013;81(3):566–72.

27. Lindgren S, Wacker D, Suess A, et al. Telehealth and autism: treating challenging behavior at lower cost. Pediatrics 2016;137(Supplement 2):S167–75.

28. Hepburn SL, Blakeley-Smith A, Wolff B, et al. Telehealth delivery of cognitive-behavioral intervention to youth with autism spectrum disorder and anxiety: a pilot study. Autism Int J Res Pract 2016;20(2):207–18.

29. Clark RR, Fischer AJ, Lehman EL, et al. Developing and implementing a tele-health enhanced interdisciplinary pediatric feeding disorders clinic: a program description and evaluation. J Dev Phys Disabil 2019;31(2):171–88.
30. Ransom DM, Butt SM, DiVirgilio EK, et al. Pediatric teleneuropsychology: feasi-bility and recommendations. Arch Clin Neuropsychol 2020. https://doi.org/10.1093/arclin/acaa103.
31. Cook RE, Schneider I, Hazlewood ME, et al. Gait analysis alters decision-making in cerebral palsy. J Pediatr Orthop 2003;23(3):292–5.
32. Narayanan UG. The role of gait analysis in the orthopaedic management of ambulatory cerebral palsy. Curr Opin Pediatr 2007;19(1):38–43.
33. Phinyomark A, Petri G, Ibáñez-Marcelo E, et al. Analysis of big data in gait biome-chanics: current trends and future directions. J Med Biol Eng 2018;38(2):244–60.
34. Gregory P, Alexander J, Satinsky J. Clinical telerehabilitation: applications for physiatrists. PM R 2011;3(7):647–56 [quiz: 656].
35. Child health screening and surveillance: a critical review of the evidence [elec-tronic resource]/report prepared by Centre for Community Child Health, Royal Children's Hospital Melbourne for the National Health and Medical Research Council. - Trove. Available at: https://trove.nla.gov.au/work/17064822. Accessed November 20, 2020.

Telemedicine for Musculoskeletal Rehabilitation and Orthopedic Postoperative Rehabilitation

Melissa E. Phuphanich, MD, MS[a], Kunal R. Sinha, MD[a],
Michael Truong[b], Quynh Giao Pham, MD[c],*

KEYWORDS

- Telemedicine • Virtual physical examination • Musculoskeletal injuries
- Postoperative orthopedics

KEY POINTS

- Telemedicine is a cost-effective platform to evaluate, manage, and rehabilitate patients with musculoskeletal pathologies and recent orthopedic surgeries.
- Telehealth visits have been shown to result in high-quality care, and patients and providers report satisfaction with these encounters.
- This article provides extensive guidance on conducting telemedicine visits, with particular emphasis on physical examination.

INTRODUCTION

Historically, telemedicine has played a significant role in reducing the cost of health care, minimizing inequalities in access to care, boosting efficiency, and managing care for patients with chronic diseases.[1] For the 100 million Americans with chronic disease receiving conventional treatment through periodic office-based visits, telemedicine has the potential to dramatically reduce health care–related costs.[2] However, widespread adoption of telemedicine has been limited by technological, legal, financial, and community adoption barriers.[3]

[a] Department of Physical Medicine and Rehabilitation, Greater Los Angeles VA Healthcare System, (117), 11301 Wilshire Boulevard, Los Angeles, CA 90073, USA; [b] University of California, San Diego, 9500 Gilman Drive, La Jolla, CA 92093, USA; [c] Pain Medicine Fellowship Training Program, Department of Medicine, Division of Physical Medicine and Rehabilitation, Greater Los Angeles VA Healthcare System, David Geffen School of Medicine at UCLA, (117), 11301 Wilshire Boulevard, Los Angeles, CA 90073, USA
* Corresponding author. Department of PM&R, (117), 11301 Wilshire Boulevard, Los Angeles, CA 90073.
E-mail address: Quynh.pham@va.gov

Phys Med Rehabil Clin N Am 32 (2021) 319–353
https://doi.org/10.1016/j.pmr.2020.12.004
1047-9651/21/Published by Elsevier Inc.
pmr.theclinics.com

The 2019 coronavirus pandemic has affected nearly every aspect of clinical rehabilitation. The widespread adoption of social distancing practices as a means of slowing the spread of novel coronavirus disease 2019 and improved reimbursement has refined and accelerated implementation of clinical telemedicine practices. Modern telemedicine makes use of online telephone and/or video consultations, telemonitoring, sensors, and online chat functions to connect patients with appropriate care options.[4] Many authors, including Laskowski and coworkers,[5] Satin and Lieberman,[6] Wahezi and coworkers,[7] and Tanaka and coworkers,[8] have established best-practices protocols for virtual musculoskeletal physical examinations. An adaptation and combination of these protocols is presented (**Table 1**).

THE VIRTUAL PHYSICAL EXAMINATION
Set Up and Preparation

Before the virtual visit, the patient should be educated on the logistics of the telehealth visit, and their home environment should be assessed. The patient's room should have adequate lighting for visualization, ample space to stand and move about in front of the camera, and a neutral blank background. Ideally, the patient should have a sturdy chair, bench, or table to safely perform all necessary examination maneuvers. If possible, an assistant should be present to ensure the patient's safety, help with positioning the camera, and assist in conducting some of the examination maneuvers. Visual instructions for the examination can be downloaded ahead of time or shown to the patient during the visit using screen sharing functions.

Patients should be instructed to wear attire conducive to visualization of all necessary structures (ie, tank top, shorts) and to performing all necessary maneuvers (ie, loose, nonrestrictive clothing). For this same reason, long hair should be tied up and accessories should be removed. If seated, the patient should be in a stable chair with no wheels. Finally, before initiating the visit, the patient's identity should be confirmed with multiple identifiers, and the examiner should note the patient's location and contact information to facilitate dispatching an emergency response team to the patient's location if necessary.

For the physical examination of the spine, upper extremities, and lower extremities during the telehealth visit, visual inspection may be used to determine sitting and standing posture, presence of muscle atrophy/hypertrophy, bony deformity, skin changes, and inflammation. Although the presence of inflammation is challenging to detect during a virtual visit, it is possible to diagnose with adequate image capture and visual comparison with contralateral limb.[9] Range of motion (ROM) assessment is done with image capture or video camera, using a goniometer or online protractor from the browser or downloaded application.

TELEHEALTH TREATMENT OPTIONS
Validity and Reliability of Physical Therapy via Telehealth

Physical therapy, the mainstay of rehabilitation treatment plans, is largely effective using telehealth and equivalent to face-to-face practices. Several systematic reviews establish equivalent outcomes (ie, improvement in physical function, disability, pain) using telerehabilitation for a variety of musculoskeletal conditions (eg, osteoarthritis, nonspecific low back pain) when compared with conventional methods of health care delivery.[17,18] One systematic review analyzed 898 studies on virtual physical therapy assessments for musculoskeletal disorders, and found good validity and excellent reliability for pain, swelling, ROM, muscle strength, balance, gait, and functional assessment; however, evidence for lumbar spine posture was inconclusive.[19,20]

Type of Examination	Patient Instructions and Clinical Relevance	Example

Table 1
Guidelines for virtual physical examination of the spine and extremities

Cervical Spine

Inspection/ ROM

Type of Examination	Patient Instructions and Clinical Relevance	Example
Inspect for asymmetry and anatomic abnormalities.	Ask the patient to hold the head in neutral position, flexion, extension, side bending, and rotation. Observe for cervical spine lordosis, head carriage, side-to-side symmetry, spinous process alignment, and scapula symmetry. Note any pain or limitation with movement.	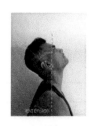 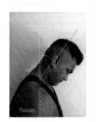 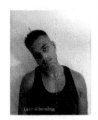 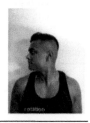

(continued on next page)

Table 1
(continued)

Type of Examination	Patient Instructions and Clinical Relevance	Example
	Cervical Spine	

Palpation

| The patient should palpate for tenderness, swelling, temperature differences, and obvious structural abnormalities. | Palpate spinous processes, interspinous/supraspinous ligaments, paracentral structures, paravertebral structures, trapezius muscles, and deltoid muscles. Ask the patient to note pain, swelling, increased warmth, muscle wasting, skin changes, or pain radiation. Identification of the most prominent cervical spinous process, C7, can help determine the relative location of pain. | 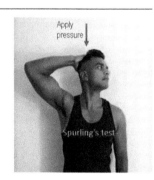 |

| | **Special Tests** | |

Cervical spine compression test (Spurling)

| Test for cervical radiculopathy. | Extend and rotate or side bend the neck to one side. Using the arm on the other side, apply a gentle downward force on top of the head. Positive test: pain/numbness in the upper limb is reproduced. | |

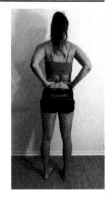

| | **Lumbar Spine** | |

Inspection/ROM

| Inspect for presence or absence of normal cervical and lumbar lordosis, and thoracic kyphosis. Inspect for side-to-side symmetry, spinous process alignment, skin creases, and pelvic symmetry. | While keeping the knee straight, bend forward, backward, to the sides, and rotate at the waist, noting any limitation of motion caused by pain, stiffness, or weakness. | |

(continued on next page)

| Table 1 |
| (*continued*) |

Lumbar Spine

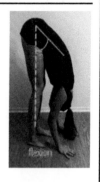

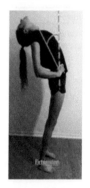

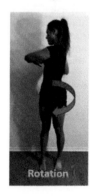

(*continued on next page*)

Table 1
(continued)

Lumbar Spine

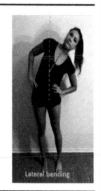

Lateral bending

Palpation

| Observe for areas of tenderness. | Facing away from camera, palpate midline (as high as possible) in the lumbar spine, noting any areas of tenderness. Then palpate the paraspinal muscles on each side. Continue to palpate the sacroiliac ligament area, quadratus lumborum, and buttock muscles. Note any local tenderness, which may suggest presence of muscle or ligament strain/injury. | 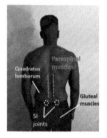 |

Gait

| Inspect for any gait abnormality, such as antalgic gait, pelvic tilt, side lean, or foot drag. | Instruct the patient to walk away from and then toward the camera. | 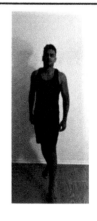 |

(continued on next page)

Table 1
(*continued*)

Lumbar Spine

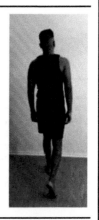

Special Tests

Straight leg raise test

| Test for lumbar root compression. | This test is done in a seated or supine position (also called the slump test).
While seated, extend the knee and passively dorsiflex the ankle using a towel or cloth.
In the supine position, with the knee extended, the leg can be raised using a towel.
Positive test: lumbar radiculopathy is suspected if pain in the leg/foot is reproduced in the ipsilateral or contralateral leg.
The straight leg raise test is equivalent in the sitting and supine position and the positive angles should be similar.[10] | 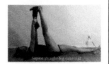

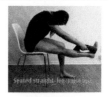 |

FABER test (Patrick test)

| Test for sacroiliac joint pathology. | While laying supine or seated, flex the knee, externally rotate the hip, and place the ankle just above the contralateral knee. Then apply downward pressure on the flexed knee while stabilizing the contralateral pelvis.
Positive test: pain in the lower back is exacerbated, suggesting sacroiliac joint pathology. | 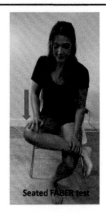
Seated FABER test |

(continued on next page)

Table 1 (continued)		
Special Tests		
		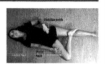
Neurologic Testing		
Lower extremity strength testing	Overall strength testing is assessed by asking patients to walk on toes, heels, and perform repeated heel raises. Sit with one knee extended, then stand up using the other leg. This unilateral sit-to-stand maneuver effectively tests for single limb muscle strength.[11]	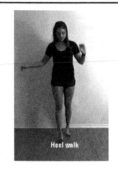 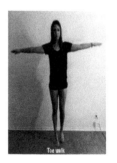 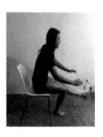

(continued on next page)

Table 1 (continued)		
Neurologic Testing		
		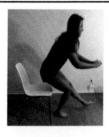 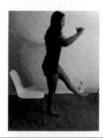
Lower extremity sensory testing	Limited sensory testing is done by using common household items, such as a soft cloth, cotton ball, make-up brush, toothpick, pen, paper clip. Comparison with the contralateral side or another dermatome is helpful to discern areas of abnormal sensation.	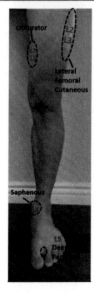

(continued on next page)

Table 1
(*continued*)

Neurologic Testing

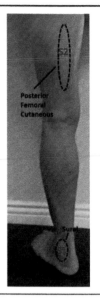

Upper extremity strength testing	Overall strength is assessed by asking patient to grip a weighted object, such as water bottle, food can, or shampoo bottle. With the elbow extended, general shoulder, elbow, and wrist strength is assessed with shoulder flexion, extension, and abduction.

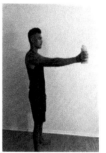

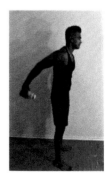

(*continued on next page*)

Table 1 (continued)		
Neurologic Testing		
		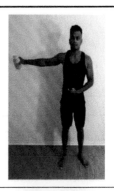
Upper extremity sensory testing	Using a soft object and a sharp object (as noted previously), test these areas for sensation changes. Note representative areas for myotome and peripheral nerve distribution.	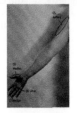
		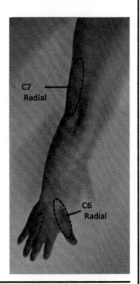
Grip and release test		
Test for myelopathy.	Close and open hand rapidly for 10 s. Although the rate varies with gender and age, inability to perform at least 20 repetitions in 10 s suggests weakness.[12]	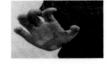

(continued on next page)

Table 1
(continued)

	Neurologic Testing

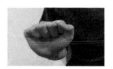

	Hip Examination

Inspection/ROM

Inspect for posture, pelvic obliquity, asymmetry.	With patient standing facing the camera, observe alignment, posture, and skin folds. On lateral view, look for posture and spine curvature. With the patient facing away from the camera, observe for symmetry of gluteal folds and skin folds. L4 is located at the level of the iliac crest.	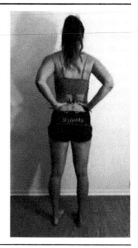
	While standing, use a sturdy chair for support to do the ROM examination. Supported by the chair, stand on one leg and perform hip abduction, adduction, flexion, extension, and internal and external rotation with hip flexed. Hip osteoarthritis may present with early limited ROM.[13]	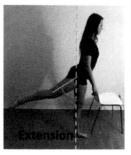

(continued on next page)

Table 1
(*continued*)

Hip Examination

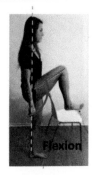

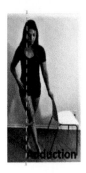

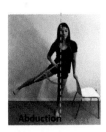

(continued on next page)

Table 1 (continued)		
Hip Examination		

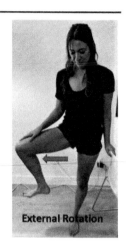

External Rotation

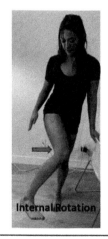

Internal Rotation

| Palpation | Palpate the groin area for local tenderness, which is present with hip flexor tendinitis, inguinal ligament strain, local nerve entrapment, and other pathologies.
If local palpation does not reproduce pain, hip joint pathology should be considered as a cause of pain.
Locate the trochanteric bursa, located over the widest area of the hip. Tenderness here suggests trochanteric bursitis.
Check distally, following the iliotibial band for additional tenderness because trochanteric bursitis is often associated with tight and painful iliotibial band. | 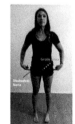 |

(continued on next page)

Table 1
(continued)

Hip Examination		
Trendelenburg test		
Gluteus medius weakness.	Facing away from the camera, stand on one leg, then the other leg. Positive test: weak gluteus medius causes pelvic drop on contralateral side.	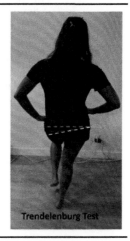
Thomas test		
Hip flexor tightness.	Lie on a table or bed, facing up. With both knees drawn up to the chest area, grab one knee with both hands and allow the other knee to fall to the table. Positive test: the thigh remains above the flat surface, signifying tight hip flexors. Measure the distance of the thigh from the table and compare with the other side.	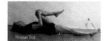
Shoulder Examination		
Inspection	Face the camera with both shoulders and arms/hands in view. Inspect the clavicles, trapezius, deltoid, AC joint, and biceps for asymmetry, atrophy, or deformity. Look for prominence of the AC joint, which could represent AC joint pathology or shoulder instability. If there is asymmetry of the shoulder with very limited ROM, suspect pathology, such as joint dislocation, bony deformity, and/or muscle atrophy and spasm.	 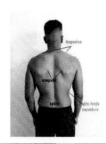

(continued on next page)

Table 1
(continued)

Shoulder Examination

ROM	Actively go through ROM with shoulders in flexion, abduction, and extension. With the arms at the side and elbow flexed to 90°, check for internal and external rotation. Have patient face toward a wall, pressing against it with both hands, to assess for scapula winging. Combination ROM is tested with scratching the back from above and below the shoulder.	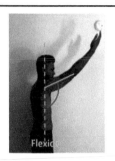
		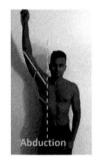
		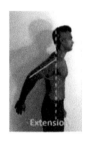
		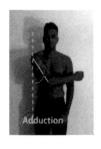

(continued on next page)

Table 1 (continued)	
Shoulder Examination	

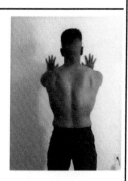

| Palpation | Palpate the clavicle anteriorly and move more laterally to the AC joint, subacromial area, noting areas of tenderness.
Inferior and slightly medial to the AC joint is the coracoid, the insertion location of the short head of the biceps before it travels through the bicipital groove. Patients with bicipital tendinitis may have pain here.
Patients with rotator cuff tendinitis may have pain over the subacromial area, where the supraspinatus tendon travels under the acromion, cushioned by the subacromial bursa. | 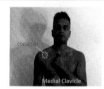
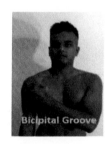
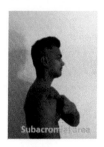 |

(continued on next page)

Table 1
(continued)

Shoulder Examination

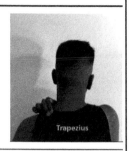

Cross body adduction test AC separation/ strain.	Flex the shoulder and adduct the arm across the body. Positive test: pain in the shoulder is reproduced with AC joint pathology.	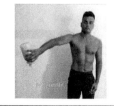

AC traction test AC separation/ strain.	Hold a weighted object while relaxing the shoulder. Positive test: visible separation of AC joint, or increased in pain over the AC joint.	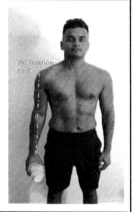

The Hawkins test Rotator cuff impingement.	With the shoulder abducted and in 90° of forward flexion, elbow flexed at 90°, palm facing the floor, use the other arm to apply downward pressure on the arm. Positive test: pain over the shoulder area suggests rotator cuff pathology.

The empty can Jobe test Rotator cuff impingement.	With the arms abducted hold the can or jar and turn it upside down. Positive test: inability to maintain this position because of pain or weakness from rotator cuff impingement.

(continued on next page)

Table 1 (continued)		
Shoulder Examination		
The belly press test Subscapularis weakness.	Press on the belly with palm and the wrist in neutral position. The elbow, forearm, and wrist should be in the same plane. Positive test: the elbow moves posteriorly and the wrist flexes, indicating weak subscapularis.	
The upper cut test Bicep tendinopathy.	Compared with other tests for bicep tendinopathy, such as the Yergason and speed tests, the upper cut test is easily performed without an assistant and has higher sensitivity and specificity.[14] This test is performed with the shoulder in neutral position, elbow flexed to 90°, fist clenched, and wrist supinated. The patient moves the wrist toward the chin while the other hand is placed over the fist to resist this "upper cut" motion. Positive test: pain or snapping sensation felt at the shoulder.	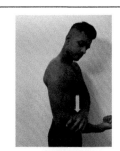
Sulcus sign test Shoulder instability.	Facing to the side of the camera, relax the shoulder with the elbow flexed at 90°. Use the other hand to grip the elbow and place downward pressure. Positive test: subluxation of the glenohumeral joint caused by shoulder instability.	

(continued on next page)

Table 1
(continued)

Shoulder Examination

Roos test Thoracic outlet syndrome.	With shoulders abducted and externally rotated, and elbow flexed, ask the patient close and open hands for 3 min. Positive test: pain, paresthesias, or weakness in the upper extremity.	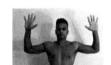 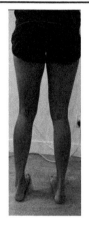

Knee Examination

Inspection/ROM	In a standing position, observe for symmetry and appreciate any redness, joint swelling, position of the patella, quadriceps atrophy, bony deformity, abnormal angulation, and swelling over pes anserine bursa or tibial tubercle. Observe for knee position, Q angle, and genu recurvatum. Inspect for popliteal swelling and hamstring atrophy. Standing on the side, check for knee flexion and extension.	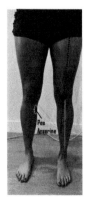

(continued on next page)

Table 1 *(continued)*		
Knee Examination		
		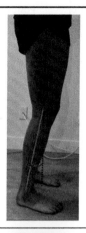
Palpation	With the knee extended and leg supported on a table or chair, feel for increased warmth compared with the unaffected knee. Palpate the patella tendon, tibial tuberosity, patella (including superior and inferior pole), medial and lateral joint line, and pes anserine bursa.	
Patella grind Patellofemoral syndrome.	Using the palm, apply downward pressure on the patella while the knee is extended. Positive test: reproducible pain suggests patellofemoral pathology.	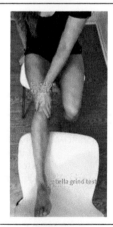
Milking the *joint fluid* Joint effusion.	Place the hand above the knee and press down while sliding the hand distally, pushing fluid to accumulation over the medial joint line. Positive test: fluid accumulation over medial joint causing skin bulge.	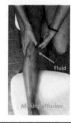

(continued on next page)

Table 1
(continued)

Knee Examination

Posterior sag sign Posterior interosseous tear.	With the knee bent at 90°, observe for posterior displacement of the proximal tibia. Positive test: the tibia sags posteriorly because of gravity if the posterior cruciate ligament is torn.	
Thessaly test Meniscus tear.	Using a table or stable structure for support, stand on the affected knee, flex to 20°, and twist side-to-side. Positive test: reproduces or increases knee pain, possibly with locking or grinding sensation.	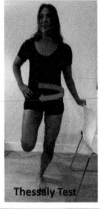
Strength test	Perform a squat to test for quadricep and hamstring strength.	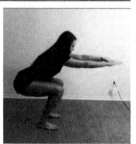

Special Considerations

Elbow examination

Inspection/ROM	Observe for carrying angle. Normal is 5°–15°. With shoulders abducted, ask patient to flex/ extend the elbow. Then with shoulders adducted, and the elbow flexed at 90°, ask patient to place palm face up (supinate) and down (pronate). Observe for swelling, redness, scaring, or bony deformity over the epicondyles and olecranon. Palpate the ulnar groove, olecranon, epicondyles, common flexor/extensor tendons, and the biceps tendon.

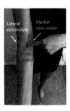

(continued on next page)

Table 1
(continued)

	Special Considerations	
Tinel test at the elbow Cubital tunnel syndrome.	With the elbow and shoulder flexed, and the shoulder abducted, have patient tap over the ulnar groove. Positive test: pain radiation to the 4th and 5th digits is suggestive of ulnar nerve compression at the cubital tunnel.	
Cozen test Lateral epicondylitis test Lateral epicondylitis.	With elbow and wrist extended, and the forearm pronated, place downward pressure on volar surface of the palm to resist wrist extension. Positive test: pain over the lateral epicondyle with these maneuvers suggests lateral epicondylitis.	
Test for medial epicondylitis (golfer's elbow, Little Leaguer's elbow) Medial epicondylitis.	With the elbow extended, wrist flexed, and forearm supinated, place downward pressure on the palmar surface of the hand to resist wrist flexion. Positive test: pain over the medial epicondyle with these maneuvers suggests medial epicondylitis.	
Inspection/ROM	With both hands resting on the table with the palms facing down, inspect the skin and nails for discoloration. Compare the fingers, wrists, and hands for symmetry. Note presence of skin folds, swelling, discoloration, bony/joint deformity, and wrist deviation. Inspect the first dorsal interossei for signs of atrophy. With the palm upward, inspect the joints, and fingers for color, soft tissue swelling, deformity, calluses, flexor tendon prominence, and thenar or hypothenar atrophy. Ask patient to perform finger flexion, extension, abduction, adduction, and opposition. Note any difficulties.	

(continued on next page)

Table 1
(continued)

	Special Considerations	
Palpation	Palpate the finger and thumb joints, wrist, thenar eminence, hypothenar, eminence, and palm for pain, swelling, nodules, or temperature changes.	
Scaphoid examination/ wrist tendons	Palpate the distal radial head (pain will be noted with distal radial fracture). With the palm facing down on the table and thumb abducted and extended, identify the 2 prominent tendons at the base of the thumb (extensor pollicis longus and extensor pollicis brevis). Then press between these 2 tendons. Pain in this area suggests scaphoid injury or fracture.	
Tinel test at wrist Carpal tunnel syndrome.	Ask the patient to place the wrist on the table with the palm facing up and flex the wrist to identify 2 tendons that are seen at the base of the hand, the flexor carpi radialis and palmaris longus tendons. Then tap over the space between these 2 tendons at the crease of the wrist. Positive test: pain, tingling, or numbness are reproduced in the first 3 digits and thenar area.	

(continued on next page)

Table 1
(continued)

	Special Considerations	
Phalen test Carpal tunnel syndrome.	Flex both wrists and press the dorsal surface of hands together for 1 min. Positive test: symptoms in the thenar area and first 3 digits are reproduced.	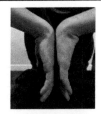
Finkelstein test De Quervain tendinitis.	Make a fist with the thumb tucked inside. Use the other hand to passively pull the wrist down (ulnar deviate). Positive test: wrist pain with this maneuver suggests pathology of the extensor pollicis brevis and abductor pollicis longus.	
OK sign Anterior interosseous nerve pathology.	Make an "OK" sign with the thumb and index finger. Positive test: inability to make a round "O" suggests weakness of the distal finger and thumb flexors, innervated by the anterior interosseous nerve.	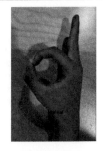 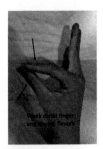
Thumb adduction test (Froment sign) Ulnar nerve pathology.	Hold a piece of paper between the thumb and index finger. Pull the paper out using the other hand. Positive test: if the thumb adductor (ulnar innervated) is weak, patient will compensate by flexing the distal interphalangeal joint (median innervated).	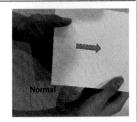

(continued on next page)

Table 1
(*continued*)

Special Considerations

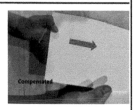

Ankle and Foot Examination

Inspection/ROM   Ask patient to walk without footwear and observe for antalgic gait, foot drop, foot slapping, and pronation or supination of the foot. Observe for proper alignment of the foot, ankle, knee, hip, and pelvis.
Inspect the foot. Note any swelling or deformity of the ankle, malleoli, tibialis anterior tendon, or Achilles tendon.

With the knee flexed to at least 30°, measure and compare ankle ROM in plantarflexion, dorsiflexion, inversion (supination), eversion (pronation), great toe, and interphalangeal flexion/extension.

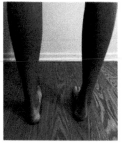

Dorsiflexion/Extension

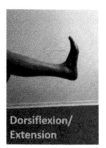

Plantarflexion/Flexion

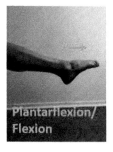

Inversion/Supination

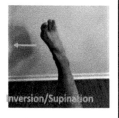

(*continued on next page*)

Table 1
(*continued*)

Ankle and Foot Examination

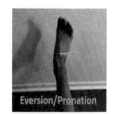

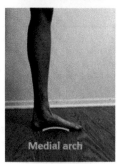

Palpate the medial and lateral malleoli, calcaneus, metatarsal heads, anterior tibialis tendon, Achilles tendon, fibular (peroneal) longus tendon, plantar fascia from heel to metatarsal, and tarsal tunnel (posterior to medial malleolus). Note any swelling, pain, or increased warmth.

Tinel test at medial ankle Tarsal tunnel syndrome.	Use fingers to firmly tap behind the medial malleolus. Positive test: burning/shooting pain in sole of the foot indicates tibial nerve entrapment at the tarsal tunnel.	
Thompson test Achilles rupture.	Kneeling on the chair and facing to the side, reach back to squeeze the calf muscle. This should cause the ankle to plantar flex. Positive test: absent ankle plantar flexion signifies Achilles tendon rupture.	
Metatarsal squeeze test Metatarsalgia, Morton neuroma, interdigital neuritis.	Squeeze the foot at the base of the toes. Positive test: pain in the toes (neuroma) or in the joint (metatarsalgia).	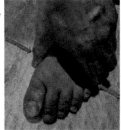

(*continued on next page*)

Table 1 (continued)		
Ankle and Foot Examination		
Thumb index squeeze test Morton neuroma, interdigital neuritis.	Using the thumb and index fingers, squeeze the area between the toes. Positive test: pain reproducible with pressure.	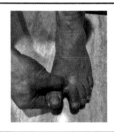

Special testing and ROM examinations were adapted from the Centers of Disease Control Normal Joint of Motion Study[15] and *Physical examination of the spine and extremities.*[16]

Abbreviations: AC, acromioclavicular; FABER, flexion, abduction, and external rotation; ROM, range of motion.

Although the evidence supporting Internet-based physical therapy for the lumbar spine is weaker, another study demonstrated that complementary technology exists to compensate for the deficits of virtual care. Kinect, a motion-sensing input device capable of detecting a patient's movement, posture, and ROM, enabled providers to deliver real-time feedback and correctional cuing.[20,21] The Kinect intervention facilitated customization of the physical exercise program, comparable with face-to-face physical therapy programs.

Validity and Reliability of Occupational Therapy via Telehealth

The existing literature examining the efficacy of virtual occupational therapy is small, but overall supportive. A systematic review reported most studies indicated high patient satisfaction and positive therapeutic effects when using telerehabilitation in occupational therapy practices, but more research is needed to confirm its effectiveness for various conditions and cost-efficiency.[22] Moreover, the American Occupational Therapy association supports telehealth methods for ergonomic evaluation.[23]

Telerehabilitation for the Postoperative Orthopedic Patient

Virtual physical therapy for the postarthroplasty patient

In particular, strong evidence establishes that virtual physical therapy management for knee arthroplasty is noninferior to standard face-to-face physiotherapy following total knee arthroplasty.[17] Systematic reviews on total knee arthroplasty patients found that telerehabilitation treatment resulted in comparable pain relief, and significantly higher extension range and quadriceps strength than face-to-face rehabilitation.[24] Perhaps the more substantial gains in functional recovery are explained by the convenience of telerehabilitation and possible increased compliance.

Less literature exists examining telerehabilitation for the upper extremity; however, the existing literature is promising. A recent study established evidence for the efficacy of telerehabilitation after shoulder arthroscopy in impingement syndrome. This research concluded that a virtual rehabilitation exercise program with ROM and strengthening of the rotator cuff and scapula stabilizers was comparable and noninferior to traditional face-to-face physical therapy.[25]

Virtual postoperative care

Research asserts telerehabilitation following orthopedic surgery has strong positive effect on clinical outcomes, and suggests that the increased intensity telerehabilitation programs can offer is a promising option for patients.[26] Several studies demonstrate effective virtual postoperative management, including dressing and suture removal, drain removal, and evaluation of the surgical wound.[27–29]

One group developed a software application with interactive steps and video instructions for patients who had undergone carpal tunnel release. Patients were able to remove their postoperative dressings, remove their sutures with or without the assistance of a friend or family member, capture a photograph of their surgical wound adequate for clinical decision-making by a health care provider, answer a question addressing their postoperative median nerve symptoms, and capture a clinically adequate video of physical examination maneuvers sufficient for motor and ROM examination. This study found that figure-eight sutures were substantially easier for patients to remove than horizontal mattress sutures, and the data collected from this novel application strongly agreed with the clinical documentation from in-person visits.[27]

Another case series established that Jackson-Pratt drains are successfully removed at home with caregiver support, an instructional infographic, and a telemedicine visit with physician guidance. The study on patients who had undergone major head and neck surgery demonstrated 100% success rate for drain removal, no reported complications, and high patient satisfaction.[28]

Virtual Chiropractic Care

Minimal literature exists on telehealth for chiropractic care, but a recent study establishes its feasibility. At the beginning of the coronavirus disease 2019 pandemic, telehealth for chiropractic services was quickly implemented at two health centers located on two campuses of a large company in California. These providers prescribed therapeutic exercises by demonstrating them to the patient, and then having the patient demonstrate the exercises back using the well-established teach-back method. Given the two-dimensional nature of video, it was necessary for providers and patients to demonstrate the exercises in at least two angles (eg, front and side).[23]

Additionally, telehealth assessment of directional movement preference for evaluation and treatment of low back pain has been shown to be equally as effective as in-person observation.[23] A study comparing the effects of Telerehabilitation-Based McKenzie Therapy and Clinic-Based McKenzie Therapy in patients with chronic low back pain showed comparable clinical outcomes.[30]

Virtual Yoga

Yoga is popular form of complementary and integrative medicine that supplements standard medical treatment, and studies provide evidence that yoga via telehealth provides comparable satisfaction and health improvement to in-person yoga. A study examining a clinical yoga program at a Veteran Affairs Medical Center reported high patient satisfaction and found 88% of participants reported some degree of subjective symptom improvement, including pain, energy level, depression, or anxiety. Those who participated via telehealth did not significantly differ from in-person participants in any measure of satisfaction, overall improvement, or improvement in any of 16 specific health problems.[31] Studies support the use of yoga in health care settings, and show that delivering yoga to a wide range of patients within a health care setting seems to be feasible and acceptable, when delivered in-person and via telehealth.[31,32]

CLINICALLY RELEVANT OUTCOMES
Patient Satisfaction

Patients consistently report high levels of satisfaction with physician visits and therapy sessions conducted via telehealth,[18,33–35] with some studies reporting significantly higher satisfaction among patients who undergo telerehabilitation compared with traditional face-to-face visits.[36,37] Patients attribute their satisfaction with telemedicine to a multitude of factors, including convenience,[38] reduced cost of care, improved communication with providers, less travel time, increased access to desired services, and decreased wait times for appointments.[39] Patients and caregivers largely rated their interactions during these visits with physicians as excellent, praising physician clarity, carefulness, skillfulness, respect, and sensitivity.[37] This favorable impression of telemedicine extends to telehealth encounters following orthopedic surgeries, including physician visits following total knee arthroplasty[40] or carpal tunnel release,[41] and rehabilitation programs following proximal humerus repair.[42] Although it is commonly believed that telehealth will mostly be favored by young affluent patients living in coastal cities, patients of advanced age[38] and patients residing in rural neighborhoods[43] have also reported high satisfaction with telemedicine. Unsurprisingly, patients tend to be least satisfied with their decreased ability to form a personal connection with their physician during a telemedicine encounter when compared with in-person visits[20,44]; however, most users also strongly agreed that they would use telehealth services again in the future.[37]

Provider Satisfaction

Crucially, providers also report a high level of satisfaction with telehealth visits.[39,45] For example, in a quality improvement study surveying 14 physiatrists who completed a total of 293 telemedicine encounters, more than 90% of physicians rated their experience as "very good" or "excellent," despite more than half of the providers having no prior experience with telemedicine.[45] Although physicians have expressed concerns regarding the limited capacity to perform a physical examination remotely,[46] potential technical failures of videoconferencing interfaces, and other such challenges of telehealth visits, most providers reported feeling that they are able to provide high-quality care to their patient during these visits,[37] and wished to continue using telehealth if reimbursement for these visits continued.[45]

Cost-Effectiveness

Telerehabilitation is a cost-effective alternative to in-person clinical encounters.[18] Most studies on this topic have focused on telemedicine for postoperative rehabilitation, which has been shown to be cost-effective for patients who undergo total hip arthroplasty[47]; total knee arthroplasty[48,49]; and other orthopedic surgeries, such as subacromial decompression.[50] These effects are particularly pronounced if travel time is considered[49] and if patients would have otherwise had to travel long distances for in-person encounters.[48] Telerehabilitation has also been shown to be cost-effective for the treatment of chronic musculoskeletal conditions, such as low back pain,[51] but less data are available for these conditions.

Quality of Care

In contrast to telerehabilitation for musculoskeletal injuries or telemedicine for postoperative follow-up visits, there is a relative paucity of data on the quality of telehealth encounters for initial consultations by orthopedic surgeons or physiatrists. One randomized controlled trial comparing initial orthopedic consultation via telehealth versus traditional face-to-face evaluation demonstrated no significant difference in percentage of patients referred for surgery or rates of complications 12 months following the initial encounter.[52] Unfortunately, most other studies on initial encounters for musculoskeletal complaints focus discussion on patient satisfaction,[46] cost-effectiveness,[53] or physician perception of quality of care rather than objective determinants of quality of care.[37] Further research is needed on this topic.

Barriers and Limitations

There are several patient-specific and provider-specific factors that may limit the expansion of telemedicine. Patients are typically amenable to participating in telehealth encounters,[43] with some strongly preferring remote visits over conventional face-to-face visits.[39] However, some patients may be unfamiliar with videoconferencing technology, and require guidance and instruction from clinic staff before their scheduled appointments.[54] Others, particularly those in rural areas or with limited financial resources, may be precluded from participating in telemedicine altogether because of lack of access to telephones, web camera–enabled devices, or high-speed Internet services.[43] Providers may also be resistant to implementing telehealth into their practices for a multitude of reasons, such as the high cost of purchasing videoconferencing hardware and software, lack of training on providing patient care via telehealth, subjective resistance to change, uncertainty regarding reimbursement for remote encounters, and a relative lack of legal guidelines regarding privacy and safe use of videoconferencing technologies.[54]

SUMMARY

Telemedicine is a cost-effective platform to evaluate, manage, and rehabilitate patients with musculoskeletal pathologies and recent orthopedic surgeries. These visits have been shown to result in high-quality care, and patients and providers report satisfaction with these encounters. This article provides extensive guidance on conducting telemedicine visits, with particular emphasis on physical examination.

CLINICS CARE POINTS

- Physical examination for most musculoskeletal conditions is effectively conducted via telemedicine.
- Virtual physical therapy is noninferior to conventional face-to-face physical therapy for a variety of musculoskeletal disorders.
- Virtual postoperative telerehabilitation has a strong positive effect on clinical outcome and is effective in management of surgical wounds, dressing changes, suture removal, and drain removal.
- Before evaluation, the examiner should note the patient's location and contact information to facilitate dispatching an emergency response team to the patient's location if needed.
- Before virtual visit, the patient should be instructed on navigating the required technology; dressing in clothing conducive to the physical examination (ie, tank top and shorts); and preparing the home environment with adequate lighting, ample space to move in front of the camera, chair or table available for support, and having household items available to aid the physical examination (eg, towel, can of soup).
- Visual instructions for the examination are downloaded ahead of time or shown to the patient during the visit using screen sharing functions.

- If possible, an assistant should be present to ensure the patient's safety, help with positioning the camera, and assist in performing some of the examination maneuvers.
- Visual inspection may be used to determine sitting and standing posture, presence of muscle atrophy/hypertrophy, bony deformity, skin changes, and inflammation.
- Although the presence of inflammation is challenging to detect during a virtual visit, it is possible to diagnose with adequate image capture and visual comparison with contralateral limb.
- Range of motion assessments are done with image capture or video camera, using a goniometer or online protractor from the browser or downloaded application.

DISCLOSURES

All authors- None.

REFERENCES

1. Bashshur RL, Shannon GW, Krupinski EA, et al. National telemedicine initiatives: essential to healthcare reform. Telemed J E Health 2009;15(6):600–10.
2. Nesbitt T. The evolution of telehealth: where have we been and where are we going? In: The role of telehealth in an evolving health care environment: workshop summary. National Academy of Sciences, Engineering, Medicine. The National Academies Press 2012;(3):6-11
3. LeRouge C, Garfield MJ. Crossing the telemedicine chasm: have the U.S. barriers to widespread adoption of telemedicine been significantly reduced? Int J Environ Res Public Health 2013;10(12):6472–84.
4. Vidal-Alaball J, Acosta-Roja R, PastorHernández N, et al. Telemedicine in the face of the COVID-19 pandemic. Aten Primaria 2020;52(6):418–22.
5. Laskowski ER, Johnson SE, Shelerud RA, et al. The telemedicine musculoskeletal examination. Mayo Clin Proc 2020;95(8):1715–31.
6. Satin AM, Lieberman IH. The virtual spine examination: telemedicine in the era of COVID-19 and beyond. Global Spine J 2020. https://doi.org/10.1177/2192568220947744.
7. Wahezi SE, Duarte RV, Yerra S, et al. Telemedicine during COVID-19 and beyond: a practical guide and best practices multidisciplinary approach for the orthopedic and neurologic pain physical examination. Pain Physician 2020;23(4):S205–38.
8. Tanaka MJ, Oh LS, Martin SD, et al. Telemedicine in the era of COVID-19. J Bone Joint Surg Am 2020;102(12). https://doi.org/10.2106/jbjs.20.00609.
9. Rotstein R, Berliner S, Fusman R, et al. The usefulness of telemedicine for the detection of infection/inflammation at the point of care. Telemed J E Health 2001;7. https://doi.org/10.1089/15305620152814719.
10. Fajolu OK, Pencle FJR, Rosas S, et al. A prospective analysis of the supine and sitting straight-leg raise test and its performance in litigation patients. Int J Spine Surg 2018;12(1). https://doi.org/10.14444/5010.
11. Thongchoomsin S, Bovonsunthonchai S, Joseph L, et al. Clinimetric properties of the one-leg sit-to-stand test in examining unilateral lower limb muscle strength among young adults. Int J Clin Pract 2020;74(9). https://doi.org/10.1111/ijcp.13556.
12. Yukawa Y, Nakashima H, Ito K, et al. Quantifiable tests for cervical myelopathy; 10-s grip and release test and 10-s step test: standard values and aging variation

from 1230 healthy volunteers. J Orthop Sci 2013;18(4). https://doi.org/10.1007/s00776-013-0381-6.

13. Metcalfe D, Perry DC, Claireaux HA, et al. Does this patient have hip osteoarthritis? The rational clinical examination systematic review. JAMA 2019;322(23). https://doi.org/10.1001/jama.2019.19413.

14. Cotter EJ, Hannon CP, Christian D, et al. Comprehensive examination of the athlete's shoulder. Sports Health 2018;10(4). https://doi.org/10.1177/1941738118757197.

15. Soucie JM, Wang C, Forsyth A, et al. Range of motion measurements: reference values and a database for comparison studies. Haemophilia 2011;17(3). https://doi.org/10.1111/j.1365-2516.2010.02399.x.

16. Hoppenfeld S. Physical examination of the spine and extremities. 1st edition. Prentice Hall: Appleton-Century-Crofts; 1976.

17. Cottrell MA, Galea OA, O'Leary SP, et al. Real-time telerehabilitation for the treatment of musculoskeletal conditions is effective and comparable to standard practice: a systematic review and meta-analysis. Clin Rehabil 2017;31(5):625–38.

18. Cottrell MA, Russell TG. Telehealth for musculoskeletal physiotherapy. Musculoskelet Sci Pract 2020;48:102193.

19. Mani S, Sharma S, Omar B, et al. Validity and reliability of Internet-based physiotherapy assessment for musculoskeletal disorders: a systematic review. J Telemed Telecare 2017;23(3):379–91.

20. Peretti A, Amenta F, Tayebati SK, et al. Telerehabilitation: review of the state-of-the-art and areas of application. JMIR Rehabil Assist Technol 2017;4(2):e7.

21. Gal N, Andrei D, Nemeș DI, et al. A Kinect based intelligent e-rehabilitation system in physical therapy. Stud Health Technol Inform 2015;210:489–93.

22. Hung Kn G, Fong KN. Effects of telerehabilitation in occupational therapy practice: a systematic review. Hong Kong J Occup Ther 2019;32(1):3–21.

23. Green BN, Pence TV, Kwan L, et al. Rapid deployment of chiropractic telehealth at 2 worksite health centers in response to the COVID-19 pandemic: observations from the field. J Manipulative Physiol Ther 2020. https://doi.org/10.1016/j.jmpt.2020.05.008.

24. Jiang S, Xiang J, Gao X, et al. The comparison of telerehabilitation and face-to-face rehabilitation after total knee arthroplasty: a systematic review and meta-analysis. J Telemed Telecare 2018;24(4):257–62.

25. Pastora-Bernal JM, Martín-Valero R, Barón-López FJ, et al. Telerehabilitation after arthroscopic subacromial decompression is effective and not inferior to standard practice: preliminary results. J Telemed Telecare 2018;24(6):428–33.

26. Agostini M, Moja L, Banzi R, et al. Telerehabilitation and recovery of motor function: a systematic review and meta-analysis. J Telemed Telecare 2015;21(4):202–13.

27. Tofte JN, Anthony CA, Polgreen PM, et al. Postoperative care via smartphone following carpal tunnel release. J Telemed Telecare 2020;26(4):223–31.

28. Go BC, Brewster R, Patel R, et al. Using telemedicine and infographics for physician-guided home drain removal. OTO Open 2020;4(2). 2473974X20933566.

29. Sandberg CEJ, Knight SR, Qureshi AU, et al. Using telemedicine to diagnose surgical site infections in low- and middle-income countries: systematic review. JMIR MHealth UHealth 2019;7(8):e13309.

30. Mbada CE, Olaoye MI, Dada OO, et al. Comparative efficacy of clinic-based and telerehabilitation application of McKenzie therapy in chronic low-back pain. Int J Telerehabil 2019;11(1):41–58.

31. Schulz-Heik RJ, Meyer H, Mahoney L, et al. Results from a clinical yoga program for veterans: yoga via telehealth provides comparable satisfaction and health improvements to in-person yoga. BMC Complement Altern Med 2017;17(1):198.

32. Field T. Yoga research review. Complement Ther Clin Pract 2016;24:145–61.

33. Lawford BJ, Delany C, Bennell KL, et al. "I was really skeptical...But it worked really well": a qualitative study of patient perceptions of telephone-delivered exercise therapy by physiotherapists for people with knee osteoarthritis. Osteoarthr Cartil 2018;26(6):741–50.

34. Moffet H, Tousignant M, Nadeau S, et al. Patient satisfaction with in-home telerehabilitation after total knee arthroplasty: results from a randomized controlled trial. Telemed J E Health 2017;23(2):80–7.

35. Tousignant M, Boissy P, Moffet H, et al. Patients' satisfaction of healthcare services and perception with in-home telerehabilitation and physiotherapists' satisfaction toward technology for post-knee arthroplasty: an embedded study in a randomized trial. Telemed J E Health 2011;17(5):376–82.

36. Cottrell MA, O'Leary SP, Raymer M, et al. Does telerehabilitation result in inferior clinical outcomes compared with in-person care for the management of chronic musculoskeletal spinal conditions in the tertiary hospital setting? A nonrandomised pilot clinical trial. J Telemed Telecare 2019. https://doi.org/10.1177/1357633X19887265. 1357633X19887265.

37. Cheng O, Law N-H, Tulk J, et al. Utilization of telemedicine in addressing musculoskeletal care gap in long-term care patients. J Am Acad Orthop Surg Glob Res Rev 2020;4(4). https://doi.org/10.5435/JAAOSGlobal-D-19-00128.

38. Shulver W, Killington M, Morris C, et al. 'Well, if the kids can do it, I can do it': older rehabilitation patients' experiences of telerehabilitation. Health Expect 2017. https://doi.org/10.1111/hex.12443.

39. Kruse CS, Krowski N, Rodriguez B, et al. Telehealth and patient satisfaction: a systematic review and narrative analysis. BMJ Open 2017. https://doi.org/10.1136/bmjopen-2017-016242.

40. Kairy D, Tousignant M, Leclerc N, et al. The patient's perspective of in-home telerehabilitation physiotherapy services following total knee arthroplasty. Int J Environ Res Public Health 2013. https://doi.org/10.3390/ijerph10093998.

41. Grandizio LC, Mettler AW, Caselli ME, et al. Telemedicine after upper extremity surgery: a prospective study of program implementation. J Hand Surg Am 2020. https://doi.org/10.1016/j.jhsa.2020.06.002.

42. Cabana F, Pagé C, Svotelis A, et al. Is an in-home telerehabilitation program for people with proximal humerus fracture as effective as a conventional face-to-face rehabilitation program? A study protocol for a noninferiority randomized clinical trial. BMC Sports Sci Med Rehabil 2016. https://doi.org/10.1186/s13102-016-0051-z.

43. Hale-Gallardo JL, Kreider CM, Jia H, et al. Telerehabilitation for rural veterans: a qualitative assessment of barriers and facilitators to implementation. J Multidiscip Healthc 2020. https://doi.org/10.2147/JMDH.S247267.

44. Hanna GM, Fishman I, Edwards DA, et al. Development and patient satisfaction of a new telemedicine service for pain management at Massachusetts General Hospital to the Island of Martha's Vineyard. Pain Med 2016. https://doi.org/10.1093/pm/pnw069.

45. Tenforde AS, Iaccarino MA, Borgstrom H, et al. Telemedicine during COVID-19 for outpatient sports and musculoskeletal medicine physicians. PM R 2020. https://doi.org/10.1002/pmrj.12422.

46. Tenforde AS, Hefner JE, Kodish-Wachs JE, et al. Telehealth in physical medicine and rehabilitation: a narrative review. PM R 2017. https://doi.org/10.1016/j.pmrj.2017.02.013.

47. Nelson M, Russell T, Crossley K, et al. Cost-effectiveness of telerehabilitation versus traditional care after total hip replacement: a trial-based economic evaluation. J Telemed Telecare 2019. https://doi.org/10.1177/1357633X19869796.

48. Tousignant M, Moffet H, Nadeau S, et al. Cost analysis of in-home telerehabilitation for post-knee arthroplasty. J Med Internet Res 2015. https://doi.org/10.2196/jmir.3844.

49. Fusco F, Turchetti G. Telerehabilitation after total knee replacement in Italy: cost-effectiveness and cost-utility analysis of a mixed telerehabilitation-standard rehabilitation programme compared with usual care. BMJ Open 2016. https://doi.org/10.1136/bmjopen-2015-009964.

50. Pastora-Bernal JM, Martín-Valero R, Barón-López FJ. Cost analysis of telerehabilitation after arthroscopic subacromial decompression. J Telemed Telecare 2018. https://doi.org/10.1177/1357633X17723367.

51. Fatoye F, Gebrye T, Fatoye C, et al. The clinical and cost-effectiveness of telerehabilitation for people with nonspecific chronic low back pain: randomized controlled trial. JMIR MHealth UHealth 2020. https://doi.org/10.2196/15375.

52. Buvik A, Bugge E, Knutsen G, et al. Quality of care for remote orthopaedic consultations using telemedicine: a randomised controlled trial. BMC Health Serv Res 2016. https://doi.org/10.1186/s12913-016-1717-7.

53. Harno K, Arajärvi E, Paavola T, et al. Clinical effectiveness and cost analysis of patient referral by videoconferencing in orthopaedics. J Telemed Telecare 2001. https://doi.org/10.1258/1357633011936435.

54. Scott Kruse C, Karem P, Shifflett K, et al. Evaluating barriers to adopting telemedicine worldwide: a systematic review. J Telemed Telecare 2018. https://doi.org/10.1177/1357633X16674087.

Telerehabilitation for Pain Management

Udai Nanda, DO[a,b,*], Jerry Luo, MD[a,b], Quinn Wonders, PharmD, BCPS[a,c],
Sanjog Pangarkar, MD[a,b]

KEYWORDS

- Telerehabilitation • Telehealth • Telemedicine • Chronic pain • Pain management
- Opioids • Whole health approach • Patient-centered care

KEY POINTS

- Telerehabilitation for pain management decreases the burden of geographic, economic, and physical barriers for patients with chronic pain disorders.
- The successful implementation of telerehabilitation for pain should include a structured set-up, interview, and examination to reduce errors and variability in patient outcomes.
- The coronavirus disease-2019 public health emergency, along with changes to the Ryan Haight Act, and reimbursement schedule has increased access to telerehabilitation for pain management.
- A whole health approach to pain management engages patients in self-care, emphasizes partnerships in a team-based approach, and supports general health and well-being.

INTRODUCTION

Timely access to medical care helps prevent and mitigate the impact chronic pain has on patients, their environment, and the health care system. In the United States, 20.4% of adults experience chronic pain and 7.4% experience high impact chronic pain, with women, non-Hispanic whites, and those older than 65 years most affected (**Fig. 1**).[1] These patients often require effective coordination of services between their medical providers to ensure communication and establish an interdisciplinary platform of care. Despite these efforts, barriers may still exist that make in-person medical care impractical, inconvenient, or unsafe. Such obstacles include the hardship of securing transportation for an appointment, which affects an estimated 3.6 million Americans

[a] Department of Physical Medicine and Rehabilitation, VA Greater Los Angeles Healthcare System, 11301 Wilshire Boulevard (W117), Los Angeles, CA 90073, USA; [b] Division of Physical Medicine and Rehabilitation, Department of Medicine, David Geffen School of Medicine at UCLA, Los Angeles, CA, USA; [c] Department of Pharmacy, VA Greater Los Angeles Healthcare System, Los Angeles, CA, USA
* Corresponding author. Department of Physical Medicine and Rehabilitation, VA Greater Los Angeles Healthcare System, 11301 Wilshire Boulevard (W117), Los Angeles, CA 90073.
E-mail address: udai.nanda@va.gov

Phys Med Rehabil Clin N Am 32 (2021) 355–372
https://doi.org/10.1016/j.pmr.2021.01.002
1047-9651/21/Published by Elsevier Inc.

each year who cannot obtain medical care owing to a lack of transportation. These individuals demonstrate a higher prevalence of medical comorbidities, including pain-related disorders.[2] To ensure access to timely care, especially in circumstances such as the coronavirus disease-2019 pandemic, virtual visits may provide the safest avenue to medical services.

Telemedicine was formally identified in the 1970s but has played a role in medical care for more than 100 years.[3] The term literally means "healing at a distance" though more recently has been defined by the World Health Organization as:

> The delivery of health care services, where distance is a critical factor, by all health care professionals using information and communication technologies for the exchange of valid information for diagnosis, treatment and prevention of disease and injuries, research and evaluation, and for the continuing education of health care providers, all in the interests of advancing the health of individuals and their communities.[4]

Telemedicine uses many of the technologies already in use by the general population for routine communication, with modifications made for the purpose of health care delivery. Telerehabilitation for pain management provides a method for the prompt delivery of pain care to a vulnerable population when there is no alternative, or to improve on conventional approaches.[5] To develop the necessary skills, medical providers should review relevant evidence-based principles and practice a structured patient-centered approach. Regulations and guidance can vary during a given time period, with medical, legal, and financial implications. For example, paying close attention to the evolving telehealth guidelines for opioid prescribing and risk mitigation strategies can prevent serious health-related consequences, maintain compliance with governmental requirements, and ensure proper billing practices for medical encounters. This article outlines telerehabilitation strategies to deliver patient-centered care with a whole health approach to pain disorders.

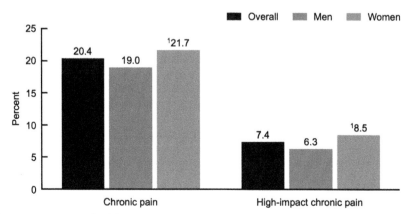

Fig. 1. Percentage of adults aged 18 and over with chronic pain and high-impact chronic pain in the past 3 months, overall and by sex, United States, 2019. (*From* Centers for Disease Control and Prevention (CDC). Zelaya CE, Dahlhamer JM, Lucas JW, Connor EM. Chronic pain and high-impact chronic pain among U.S. adults, 2019. NCHS Data Brief, no 390. Hyattsville, MD: National Center for Health Statistics. 2020.)

OVERVIEW

As technological innovations have fostered development in the field of telerehabilitation, the coronavirus pandemic has spurred rapid transformation in health care. Before understanding how to best implement telerehabilitation for the purposes of pain management, it is useful to revisit the general principles of telemedicine. The roles and capabilities of telemedicine are dynamic, and the World Health Organization has identified 4 central pillars:

1. "To provide clinical support
2. To overcome geographic barriers
3. The utilization of various types of information and communication technologies
4. To improve health outcomes."[6]

Adapting these principles to the telerehabilitation of pain is particularly challenging given the sheer number and complexity of chronic pain syndromes. The nature of this complexity is captured by the newly revised definition of pain by the International Association for the Study of Pain as "an unpleasant sensory and emotional experience associated with, or resembling that associated with, actual or potential tissue damage."[7]

The International Association for the Study of Pain attempts to provide a contextual basis for this definition by laying out several important reflections. Fundamentally, pain is a separate phenomenon from nociception, meaning that the experience of pain cannot be ascribed to sensory neuron depolarizations alone. Beyond this elementary biological basis, pain is also impacted by both psychological and social factors. Furthermore, the conceptualization of pain as an experience is one that is learned from and shaped by a culmination of life experiences. Last, and perhaps most important from the perspective of a provider, a patient's pain should be respected regardless of whether or not objective findings are present.[7]

Managing pain through telerehabilitation has many challenges and, despite advancements in technology, such as video teleconferencing, has several drawbacks. These limitations include interpreting nonverbal cues, rapport building, and performing an in-depth physical examination, all of which are necessary components for pain management. Therefore, approaching the diagnosis of pain etiologies by telemedicine requires a systematic approach, including a focused pain history, physical observation, and a mental health assessment. Combining these elements with a knowledge of pain physiology can assist in identifying the pain generator and assist in designing a therapeutic blueprint. The treatment of pain should also be met systematically. Therapeutic measures should concentrate on evidence-based approaches that minimize risk, provide holistic and integrated care, and enrich function and quality of life.

A GENERAL APPROACH TO THE TELEDIAGNOSIS OF CHRONIC PAIN

A virtual evaluation will likely be a new experience for most patients. To improve a patient's response to this format, a few general considerations should be taken into account before and during a visit. The office space of the telehealth provider should be professional, use appropriate lighting, and be equipped with a high-quality camera and microphone to best imitate a face-to-face evaluation. Additionally, from an individual standpoint, the telehealth provider should look into the camera rather than at their computer screen to better facilitate eye contact. The provider should also pay close attention to delay in terms of audio and video input and output to allow patients to fully express their thoughts without interruption. Physicians rely on their skills of observation on a daily basis, but it may be even more important when transitioning to a virtual environment. Subtle changes in language, tone, sound, facial expression, and movement can all be windows into the thoughts and feelings of a patient. Last, an expression of compassion toward the patient comes as second nature in an in-person evaluation; however, much of this nuance may be lost in a video format. It is, therefore, important for the telehealth provider be attentive and convey empathy during the session.

EVALUATION
Clinical History

Similar to a traditional in-person evaluation, the initial telemedicine evaluation for a chronic pain complaint begins with the clinical history (**Box 1**). The clinical history not only localizes the pain, but also distinguishes whether the pain is somatic, visceral, neuropathic, or mixed in etiology. The history also provides invaluable information in terms of what measures have previously been attempted in alleviating the pain complaints and can, therefore, guide consideration for future therapies. Qualitative tools should also be used to augment the clinical history by assessing the impact of pain on the patient's physical, emotional, and social functioning. Last, a thorough assessment will include a consideration of the patient's cultural background, personality, and psychological status. Within the context of telemedicine, patients can be sent a battery of validated assessment tools gauging pain and psychosocial factors before their visit.

As mentioned elsewhere in this article, pain is a highly subjective experience and requires the identification of a metric that can be monitored over time and serve as a measure for response to treatment. There are many tests available that assess a patient's pain intensity and include single metric questions and comprehensive surveys. The tools discussed in this article can be provided to a patient before their scheduled appointment and reviewed at the time of the visit.

Box 1
Pain clinical history prompts

- What is the intensity of pain or discomfort on a 0 to 10 scale?
- When did the pain start?
- Was there any preceding injury or surgery before the onset of pain?
- Where is the pain located?
- Does the pain radiate or change with activity?
- What is the quality of pain (sharp, dull, throbbing, aching, tingling, numbness, burning, shooting)?
- What activity or posture provokes the pain?
- What alleviates the pain?
- What medications have you tried, and did they help?
- What therapies have you tried?
- What additional modalities have you tried?
- How does the pain affect your day-to-day activities?

Unidimensional Self-Report Scales

Unidimensional self-report scales typically operate on a "0 to 10" scale or in a derivative fashion. These scales are simple, valid, and reliable in both clinical and research settings.[8] Examples include the Numeric Rating Scale, Verbal Rating Scale, visual analogue scale, and Wong-Baker FACES pain rating scale (**Figs. 2** and **3**).

Multiple Dimension Instruments

These tools provide a more comprehensive evaluation of a patient's subjective pain experience oftentimes by taking in account the impact of pain on quality of life and function. Examples include the commonly used McGill Pain Questionnaire (**Fig. 4**) and Brief pain inventory (**Fig. 5**), which incorporates the impact of chronic pain on day to day functioning.

Physical Examination

Perhaps the most obvious limitation of a telehealth visit is the inability to perform a direct physical examination. For pain conditions, a thorough physical examination is integral to making an accurate diagnosis. It is, therefore, imperative to understand the strengths and limitations of the virtual examination. In general, the virtual examination for a pain visit follows a standard in-person examination. The telehealth provider should localize the presenting symptoms to the appropriate anatomic body part by history and proceed with inspection, palpation, range of motion, and special testing.

Inspection

Valuable information can be gleaned from simple observation. To facilitate observation via camera, the patient should be instructed to wear a short-sleeved shirt and shorts for the virtual examination. Next, correct laterality should be determined because the video feed may be mirrored. Therefore, before beginning any virtual examination, the patient should be asked to indicate which side is right and which side is left. Once the logistics are established, the inspection can begin.

The provider should initiate the observation portion of the examination by assessing general appearance. Hygiene, grooming, and affect are all characteristics that can be

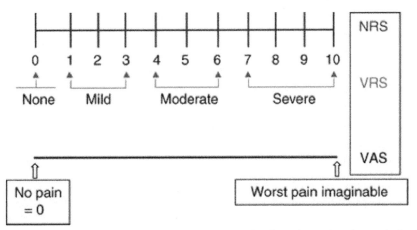

Fig. 2. Numeric rating scale (NRS), verbal rating scale (VRS), and visual analog scale (VAS). (*From* Breivik H, Borchgrevink PC, Allen SM, et al. Assessment of pain. British Journal of Anaesthesia. 2008;101(1):17-24. https://doi.org/10.1093/bja/aen103.)

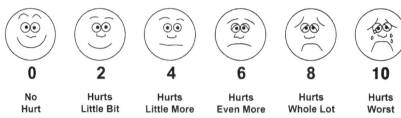

0	2	4	6	8	10
No Hurt	Hurts Little Bit	Hurts Little More	Hurts Even More	Hurts Whole Lot	Hurts Worst

Fig. 3. Wong-Baker FACES Pain Rating Scale. Explain to the person that each face represents a person who has no pain (hurt), or some, or a lot of pain. Face 0 doesn't hurt at all. Face 2 hurts just a little bit. Face 4 hurts a little bit more. Face 6 hurts even more. Face 8 hurts a whole lot. Face 10 hurts as much as you can imagine, although you don't have to be crying to have this worst pain. Ask the person to choose the face that best depicts the pain they are experiencing. (*From* Wong-Baker FACES Foundation (2020). Wong-Baker FACES® Pain Rating Scale. Retrieved [11/7/20] with permission from http://www.WongBakerFACES.org.)

adequately assessed by the virtual examination and may provide significant insight into a patient's mood and state of mind. After assessing general appearance, the provider should locate the anatomic region of interest as determined by the clinical history. Any obvious asymmetry from right to left, atrophy, hypertonicity, anatomic deformity, discoloration, or presence of swelling should be noted.

Palpation

The difference between pain as a subjectively reported symptom versus tenderness, which is objectively inferred by a health care provider, often relies upon palpation. Within a virtual examination, the provider must rely on the patient to report the findings of palpation. Palpation as a means to obtain objective data is therefore limited in a virtual examination because it is difficult to determine how much pressure is being applied by the patient or assistant during palpation. Despite this limitation, palpation is useful in determining the focal point of a patient's pain; the provider can instruct a patient or family member toward anatomic landmarks. Palpation is also useful in the assessment of abnormal findings to gauge temperature, which may be increased with inflammation. Swelling can be palpated to determine underlying mobility, edema, or induration. Areas of erythema can be palpated to determine blanching; last, areas of asymmetry can be palpated to determine whether soft tissue laxity or osseous reducibility exists.

Range of motion

Before assessing for range of motion, patients should be instructed to position themselves or the camera to allow for a full body view. Additionally, providers should assess whether there exists enough space for the patient to safely move without restriction such that all planes of motion can be captured. Unfortunately, for the virtual physical examination, only active range of motion can be assessed. Passive range of motion can, however, be assessed with the assistance of a family member, friend, or assistant.

For any given joint, all planes of motion should be tested to their fullest extent. Careful attention should be paid to the smoothness of action and any restrictions to the degree of expected motion. Any deviations from full range of motion should be assessed for a limitation owing to pain or to an intrinsic defect of the joint itself. It is important to keep in mind that any patient that can actively resist gravity with respect to a particular joint movement is displaying at least a grade 3/5 motor strength for that muscle.

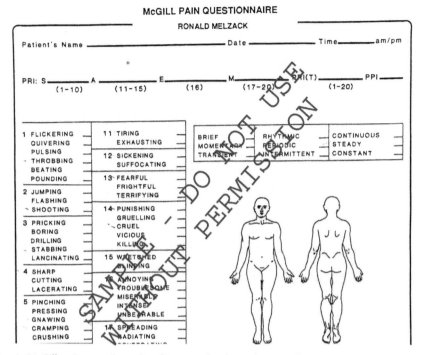

Fig. 4. McGill pain questionnaire. (*From* Melzack R. The McGill Pain Questionnaire: major properties and scoring methods. Pain 1975; 1:277-99; Mapi Research Trust, Lyon, France, https://eprovide.mapi-trust.org, with permission.)

Special testing

Last, in the absence of a nonclinician assistant, consideration must be placed for a patient's functional level when deciding upon which special tests to perform. There are several special tests that can be performed by the patient alone with adequate instruction and guidance from the telehealth provider. In general, the smaller the joint under consideration, the greater the feasibility of a nonassisted special test. For example, special testing of the hands including Phalen's test, Tinel's sign, Finkelstein test, and the CMC grind can generally be easily imitated by the patient. Special testing of the larger joints such as the lumbar spine or the hips requires an assistant, but can be achieved with guidance.[9]

Telehealth provider considerations

Throughout the virtual examination, it is critical to the success of a telehealth visit that the provider constantly be attuned to the subtle changes of a patient. Changes in facial expression, grimaces, and breathing patterns all provide insight into what a patient may be feeling without the need for verbal expression. The subtle reactions of a patient to any active or special testing maneuvers can not only guide the clinician, but also solidify the diagnosis.

Mental Health Assessment

A chronic pain evaluation is not complete without, at a minimum, a psychosocial screen. The simultaneous treatment of comorbid mental health disorders has been demonstrated to improve chronic pain symptoms.[10,11] Additionally, the psychosocial factors of any individual experiencing chronic pain cannot be understated and are

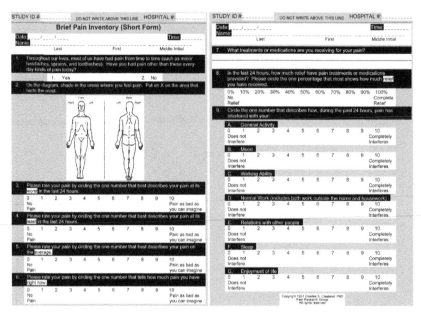

Fig. 5. Brief pain inventory. (Copyright ©2009. MD Anderson Cancer Center. Reproduced from Cleeland CS. The Brief Pain Inventory User Guide. Available from: https://www.mdanderson.org/documents/Departments-and-Divisions/Symptom-Research/BPI_UserGuide.pdf.)

predictive of morbidity.[12] Therefore, validated screening tools for mental health disorders, patterns in cognition, and alcohol or substance use disorder is an absolute necessity. The surveys described in this article can be combined in a single packet with the aforementioned unidimensional and multidimensional instruments for pain and delivered to the patient before evaluation by the telehealth provider.

Mental Health Screening Tools
Depression: Patients Health Questionnaire-9
Anxiety: General Anxiety Disorder-7
Post-traumatic stress disorder: Primary Care PTSD for DSM-V
Bipolar disorder: Mood Disorder Questionnaire
Pain catastrophizing scale
Alcohol or substance use screening tools
CAGE Adapted to Include Drugs

TREATMENT
Pharmacologic

Pharmacologic treatments for pain and rehabilitation in telemedicine are selected in a similar fashion to in-person visits. According to the diagnosis, treatments may be chosen for somatic, visceral, neuropathic, and mixed pain etiologies. Common medications that are used in pain and rehabilitation include nonsteroidal anti-inflammatory drugs (NSAIDs), opioids, acetaminophen, and medications for muscle spasm and neuropathic pain. NSAIDs provide analgesic and anti-inflammatory properties by preventing the creation of proinflammatory prostaglandins.[13] NSAIDs also bind and block the cyclo-oxygenase-2 enzyme to decrease prostanoid production and relieve pain. **Table 1** includes common NSAID medications and dosing. Opioids produce pain relief

Table 1
Common NSAID dosing

Medication	Starting Dose	Usual Dosing Range	Other
Aspirin	325 mg 3 times a day	325–650 mg 4 times a day	Doses of 3600 mg/d are needed for anti-inflammatory activity
Celecoxib	100 mg/d	100 mg twice daily or 200 mg/d	
Diclofenac XR	100 mg/d	100–200 mg/d	
Diclofenac IR	50 mg twice a day	50–75 mg twice a day	
Etodolac	300 mg twice a day	400–500 mg twice a day	
Ibuprofen	200 mg 3 times a day	1200–3200 mg/d in 3 to 4 divided doses	Available OTC and Rx
Indomethacin	25 mg twice a day	Titrate dose by 25–50 mg/d until pain controlled or maximum dose of 50 mg 3 times a day	
Indomethacin SR	75 mg SR once daily	Can titrate to 75 mg SR twice daily if needed	
Ketoprofen	50 mg 3 times a day	50–75 mg 3 to 4 times a day	
Meloxicam	7.5 mg/d	15 mg/d	
Naproxen	250 mg twice a day	500 mg twice a day	Available OTC and Rx
Naproxen sodium	220 mg twice a day	220–550 mg twice a day	
Naproxen sodium CR		375–750 mg twice a day	
Salsalate	500 mg twice a day	500–1000 mg 2 to 3 times a day	

Abbreviations: CR, controlled release; IR, immediate release; OTC, over-the-counter; Rx, prescription; SR, sustained release; XR, extended release.

Data from Buys LM, Wiedenfeld SA. Osteoarthritis. In: DiPiro JT, Talbert RL, Yee GC, Matzke GR, Wells BG, Posey L. eds. Pharmacotherapy: A Pathophysiologic Approach, 10e. McGraw-Hill; Accessed October 06, 2020. https://accesspharmacy.mhmedical.com/content.aspx?bookid=1861&sectionid=133893029.

by binding mu, kappa, and delta opioid receptors in the central nervous system to block the release of neurotransmitters that propagate pain signals. **Table 2** provides a summary of common oral opioids.[14] Of note, the Centers for Disease Control and Prevention and the Veterans Administration/Department of Defense do not recommend long-term opioid treatment for most patients with chronic pain.[15,16] If opioids are used, proper safety precautions should be in place, including long-term opioid consents, naloxone kit prescribing, prescription drug monitoring program review, and urine toxicology screening. Urine toxicology screening may be performed at an appropriate health care facility or laboratory to ensure confirmation screening, urine specific gravity, and the presence of adulterants.

Medication monitoring will need to be planned before prescribing pharmacologic treatments. **Table 3** includes common adverse drug reactions and monitoring parameters. For example, if laboratory monitoring is not feasible, alternative treatments should be chosen. Many pharmacies can also mail prescriptions to patient's residences and provide telephonic medication counseling.

Pharmacologic treatments can be provided by remote prescribing only after a patient–provider interaction. The Ryan Haight Online Pharmacy Consumer Protection

Table 2
Common opioid dosing

Medication	Usual Dosing Range	Other
Morphine	PO 5–30 mg every 4 h SR 15–30 mg every 12 h (may need to be every 8 h in some patients)	Drug of choice in severe pain, use with caution in renally compromised patients
Hydromorphone	PO 2–4 mg every 4–6 h	Use in severe pain
Codeine	PO 15–60 mg every 4–6 h	Use in mild to moderate pain
Hydrocodone	PO 5–10 mg every 4–6 h	Use in moderate/severe pain
Oxycodone	PO 5–15 mg every 4–6 h CR 10–20 mg every 12 h	Use in moderate/severe pain
Fentanyl	Transdermal 25 μg/h every 72 h Transmucosal, intranasal, and sublingual dosing based off of individual product	Do not use transdermal patch in acute pain Follow product-specific initiation and titration dosing recommendations
Methadone	PO 2.5–10 mg every 8–12 h	Effective in severe chronic pain Equianalgesic dose of methadone when compared with other opioids will decrease progressively the higher the previous opioid dose. Methadone prescribed for maintenance or detoxification treatment and must be dispensed under a Substance Abuse and Mental Health Services administration–certified opioid treatment program
Buprenorphine	Transdermal delivery systems 5, 7.5, 10, 15, 20 μg/h every 7 d Buccal film 75 μg every 12 h to 900 μg every 12 h	Second-line agent for moderate-to-severe pain May precipitate withdrawal in opiate-dependent patients Detailed manufacturer dosing conversion recommendations exist Buprenorphine products that contain naloxone (Suboxone) should be considered in patients with OUD). The prescribers of buprenorphine/naloxone products for OUD require a Drug Enforcement Agency waiver
Tramadol	PO 50–100 mg every 4–6 h ER PO 100 mg every 24 h	Maximum dose for nonextended release, 400 mg/24 h; maximum for extended release, 300 mg/24 h Decrease dose in patient with renal impairment and in the elderly

Abbreviations: CR, controlled release; ER, extended release; OUD, opioid use disorder; PO, oral; SR, sustained release.

Data from Herndon CM, Strickland JM, Ray JB. Pain Management. In: DiPiro JT, Talbert RL, Yee GC, Matzke GR, Wells BG, Posey L. eds. Pharmacotherapy: A Pathophysiologic Approach, 10e. McGraw-Hill; Accessed October 06, 2020.2020. https://accesspharmacy.mhmedical.com/content.aspx?bookid=1861&sectionid=146063604.

Table 3
Adverse drug reactions and monitoring parameters

Medication	Adverse Drug Reactions	Monitoring Parameters	Comments
Acetaminophen	Hepatotoxicity	Total daily dose limits	Use caution with multiple acetaminophen-containing products—total 4 g per 24-h limit
Opioids	Sedation, constipation, nausea, dry mouth, hormonal changes	Periodic assessment of renal (serum creatinine, eGFR) and hepatic (LFTs) function If methadone is used, EKG should be obtained before initiating treatment, at 30-d follow-up, and at least annually thereafter	Risks of addiction, dependence, and drug diversion
NSAIDs	Dyspepsia, cardiovascular events, GI bleeding, renal impairment	BUN/creatinine, hemoglobin/hematocrit, blood pressure	Risks higher in those older than 75 y of age

Abbreviations: BUN, blood urea nitrogen; eGFR, estimated glomerular filtration rate; EKG, electrocardiogram; GI, gastrointestinal; LFT, liver function test.

Data from Buys LM, Wiedenfeld SA. Osteoarthritis. In: DiPiro JT, Talbert RL, Yee GC, Matzke GR, Wells BG, Posey L. eds. Pharmacotherapy: A Pathophysiologic Approach, 10e. McGraw-Hill; Accessed October 06, 2020. https://accesspharmacy.mhmedical.com/content.aspx?bookid=1861&sectionid=133893029.

Act of 2008 requires an in-person patient examination before delivering, distributing, or dispensing controlled substances. The Ryan Haight Act was drafted in response to Internet pharmacies that were dispensing controlled substances online without prescribers seeing and evaluating the patient.[17]

In March of 2020, the Drug Enforcement Agency (DEA) detailed exceptions to the Ryan Haight Act to allow controlled substance prescribing via telehealth without a prior in-person visit and examination.[18] The designation of a Department of Health and Human Services public health emergency allows DEA-registered practitioners to issue controlled substances without a prior in-person evaluation if the following conditions are met: (1) the prescription is issued for a legitimate medical purpose in the normal course of the professional practice, (2) the telehealth platform uses audio-visual, real-time, 2-way communication, and (3) the practitioner is acting in accordance with applicable federal and state laws. The public health emergency exception applies to all schedule II through V controlled substances in all areas of the United States. The exemption rules remain in effect for as long as the public health emergency is in place. The designation of a public health emergency may also activate Section 1135 Waiver of the Social Security Act, which, for example, may waive or modify Medicare, Medicaid, Children's Health Insurance Program, and Health Insurance Portability and Accountability Act requirements to allow health care services to meet individuals' needs.[19] **Fig. 6** outlines the process of providing controlled substances to patients via telehealth as per DEA regulations. For additional information, the DEA has also published a coronavirus disease-2019 related informational webpage at www.deadiversion.usdoj.gov/coronavirus.html.[20]

Part I: Evaluating the Patient

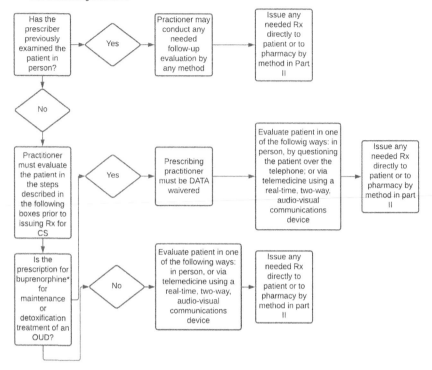

Part II: Delivering the Rx to the Pharmacy

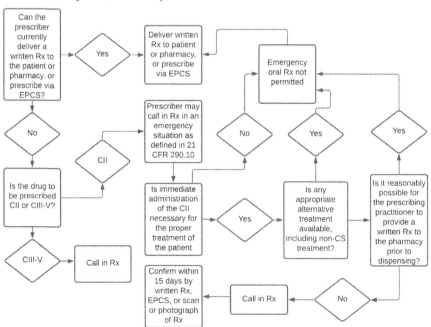

Nonpharmacologic

The management of chronic pain frequently requires a multidisciplinary approach that takes advantage of pharmacologic and nonpharmacologic modalities. The nonpharmacologic modalities are well-suited for a telerehabilitation approach. Evidence-based, nonpharmacologic therapies for the management of pain are generally encompassed within 3 broad categories: psychological and behavioral therapies, exercise and movement therapies, and manual therapies. Of these 3 categories, the psychological and behavioral therapies have an advantage in terms of evidence as well as ease of delivery. Although the exercise and movement therapies contain several therapies such as Tai Chi and yoga that are beneficial for chronic pain, there currently is insufficient evidence supporting its use via telemedicine.[21,22] Last, the manual therapies require a hands-on approach by a licensed provider and therefore fall out of the scope of telerehabilitation.

The overall philosophy of the psychological and behavioral therapies are similar in that they are all biopsychosocial interventions. As a result, their delivery to patients also follow similar schemata.[23] These therapies are time-limited protocols that are delivered by a trained expert in a standardized format and rely on goal-oriented lessons, active participation, and the tracking of progress by objective metrics.[24] Three well-known psychological and behavioral therapies that have found sufficient evidence in the treatment of chronic pain via telemedicine are cognitive behavioral therapy (CBT), acceptance and commitment therapy (ACT), and mindfulness-based stress reduction.

Cognitive behavioral therapy

CBT is a form of active psychotherapy that uses the interconnected nature of thoughts, behaviors, and feelings as a model to effect change. Within the context of pain management, the goal of CBT is to diminish both the maladaptive patterns of thoughts and behaviors that drive feelings of pain.[25] In a 2012 Cochrane review of randomized clinical trials addressing chronic pain with CBT versus usual treatment or wait-listed controls, CBT was found to have small effects on decreasing pain and disability, as well as moderate effects on easing catastrophizing thoughts.[26]

CBT with the use of video chat can easily be practiced within the comfort of a patient's home. The application of CBT through technological innovations has also shown to be beneficial in the management of chronic pain through randomized clinical trials. In the 2017 Cooperative Pain Education and Self-management (COPES) trial, interactive voice response CBT was found to be noninferior to in-person CBT in the management of chronic back pain. Patients randomized to the interactive voice response CBT arm were provided a self-help manual as well as weekly prerecorded feedback from their therapist based on their outcome metrics. At the conclusion of the 3-month trial, the primary outcome of average pain measured by the Numeric Rating Scale was −0.77 for the interactive voice response CBT arm and

Fig. 6. DEA-compliant prescribing of controlled substances via telehealth. C, schedule; CS, controlled substance; DATA, Drug Addiction Treatment Act of 2000; EPCS, electronic prescriptions for controlled substances; OUD, opioid use disorder; Rx, prescription. Note: aMethadone cannot be prescribed for maintenance or detoxification treatment and must be administered or dispensed directly to the patient for that purpose. 21 CFR 1306.07(a). (*From* How To Prescribe Substances To Patients During The COVID-19 Public Health Emergency. Drug Enforcement Agency: 2020. https://www.deadiversion.usdoj.gov/GDP/(DEA-DC-023)(DEA075)Decision_Tree_(Final)_33120_2007.pdf. Accessed November 12, 2020.)

−0.80 for the in-person CBT arm with a mean difference between groups of 0.07 (95% confidence interval, −0.67 to −0.80). Interestingly, patients in the virtual arm of the study also participated in more sessions than the in-person arm (mean difference, 2.3; $P<.001$).[27]

Acceptance and commitment therapy

ACT is a subset of CBT and is a relatively newer form of behavioral psychotherapy. The major aim of ACT is to promote psychological flexibility, examining thoughts as they come and go rather than wrestling with negative feelings. In contrast, CBT attempts to change fundamental beliefs. In this way, ACT can be thought of as a more passive engagement as compared with CBT.[28] In a 2017 systematic review and metanalyses of 11 randomized controlled trials with a total sample size of 863, participation in ACT compared with control conditions was found to have medium to large effect sizes on pain acceptance and psychological flexibility, as well as small to medium effect sizes on improved functioning, anxiety, and depression.[29]

A 2017 randomized noninferiority trial of 129 veterans demonstrated that ACT delivered by a video teleconferencing platform was as effective as in-person therapy in terms of the primary outcome of pain interference. This study also supported noninferiority of video teleconferencing delivery in regard to several secondary outcomes including mental and physical health quality of life.[30] Given the benefits of ACT for managing chronic pain as well as improving function and overall quality of life, transitioning toward a video-based platform is an option in situations of poor access to therapy.

Mindfulness-based stress reduction

Mindfulness-based stress reduction seeks to reframe a patient's relationship to pain through detached self-observation.[31] Mindfulness-based interventions have the benefit of being simple to use and least reliant on technology. Instructions and protocols can be delivered to patients through a variety of mediums, including written instructions, telephone, video conferencing, and smartphone applications. Compared with CBT and ACT, there is less evidence supporting the use of mindfulness-based stress reduction for chronic pain. There are, however, meta-analyses demonstrating that mindfulness interventions for chronic pain do have small beneficial effects on pain symptoms as well as mental and physical health quality of life metrics.[32,33] Tele-mindfulness interventions have also demonstrated significant improvements in key aspects of chronic pain syndromes, including pain catastrophizing, suffering levels, and mental health.[34]

Exercise therapies

Exercise-based therapy and physical therapy oftentimes form the foundation for conservative treatment of musculoskeletal pain. Moreover, regular physical activity is widely accepted to be essential for overall quality of life, mood, and function. A 2017 Cochrane review examining physical activity and exercise-based interventions for chronic pain suggests that exercise interventions yield improved pain severity, physical function, and quality of life, albeit with a low level of evidence. Importantly, these findings were also in the setting of minimal adverse events.[35] Similar findings were found in a telemedicine approach. A 2017 systematic review with a total sample size of 3575 concluded that compared with no intervention, telemedicine-based exercise intervention was beneficial for reducing pain in patients experiencing chronic pain.[36] Although there is a lack of strong evidence for the treatment of chronic pain with an exercise-based intervention, patients should be encouraged to maintain mobility through appropriate exercise and activity. Last, we defer the discussion of any specific physical therapies or exercises, because the musculoskeletal pain conditions that would benefit from physical medicine typically require a highly individualized movement regimen.

SUMMARY

Telerehabilitation for pain management uses communication technology to minimize barriers posed by geographic separation. Access to such technology has proven critically important during the coronavirus disease-2019 pandemic, but has also been useful in patients with chronic pain disorders who are unable to travel because of physical limitations. The evaluation and treatment of such disorders requires a whole health approach that individualizes treatment options and delivers care through a biopsychosocial approach. Although circumstances surrounding the need for telerehabilitation use may vary, including lack of reliable transportation to a medical facility, physical limitation precluding transport, or mitigation of person-to-person transmission of an illness, the goals of care are unchanged from an in-person patient–provider experience. Telerehabilitation can be successfully implemented in pain management with appropriate consideration for staging an evaluation, a structured approach to the visit, the use of standard clinical metrics, and the appropriate application of pharmacologic and nonpharmacologic treatments.

CLINICS CARE POINTS

- During the coronavirus disease-2019 pandemic, there have been temporary policy changes for telehealth to allow Health Insurance Portability and Accountability Act flexibility, expansion of covered services, and reimbursement equivalent to in-person visits.

- Telerehabitation for pain management can be offered in conjunction with, or in lieu of, in-person interaction. For example, a hybrid model may include an initial in-person consultation with options for virtual and/or in-person follow up visits.

- Confirm the patient's location, telephone number, emergency contact, and proximity to others during the initial stages of the visit in case communication becomes compromised or emergency medical services need to be rendered.

- If the patient lacks access to a secure environment, options should be provided to them to ensure their comfort, privacy, and safety.

- Avoid clothing with stripes or patterns because they can cause video distortion.

- When available, a designated individual may accompany the patient to assist with camera operation during the physical examination.

DISCLOSURE

The authors have nothing to disclose.

REFERENCES

1. Zelaya CE, Dahlhamer JM, Lucas JW, et al. Chronic pain and high-impact chronic pain among U.S. adults, 2019. NCHS Data Brief, no 390. Hyattsville (MD): National Center for Health Statistics; 2020.
2. Wallace R, Hughes-Cromwick P, Mull H, et al. Access to health care and nonemergency medical transportation: two missing links. Transportation Res Rec 2005;1924:76–84.
3. Strehle EM, Shabde N. One hundred years of telemedicine: does this new technology have a place in Paediatrics? Arch Dis Child 2006;91(12):956–9.

4. WHO. A health telematics policy in support of WHO's Health-For-All strategy for global health development: report of the WHO group consultation on health telematics, 11–16 December, Geneva, 1997. Geneva: World Health Organization; 1998.

5. Craig J, Patterson V. Introduction to the practice of telemedicine. J Telemed Telecare 2005;11(1):3–9.

6. Ryu S. Telemedicine: Opportunities and Developments in Member States: Report on the Second Global Survey on eHealth 2009 (Global Observatory for eHealth Series, Volume 2). Healthc Inform Res 2012;18(2):153–5.

7. Raja SN, Carr DB, Cohen M, et al. The revised International Association for the Study of Pain definition of pain: concepts, challenges, and compromises. Pain 2020. https://doi.org/10.1097/j.pain.0000000000001939.

8. McDowell I. Measuring health: a guide to rating scales and questionnaires. 3rd edition. New York: Oxford University Press; 2006.

9. Verduzco-Gutierrez M, Bean AC, Tenforde AS, et al. How to Conduct an Outpatient Telemedicine Rehabilitation or Prehabilitation Visit. J Inj Funct Rehabil 2020; 12:714–20.

10. Howe CQ, Sullivan MD. The missing 'P' in pain management: how the current opioid epidemic highlights the need for psychiatric services in chronic pain care. Gen Hosp Psychiatry 2014;36:99–104.

11. Cherkin DC, Sherman KJ, Balderson BH, et al. Effect of mindfulness-based stress reduction vs cognitive behavioral therapy or usual care on back pain and functional limitations in adults with chronic low back pain: a randomized clinical trial. JAMA 2016;315(12):1240–9.

12. Jensen MP, Moore MR, Bockow TB, et al. Psychosocial factors and adjustment to chronic pain in persons with physical disabilities: a systematic review. Arch Phys Med Rehabil 2011;92(1):146–60.

13. Buys LM, Wiedenfeld SA. Osteoarthritis. In: DiPiro JT, Talbert RL, Yee GC, et al. eds Pharmacotherapy: a pathophysiologic approach, 10th edition. McGraw-Hill. Available at: https://accesspharmacy.mhmedical.com/content.aspx?bookid=1861&sectionid=133893029. Accessed October 06, 2020.

14. Herndon CM, Strickland JM, Ray JB. Pain Management. In: DiPiro JT, Talbert RL, Yee GC, et al, editors. Pharmacotherapy: a pathophysiologic approach. 10th edition. McGraw-Hill; 2020. Available at: https://accesspharmacy.mhmedical.com/content.aspx?bookid=1861&sectionid=146063604. Accessed October 06, 2020.

15. Dowell D, Haegerich TM, Chou R. CDC guideline for prescribing opioids for chronic pain — United States, 2016. MMWR Recomm Rep 2016;65(No. RR-1):1–49.

16. U.S. Department of Veterans Affairs. VA/DoD clinical practice guideline for opioid therapy for chronic pain. February 2017. Available at: https://www.healthquality.va.gov/guidelines/Pain/cot/VADoDOTCPG022717.pdf#.

17. RYAN HAIGHT ONLINE PHARMACY CONSUMER PROTECTION ACT OF 2008. Vol. 154. Congressional Record; 2008. 110th Congress Public Law 425. Available at https://www.congress.gov/bill/110th-congress/house-bill/6353/text.

18. COVID-19 Information Page. 2020. Available at: Deadiversion.usdoj.gov; https://www.deadiversion.usdoj.gov/coronavirus.html. Accessed October 30, 2020.

19. 1135 Waivers. cms.gov. 2017. Available at: https://www.cms.gov/Medicare/Provider-Enrollment-and-Certification/SurveyCertEmergPrep/1135-Waivers. Accessed October 4, 2020.

20. COVID-19 Information Page. 2020. Available at: Deadiversion.usdoj.gov; https://www.deadiversion.usdoj.gov/coronavirus.html. Accessed November 6, 2020.
21. Kligler B, Bair MJ, Banerjea R, et al. Clinical policy recommendations from the VHA state-of-the-art conference on non-pharmacological approaches to chronic musculoskeletal pain. J Gen Intern Med 2018;33(Suppl 1):16–23. Available at: https://www.ncbi.nlm.nih.gov/pmc/articles/PMC5902342/.
22. Mathersul DC, Mahoney LA, Bayley PJ. Tele-yoga for chronic pain: current status and future directions. Glob Adv Health Med 2018;7. 2164956118766011 Available at: https://www.ncbi.nlm.nih.gov/pmc/articles/PMC5888810/.
23. Day MA, Thorn BE, Burns JW. The continuing evolution of biopsychosocial interventions for chronic pain. J Cogn Psychotherapy 2012;26(2):114–29. Available at: https://connect.springerpub.com/content/sgrjcp%3A%3A%3A26%3A%3A%3A2%3A%3A%3A114.full.pdf?implicit-login=true&sigma-token=IFGBw5_6ykj4YFVIxRCRXtkax-NoIGd18uqn0xjlgE4.
24. Murphy JL, McKellar JD, Raffa SD, et al. Cognitive behavioral therapy for chronic pain among veterans: therapist manual. Washington, DC: U.S. Department of Veterans Affairs; 2014.
25. Hylands-White N, Duarte RV, Raphael JH. An overview of treatment approaches for chronic pain management. Rheumatol Int 2017;37(1):29–42. Available at: https://pubmed.ncbi.nlm.nih.gov/27107994/.
26. Williams AC, Eccleston C, Morley S. Psychological therapies for the management of chronic pain (excluding headache) in adults. Cochrane Database Syst Rev 2012;11(11). CD007407. Available at: https://pubmed.ncbi.nlm.nih.gov/23152245/.
27. Heapy AA, Higgins DM, Goulet JL, et al. Interactive voice response-based self-management for chronic back pain: the COPES noninferiority randomized trial. JAMA Intern Med 2017;177(6):765–73. Available at: https://pubmed.ncbi.nlm.nih.gov/28384682/.
28. Graham CD, Gouick J, Krahé C, et al. A systematic review of the use of Acceptance and Commitment Therapy (ACT) in chronic disease and long-term conditions. Clin Psychol Rev 2016;46:46–58. Available at: https://www.sciencedirect.com/science/article/pii/S0272735815301124?via%3Dihub.
29. Hughes LS, Clark J, Colclough JA, et al. Acceptance and commitment therapy (ACT) for chronic pain: a systematic review and meta-analyses. Clin J Pain 2017;33(6):552–68. Available at: https://pubmed.ncbi.nlm.nih.gov/27479642/.
30. Herbert MS, Afari N, Liu L, et al. Telehealth versus in-person acceptance and commitment therapy for chronic pain: a randomized noninferiority trial. J Pain 2017;18(2):200–11. Available at: https://pubmed.ncbi.nlm.nih.gov/27838498/.
31. Kabat-Zinn J. An outpatient program in behavioral medicine for chronic pain patients based on the practice of mindfulness meditation: theoretical considerations and preliminary results. Gen Hosp Psychiatry 1982;4(1):33–47. Available at: https://pubmed.ncbi.nlm.nih.gov/7042457/.
32. Hilton L, Hempel S, Ewing BA, et al. Mindfulness meditation for chronic pain: systematic review and meta-analysis. Ann Behav Med 2017;51(2):199–213. Available at: https://pubmed.ncbi.nlm.nih.gov/27658913/.
33. Chiesa A, Serretti A. Mindfulness-based interventions for chronic pain: a systematic review of the evidence. J Altern Complement Med 2011;17(1):83–93. Available at: https://pubmed.ncbi.nlm.nih.gov/21265650/.
34. Gardner-Nix J, Barbati J, Grummitt J, et al. Exploring the effectiveness of a mindfulness-based chronic pain management course delivered simultaneously

to on-site and off-site patients using telemedicine. Mindfulness 2014;5:223–31. Available at: https://link.springer.com/article/10.1007/s12671-012-0169-3#citeas.

35. Geneen LJ, Moore RA, Clarke C, et al. Physical activity and exercise for chronic pain in adults: an overview of Cochrane Reviews. Cochrane Database Syst Rev 2017;4(4). CD011279. Available at: https://pubmed.ncbi.nlm.nih.gov/28436583/.

36. Adamse C, Dekker-Van Weering MG, van Etten-Jamaludin FS, et al. The effectiveness of exercise-based telemedicine on pain, physical activity and quality of life in the treatment of chronic pain: a systematic review. J Telemed Telecare 2018; 24(8):511–26. Available at: https://pubmed.ncbi.nlm.nih.gov/28696152/.

Telerehabilitation for Headache Management

Don McGeary, PhD, ABPP[a],*, Cindy McGeary, PhD, ABPP[b]

KEYWORDS

- Headache • Telerehabilitation • Telemedicine • Assessment • Treatment

KEY POINTS

- Headache is underassessed and undertreated throughout the world and represents one of the most burdensome health conditions.
- Research supports multiple effective strategies for headache rehabilitation, but the evidence supporting translation of these strategies into a telemedicine format is limited.
- Behavioral interventions have the strongest existing support for headache telerehabilitation, but the level of evidence supporting their use is still weak.
- Risks of headache telerehabilitation include privacy concerns, diminished oversight of treatment regimen, and incomplete assessment.

INTRODUCTION AND BACKGROUND

Headache represents one of the most prevalent and burdensome health conditions worldwide. Studies of headache epidemiology report worldwide headache prevalence rates of approximately 20%,[1,2] and the 2010 Global Burden of Disease survey identified headache as the second most common health problem in the world and the second most burdensome health condition in the United States after back pain.[3,4] Over the past several decades there have been significant advances in the medical and nonpharmacologic management of headache, but many patients with headache are unable to take advantage of these rehabilitation treatments because of a lack of access to specialty care and headache-related disability that precludes travel to care facilities. Telerehabilitation offers a promising and potentially effective mechanism for extending headache rehabilitation services beyond the clinic, with particular benefit for individuals with chronic disabling headache. This narrative review describes the existing research on telerehabilitation for headache and recommendations for

[a] Department of Rehabilitation Medicine, University of Texas Health Science Center, 7703 Floyd Curl Drive, San Antonio, TX 78229, USA; [b] Department of Psychiatry, University of Texas Health Science Center, 7703 Floyd Curl Drive, San Antonio, TX 78229, USA
* Corresponding author.
E-mail address: mcgeary@uthscsa.edu
Twitter: @DonMcGeary (D.M.)

Phys Med Rehabil Clin N Am 32 (2021) 373–391
https://doi.org/10.1016/j.pmr.2021.01.005
1047-9651/21/© 2021 Elsevier Inc. All rights reserved.

improving the translation of effective rehabilitation strategies for headache into the telehealth environment.

Headache Prevalence

Primary headache conditions

Migraine (MA) and tension-type headache (TTH) are the 2 most common forms of headache, with global prevalence estimates of 15% and 22% respectively[3]; diagnostic criteria for primary headache are summarized in **Table 1**. Migraine headache was recently identified as the second greatest cause of worldwide disability,[4] and studies of headache prevalence in the United States estimate that approximately 1 in every 6 US adults has migraine headaches, with more than 15% of women and almost 10% of men reporting migraine within a 3-month period (mostly affecting middle-aged adults).[5] Examination of multiple data sources on migraine headache experience show that individuals with migraine spend almost 9% of their lives each year with active migraine symptoms, resulting in significant burden and disability.[6] Worldwide, TTH affects almost 2 billion people, with little change in its incidence from 1990 to 2006.[4] European studies of TTH estimate that up to 42% of individuals worldwide experience TTH, with general costs to European countries of €13.8 billion,[7] and studies in the United States reveal that up to 40% of American adults experience TTH each year.[2,8,9] Like migraine, TTH is more common in women and middle-aged adults, with a 1-year prevalence of around 33% for recurrent or frequent TTH.[10,11] Chronic TTH, although more common than chronic migraine, is infrequently assessed and undertreated in clinical care despite significant burden and disability associated with these headaches.[10,12]

Secondary headache and headache in nonadult populations

Secondary headache (ie, headaches attributable to other medical causes) is increasingly recognized as a source of significant headache burden and prevalence (common secondary headaches are summarized in **Table 2**). These headaches include headache associated with human immunodeficiency virus (HIV), headache attributable to injuries to the head or neck, and headache associated with medication overuse (although some epidemiologic studies count medication overuse headache under the primary headache that led to medication overuse; eg, migraine and TTH). Individuals with HIV are at increased risk for headache and may be vulnerable to primary

Table 1	
International Classification of Headache Disorders characteristics for primary headaches	
Primary Headache	**Clinical Characteristics**
Migraine	Headache lasting 4–72 h At least 2 of the following: unilateral, pulsating, moderate/severe pain, aggravation with activity At least 1 of the following during episodes: nausea/vomiting or photophobia/phonophobia With or without aura
TTH	Headache lasting 30 min to 7 d At least 2 of the following: bilateral, pressing/tightening, mild/moderate pain, not aggravated with activity Both of the following during episodes: no nausea/vomiting, no more than 1 of photophobia or phonophobia

Data from Headache Classification Committee of the International Headache Society (IHS) The International Classification of Headache Disorders, 3rd edition. Cephalalgia, 2018. 38(1): p. 1-211.

Table 2
International Classification of Headache Disorders characteristics for select secondary headaches

Secondary Headache	Clinical Characteristics
Posttraumatic headache	Headache developed within 7 d of an injury to the head or regaining consciousness after an injury
Cranial or cervical vascular headache	Headache caused by a cranial or cervical vascular event
Headache attributed to infection	A9.3 headache attributed to HIV

Data from Headache Classification Committee of the International Headache Society (IHS) The International Classification of Headache Disorders, 3rd edition. Cephalalgia, 2018. 38(1): p. 1-211.

headaches such as MA and TTH or to the development of headache associated with disease processes because of immunocompromise.[13] Focused studies of headache in HIV infection have found that 30% of individuals with HIV experience headache, although this estimate has diminished to 4% with the success of contemporary pharmacotherapies for HIV.[14,15] Headache associated with injuries to the head or neck (also known as posttraumatic headache) likely account for 4% of all known headache disorders, affecting close to 70 million people with traumatic brain injury worldwide.[16–18] Medication overuse headache (MOH), defined as headache attributable to overuse of medication for primary headache (often concerning increased use of abortive medications), affects between 1% and 2% of individuals worldwide, with the greatest risk attributed to individuals with more than 7 headache days per month, less than 50 years of age, and comorbid medical and/or psychiatric disorders.[19] MOH can have significant impact on individuals' quality of life and, because of its complexity, can be very difficult to treat. Overuse of numerous medications for headache can lead to MOH, and people with primary headaches and medical comorbidities are at increased risk for these secondary headaches.[19]

Headache burden is not limited to adults, and there is increasing recognition that children and adolescents experience high rates of headache and related disability. Although still understudied, emerging research has begun to highlight the significant burden of headache in children and adolescents. European studies found that up to 75% of adolescents between the ages of 10 and 18 years reported problems with headache, 24% of whom reported MA and 22% reported TTH (compare with Refs.[20–22]). Children and adolescents with headache are at increased risk for burdensome psychiatric comorbidities (eg, depression, anxiety[23,24]), which may increase suicide risk in this vulnerable population.[24] Young people with headache may also experience disruptions in school and social functioning, and those who receive treatment (many do not) generate high health care costs.[25]

Current Evidence for Headache Rehabilitation

Ongoing research has led to significant advances in the treatment of headache that mitigate the burden, especially for chronic headache, for patients who are able to access them. Primary headaches (eg, MA and TTH) are likely to benefit from physical therapy,[26] which is particularly effective when combined with pharmacotherapies, botulinum neurotoxin injection, and/or other physiotherapy modalities (transcranial magnetic/electrical stimulation[27,28]). The significant overlap between headache and psychiatric comorbidities has led to an abundance of research focusing on the efficacy of nonpharmacologic psychotherapeutic approaches for headache management (most using a cognitive behavior therapy [CBT] approach). Physical rehabilitation and psychosocial interventions for primary headache are associated with improved psychological comorbidities, decreased headache days per month, decreased mean number of headache episodes, and improved headache intensity.[29–32] There is emerging evidence supporting mindfulness-based interventions for primary headache management, which, when combined with other rehabilitation modalities, can lead to durable long-term treatment benefit,[33] and complementary and integrative health strategies (eg, acupuncture, massage, tai chi, meditation, biofeedback) also show strong promise in headache rehabilitation.[34–36] Emerging research is also starting to examine the outcomes of rehabilitation in understudied headache populations, including secondary headache and child/adolescent populations, and outcomes in these subpopulations are generally positive.[37]

Complications and Obstacles to Evidence-Based Headache Rehabilitation

Despite the significant burden of headache and abundant evidence supporting various rehabilitation strategies for primary and secondary headache, individuals with headache in the United States and throughout the world are significantly under-assessed and undertreated.[2] Patients with headache in Western countries rarely seek and/or receive medical attention for their headaches, and fewer than 10% are prescribed frontline pharmacotherapies.[38] Patients often lack access to health care providers who are knowledgeable and trained in headache management,[39] and those with lower socioeconomic status often lack the resources (eg, money/insurance, time, transportation) to use in-office care.[40] Without access to adequate education, consultation, or screening for headache, individuals are likely to underestimate their need for treatment and develop sufficient headache disability to functionally limit their ability to leave their homes to seek care.[40] Of the 40% of patients with headache who successfully seek and begin treatment, fewer than one-fourth of patients with disabling headache follow through with care recommendations because of economic limitations,[41,42] disability,[43,44] and lack of time to travel for treatment appointments.[45,46]

Clinical Relevance of Telerehabilitation for Headache Management

Telemedicine offers a significant opportunity to extend care to those who cannot otherwise access it, often at a lower cost and higher rate of use than in-person care. As described earlier, studies on headache interventions have documented the efficacy and effectiveness of numerous pharmacologic and nonpharmacologic interventions, offering a strong foundation for telehealth translation. Nonpharmacologic telerehabilitation offers significant opportunity to maintain and extend the benefits of pharmacotherapies with minimal additional risks to the patient and clinical outcomes that are noninferior to in-person care.[47] Furthermore, telemedicine-based headache management seems to provide the same patient satisfaction as in-person care. In a survey study of 279 people who participated in a randomized trial of telemedicine versus traditional neurologic outpatient consultation for headache, the proportion of patients who were satisfied with telemedicine treatment (86%) was comparable with those who were satisfied with traditional care (88%[48]). Both study groups reported equivalent treatment outcomes and there were no between-groups differences in treatment adherence.[49] After accounting for travel costs, lost work time, and longer wait times for in-office care appointments, the investigators estimated that telemedicine headache management saved patients between €120 and €480.[50] A study of telemedicine for headache treatment in a US pediatric sample found that 100% of families participating in the telemedicine clinic were satisfied with the care and found it cheaper (saving an average of $486 per family on care expenses) and more convenient (saving 6.8 hours in travel time) compared with in-office care.[51]

To maximize the likelihood of successful implementation of headache telerehabilitation, a few questions remain. The coronavirus disease 2019 (COVID-19) pandemic led to widespread recognition of the need for distance-technology platforms to add meaningful infrastructure for extended service delivery without the limitations of in-office care. As noted earlier, telemedicine-based care can decrease the cost and increase the convenience of treatment, leading some to suggest that telemedicine may eventually become a first option for treating patients.[52] Until recently, uptake of telemedicine was fragmented and slow because of weak technological infrastructure, unclear guidelines and practices for care reimbursement, weak integration of telemedicine into health care systems, and lack of trust and familiarity with telemedicine among treatment providers.[53–55] Large, centralized medical systems such as the US Department of Defense and the Department of Veterans' Affairs have developed robust telemedicine infrastructures and have already begun adoption of telemedicine programs for headache rehabilitation,[56] but smaller systems and stand-alone medical practices may lack the resources to implement a robust telerehabilitation program.

In 2020, federal legislation was enacted in the United States to encourage permanent expansion of telemedicine after the coronavirus pandemic in order to preserve the convenience and wide reach of telemedicine platforms that were developed in response to COVID-19.[57,58] The Coronavirus Aid, Relief, and Economic Security Act (CARES) resulted in sweeping changes to privacy/Health Insurance Portability and Accountability Act (HIPAA) regulations (including loosening restrictions on delivery of care across state lines) and how third-party payors reimburse telemedicine encounters, leading to a surge in telemedicine service availability nationwide. A recent study of telemedicine service use found significant growth in telemedicine after passage of CARES accompanied by increased rates of home-based management of chronic health conditions and decreased emergency department visits.[59] Individuals who accessed telemedicine services in the COVID-19 era used them to manage non-COVID health concerns.[59] However, telerehabilitation for headache is woefully underdeveloped and underused because of:

- Lack of studies confirming noninferiority of telemedicine versus in-office rehabilitation for headache
- Incomplete information about effective training for headache telerehabilitation providers
- Ongoing concerns about the contribution of nonspecific treatment factors (eg, physical presence of a provider, patient-provider relationship) to telemedicine-based treatment outcomes[60]

Research and development are sorely needed to grow the body of evidence-based telerehabilitation resources for headache management. Fortunately, there are some existing research and clinical programs that can serve as a foundation for this development.

CURRENT EVIDENCE ON TELEREHABILITATION FOR HEADACHE MANAGEMENT
Guidelines for Headache Rehabilitation

Multicomponent clinical care pathways represent the strongest blueprints for expedient and effective rehabilitation of disabling or chronic headache. The Italian Consensus Conference on Pain in Neurorehabilitation outlined a multidisciplinary pathway for headache management that begins with recommendations for headache assessment and culminates in multimodal rehabilitation options based on the headache phenotype and assessment outcomes.[61] The Ontario Protocol for Traffic Injury Management Collaboration (OPTIMa) recommends beginning with a diagnostic assessment to confirm headache phenotype and rule out of other disorders, followed by collaborative treatment planning with the patient, multimodal care, and reassessment at regular intervals throughout treatment to determine the need for changes in treatment or additional referrals.[62,63] The United States Veterans' Health Administration has established national Headache Centers of Excellence that research, develop, and implement clinical practice guidelines of headache rehabilitation for US veterans, including resources for diagnosis, assessment, and effective rehabilitation.[64] The American Headache Society (AHS) and the International Headache Society (as well as numerous other professional organizations) have curated clinical practice guidelines and policy position statements for headache management, which are summarized in **Table 3**. Across all care pathways and guidelines, subject matter experts agree that rehabilitation resources for headache should include resources for headache assessment and monitoring, educational resources for headache self-management, and efficacious rehabilitation strategies. Thus, this article covers existing practices and evidence for telerehabilitation headache management across these domains.

Telemedicine Resources for Headache Evaluation and Monitoring

The greatest amount of research on telerehabilitation for headache covers the use of distance technology (including wearable technology and mobile devices) for headache assessment and monitoring. Video-based telemedicine can be used to observe patients and their home environments and video observation can be supplemented with telemedicine peripheral devices (eg, teleophthalmoscopes, Bluetooth-linked biofeedback) to provide additional data during video observation.[65] Most headache telemedicine research focuses on the use of electronic monitoring and digital diaries for headache assessment. Digital headache diaries are available in various formats and some can be customized to include secondary variables that add dimension to headache monitoring (eg, sleep tracking, stress monitors; **Fig. 1** shows an example developed for one of the authors' headache studies). Wearable devices are increasingly used in conjunction with headache diaries to passively gather biofeedback and activity data that can be used for adding dimensions to headache assessment and treatment. For example, modern wrist-worn activity monitors include heart-rate monitoring to passively track stress and accelerometers to track activity, which can be combined with diary entries to examine how patients are responding to headache episodes.

Research on digital headache diaries supports the acceptability of telemedicine headache tracking but raises concerns about adherence to and reliability of headache diary entries.[66,67] Headache assessment completed through digital and mobile health applications is vulnerable to incompletion of entries or failure to complete entries as instructed, especially for younger individuals and those who use free (vs paid) diaries.[66] Commercially available headache diary applications rarely include medical/scientific headache experts in application development and the resulting diaries consequently fail to include a comprehensive battery of evidence-based domains for headache assessment.[67] Clinical experts and researchers who develop their own electronic and mobile health headache diaries generate scientifically comprehensive diaries but often lack usability functions and patient training resources to ensure adequate completion of the diaries.[67,68]

Table 3
Select clinical practice guidelines for headache management

Source	Guideline Topic	Link
IHS	International Classification of Headache Disorders, Third Edition	https://ihs-headache.org/en/resources/guidelines/
AHS	Migraine treatment in adults Migraine treatment in children Migraine assessment Treatment of cluster headache Drug combinations in headache pharmacotherapy	https://americanheadachesociety.org/resources/guidelines/guidelines-position-statements-evidence-assessments-and-consensus-opinions/
Association of American Family Physicians	Acute and chronic headache management Diagnosis of migraine Migraine prophylaxis Pharmacotherapy for migraine Pharmacotherapy for cluster headache Complementary and integrative health for headache Diagnosis of chronic daily headache Complications in headache treatment	https://www.aafp.org/afp/topicModules/viewTopicModule.htm?topicModuleId=10
American Academy of Neurology	Acute migraine treatment in children Pharmacotherapy for pediatric migraine Botox for headache Pharmacotherapy for adult migraine Pharmacotherapy for cluster headache Headache evaluation	https://www.aan.com/Guidelines/home/ByTopic?topicId=16
Departments of Defense/Veterans Affairs	Management of headache Clinical algorithm Patient summary Provider pocket card	https://www.healthquality.va.gov/guidelines/Pain/headache/

Professional organizations for headache research and clinical care rarely offer digital headache diary applications, making it difficult to identify reliable and comprehensive mobile health and Web-based diaries for use in headache telerehabilitation. Hundert and colleagues[69] reviewed 38 digital applications in 2014 and found that only 3 met predetermined criteria for required for a scientifically and clinically acceptable headache diary (iHeadache, ecoHeadache, Diary Pro), all 3 of which are still available at the time of this narrative review. A more recent review noted that there are now more than 100,000 digital and mobile applications for tracking headache and other medical conditions, but most of these were developed without the input of clinical or patient stakeholders and there is no available resource providing guidance on how to choose reliable and valid commercial diaries, leading many clinicians and researchers to develop their own.[70] Research is strongly encouraged to speed the

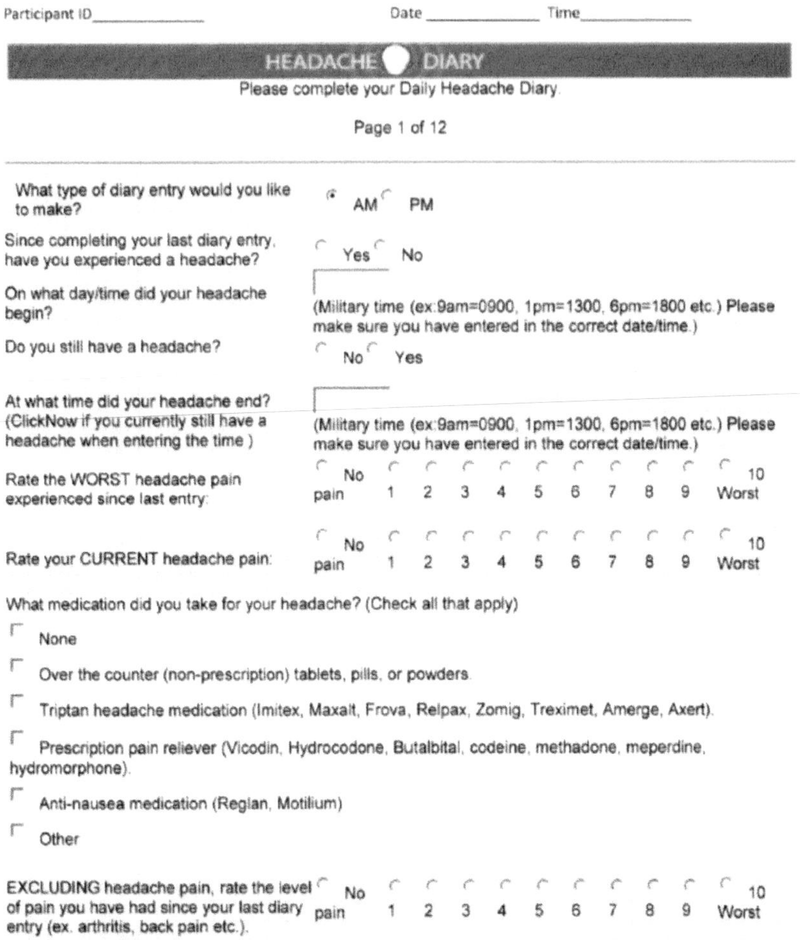

Participant ID_____   Date _____ Time_____

HEADACHE ● DIARY
Please complete your Daily Headache Diary.

Page 1 of 12

___

What type of diary entry would you like to make?
● AM ○ PM

Since completing your last diary entry, have you experienced a headache?
○ Yes ○ No

On what day/time did your headache begin?
[   ]
(Military time (ex:9am=0900, 1pm=1300, 6pm=1800 etc.) Please make sure you have entered in the correct date/time.)

Do you still have a headache?
○ No ○ Yes

At what time did your headache end? (ClickNow if you currently still have a headache when entering the time.)
[   ]
(Military time (ex:9am=0900, 1pm=1300, 6pm=1800 etc.) Please make sure you have entered in the correct date/time.)

Rate the WORST headache pain experienced since last entry:
○ No pain ○ 1 ○ 2 ○ 3 ○ 4 ○ 5 ○ 6 ○ 7 ○ 8 ○ 9 ○ 10 Worst

Rate your CURRENT headache pain:
○ No pain ○ 1 ○ 2 ○ 3 ○ 4 ○ 5 ○ 6 ○ 7 ○ 8 ○ 9 ○ 10 Worst

What medication did you take for your headache? (Check all that apply)

☐ None

☐ Over the counter (non-prescription) tablets, pills, or powders

☐ Triptan headache medication (Imitex, Maxalt, Frova, Relpax, Zomig, Treximet, Amerge, Axert).

☐ Prescription pain reliever (Vicodin, Hydrocodone, Butalbital, codeine, methadone, meperdine, hydromorphone).

☐ Anti-nausea medication (Reglan, Motilium)

☐ Other

EXCLUDING headache pain, rate the level of pain you have had since your last diary entry (ex. arthritis, back pain etc.).
○ No pain ○ 1 ○ 2 ○ 3 ○ 4 ○ 5 ○ 6 ○ 7 ○ 8 ○ 9 ○ 10 Worst

Fig. 1. Example of a digital headache diary.

___

development of telerehabilitation resources with the usability benefits of commercially available digital headache diaries and the clinical validity of those developed for research.

One of the most understudied but promising applications of telemedicine for headache assessment is the use of telemedicine resources for specialty headache consultation. For example, the European Headache Federation (EHF) used an expert panel to establish a specialty headache consultation program across Europe that included an online digital consultation form and a portal for sharing clinical report and imaging/laboratory results.[71] The resulting EHF consultation process allowed medical providers without headache expertise to access headache consultation expertise across Europe that would not otherwise be locally available. A study of inpatient neurologic specialty consultation using telemedicine visits found that telemedicine allowed convenient specialty consultation with clinical determinations/recommendations that matched in-person consultation and produced similar outcomes and morbidity/mortality to in-person consultation.[72] Patients who receive care informed by telemedicine consultation for headache report high levels of satisfaction with their care and benefit from significantly lower health care costs because of decreases in the travel and time away from work often required for in-person expert consultation.[50] As headache tele-rehabilitation continues to grow, expert consultation should become more widely available and nonexpert health care providers managing patients with headache are encouraged to take advantage of these resources.

Telemedicine Resources for Patient Education

Patient education is acknowledged as a primary component of effective headache management, and professional organizations such as the AHS recommend that clinicians educate their patients about their headache and treatment options, including pharmacotherapies, lifestyle change, and self-management.[73] Telemedicine and other electronic health (e-health) strategies offer a broad scope of resources for patient education. Digital patient education resources can be delivered to patients in multiple formats through both asynchronous (eg, information made available online that patients can access when they choose) and synchronous (eg, during an in-person videoteleconference contact) mechanisms. Various professional organizations worldwide offer libraries of research publications, webinars, infographics, and audio media designed to teach patients and nonspecialty providers about different headache phenotypes and how behavioral and lifestyle factors affect headache (some education options are summarized in **Table 4**).

Developing education resources for patients with headache is a key component of patient-centered care, and there is some evidence showing that effective education strategies can improve headache symptoms and decrease health care costs.[74] Providers can use Web site resources, email, and automated text/push messaging to asynchronously encourage headache self-management and home skills practice.[68,75] Synchronous contacts through real-time text messaging, telephone, and videoteleconferencing allow patients more opportunity to communicate with their providers about their care.[75] Education about medication use is vital to prevent MOH and can

Table 4		
Summary of available United States online patient and provider headache education resources		
Source	**Resources**	**Web Site**
National Headache Foundation	Publications Webinars Podcast Topic sheets Clinical brochures	https://headaches.org/resources/#headache-tools
AHS	Infographics Professional education Practice guidelines Video library Fact sheets	https://americanheadachesociety.org/education-training/ https://americanheadachesociety.org/resources/
American Migraine Foundation	Downloadable patient guides	https://americanmigrainefoundation.org/patient-guides/
International Health Society	Diagnostic tools Practice guidelines Research publications	https://ihs-headache.org/en/resources/

prevent relapse for individuals in treatment of MOH; for some, education alone may be sufficient to effectively address MOH.[19,76,77] Studies on the efficacy of distance technologies for encouraging self-management of headache report positive outcomes, but available studies are methodologically weak and more research is needed to confirm efficacy.[68]

Telemedicine Resources for Clinical Rehabilitation: Behavioral Therapies

Of all headache treatment options, behavioral headache management has received the most attention for telerehabilitation of headache. There are numerous variations of behavioral headache programs, although most include stress management training, headache monitoring and trigger management, cognitive therapy for pain and psychiatric comorbidities, and adjunctive biofeedback.[78] Telemedicine and mobile technologies allow health care providers to expand the scope and scale of behavioral management, but research on behavioral telerehabilitation of headache is nascent.[79] A 2016 systematic review of electronic behavioral headache treatments found that most contemporary studies examined computer-based interventions using CBT and/or relaxation modalities.[80] Subsequent meta-analytical studies of electronic behavioral health for various chronic pain conditions found that distance technologies can produce significant improvements in chronic pain, pain cognitions, and comorbid mood conditions that likely affect pain (eg, depression[81]), although the body of controlled research supporting telehealth for pain management was small at the time of this narrative review.[82] Studies of individuals with neurologic disorders found that digital CBT interventions lead to large improvements in mood, fatigue, and self-efficacy,[83] but surprisingly little is known about digital CBT for headache. Despite significant meta-analytical support for behavioral headache interventions for adults and children,[84,85] there have only been 2 published meta-analyses of behavioral headache telerehabilitation since 2016 describing a weak and underdeveloped body of research.[68,80]

Telemedicine Resources for Clinical Rehabilitation: Physical Rehabilitation

Exercise and physical therapy have well-documented benefits for individuals with chronic primary and secondary headache. One recent meta-analysis examined outcomes from 6 randomized controlled trials of suboccipital physical therapy for TTH, noting a large short-term treatment effect,[86] and randomized trials of physical therapy combined with other treatments found significant short-term improvement in headache frequency and pain intensity for adults with migraine[27] and young adults with TTH.[87] Emerging evidence supporting the efficacy of physical therapy delivered using distance technologies for chronic musculoskeletal pain conditions has led to strong pushes for the development and implementation of telerehabilitation assessment and treatment resources in physical and occupational therapy.[88] There is growing evidence showing that physical therapy can be effectively delivered in a telemedicine format resulting in improved clinical outcomes, decreased travel costs (especially among rural-dwelling patients who must travel great distances for care), and high levels of patient satisfaction.[89] Early concerns about regulatory obstacles to telemedicine-based physical therapy in the United States were overcome with passage of CARES and loosening of HIPAA restrictions, allowing physical and occupational therapists to engage, bill, and seek reimbursement for telerehabilitation services in most states.[90] Professional organizations worldwide have developed special interest groups for telemedicine translation of physical rehabilitation, but there are no available published studies of telemedicine-based physical or occupational therapy describing the efficacy, safety, or limitations of these services for individuals with headache.

Telemedicine Resources for Clinical Rehabilitation: Complementary Health

Complementary and integrative health (CIH; also referred to as complementary and alternative medicine [CAM]) has grown as a desirable and potentially effective approach for wellness and management of numerous chronic health conditions. Most Americans with headache report using CIH (acupuncture, yoga, meditation, movement therapies, chiropractic, diet/neutraceuticals, and mindfulness) to manage their headache, and CIH use across other Western countries ranges from 28% to 82%.[91] The quality of existing data supporting CIH for TTH is good (especially for manipulative and movement therapies[92,93]), whereas migraine study quality is low (although evidence for acupuncture in migraine is strong[93]). Research on telemedicine adaptation of CIH is in its infancy, but emerging studies show promise. For example, studies of yoga delivered by videoteleconference (ie, teleyoga) show high levels of satisfaction for individuals with chronic pain and psychiatric diagnoses.[94] Preliminary evidence from teleyoga studies show improvement in pain, energy, and mood,[94–96] with additional evidence showing that teleyoga may be noninferior to in-person yoga.[97]

Of all CIH options, mindfulness offers the best opportunity for telerehabilitation translation as a self-management skill. A few studies have examined synchronous and asynchronous mindfulness interventions for nonheadache conditions such as posttraumatic stress disorder and clinical depression. Telemedicine mindfulness through so-called smart messaging resulted in improved depression and motivation in a sample of 51 patients with cancer,[98] and a sample of 24 United States veterans with posttraumatic stress disorder reported improved mindfulness skills after telemedicine-based mindfulness training.[99] However, there is a dearth of research covering the application of telemedicine CIH for headache, but the results of telemedicine mindfulness for other conditions is promising.

Telemedicine Resources for Clinical Rehabilitation: Adjunctive Treatments

Telemedicine allows the home-based implementation of treatment resources that were previously limited to office-based and hospital-based visits. Videoteleconferencing can be used to aid in patient assessment and monitoring, and electronic and mobile health applications allow patients to use treatment resources wherever they are. Biofeedback (ie, any device providing information about physiologic processes) is often recommended as a core adjunct to headache management, and technical innovations have led to decreased cost and increased availability of physiologic monitors for patients with headache to use at home.[100,101] Smartphones and wearable technologies (eg, Fitbit) help patients and their providers track activity, often using passive tracking that increases adherence to monitoring.[102] Recent studies describe the feasibility, acceptability, and preliminary outcomes of telemedicine biofeedback for patients with stroke, wheelchair users, and individuals with chronic pain (compare with Ref.[103]), but there are no available studies describing outcomes of biofeedback-assisted headache management through distance technology and more research is needed to confirm their value.[67]

Technological advances now offer novel mechanisms for monitoring adherence to medication.[70] For example, cell phone–assisted remote observation of medication adherence can be used to observe and track patient medication use from afar,[104] which can improve outcomes of prophylactic pharmacotherapies and decrease risk for MOH. Providers can use videoteleconferencing to review medications with patients and instruct administration in real time or use digital medication diaries or other electronic medication monitoring applications to track pharmacotherapy; however, patients vary in their response to adherence technology so multiple options should be available.[105] Patients may benefit from peer support as an adjunct to care through online portals such as Facebook. Online peer support can promote physical activity and allow patients opportunities to talk with other people experiencing similar difficulties. However, these online resources are rarely monitored or supervised for content and research on the effective application of online peer support for headache is sparse.[106]

CONTROVERSIES IN TELEREHABILITATION FOR HEADACHE MANAGEMENT

Despite its benefits, translation of headache management into telemedicine is controversial. There is significant concern about risks to confidentiality caused by implementation of novel data management resources and transition of care into nonoffice locations, including the following:

- Data risk for online interactions and wearable/mobile assessment data[107,108]
- Unanticipated observation of care by others who may overhear private clinical interactions[109]
- Inadvertent recording of care by voice assistant devices[109]
- Personal data shared by third-party digital health applications[108]

Headache management interventions translated into a telerehabilitation format rarely include information about training providers on the effective use of the new telemedicine format. Failure to train providers on telerehabilitation may promote underuse or misuse of telerehabilitation, which can deleteriously affect care quality and the patient-provider relationship.[107,110,111] Although telerehabilitation can extend care beyond the office, it may also limit resources that can be used to assess and treat patients. For example, diagnostic assessment may suffer because of the provider's inability to use some diagnostic tools at a distance, leaving providers with incomplete assessments.[110,111] Patients may have difficulty understanding, accessing, and using telerehabilitation resources for headache management, and those without a home computer or mobile smartphone device are often excluded from these care options entirely.[107,110] Patients who can access telerehabilitation for headache management are at risk for diminished treatment outcomes or adverse events because of the inability of providers to fully teach, observe, and monitor rehabilitation practices (ie, lack of in-person observation for physical rehabilitation exercises may lead to injury[66,109]).

Fortunately, there are recommendations that can help mitigate many of these concerns. Developers and researchers should carefully consider market and society demands as well as training and usability requirements for new headache telerehabilitation assessments and interventions.[67] The United States General Services Administration Technology Transformation Service offers excellent guidelines, best practices, and tools for enhancing usability of digital products through its Web site at https://www.usability.gov. Telerehabilitation development should include clinical headache management experts and patient stakeholders to ensure that digital content is relevant. Stakeholder involvement should also include development of provider and patient training resources to maximize effective use of telerehabilitation and minimize risks. Providers who use telerehabilitation for headache management should consider slowing down the pace of their conversations with patients early in care and potentially offering more frequent follow-up contacts to enhance the patient-provider relationship.[110] They may also consider opportunities to use telephone contacts to extend care to patients without the socioeconomic or technical resources to access and use other forms of telerehabilitation.[107,112]

DISCUSSION

Telerehabilitation holds great promise for headache management, and the existing body of research on headache and other conditions serves as an excellent foundation for growth of these resources. Videoteleconferencing and distance technologies add accessibility and breadth for clinicians, making educational resources, headache assessment, and treatment options available to patients with headache without the hassle or expense of travel for in-person care. Studies of telerehabilitation for other pain conditions show robust support for nonpharmacologic interventions, CIH, and treatment adjuncts, but the existing research for headache is nascent and underdeveloped. Questions remain about the risks of using telerehabilitation for headache, but there are excellent resources available to help developers, researchers, and clinicians plan for and address these concerns as new telerehabilitation options develop. Further research is needed to confirm the safety and efficacy of telerehabilitation for headache management, but the future seems bright for the implementation, use, and outcomes of these approaches.

CLINICS CARE POINTS

- Telerehabilitation for headache is largely unproved, but there are some studies showing significant promise for telemedicine-based headache management.
- Providers can use distance technologies to supplement all phases of headache rehabilitation, including assessment, consultation, treatment, and monitoring.
- Web-based patient education products for headache are already freely available through multiple headache and neurology professional organizations.
- Providers who plan to use or develop novel headache telerehabilitation content should ensure that patient and provider stakeholders contribute to development.

DISCLOSURE

The authors have nothing to disclose.

REFERENCES

1. Dowson A. The burden of headache: global and regional prevalence of headache and its impact. Int J Clin Pract Suppl 2015;(182):3–7.
2. Saylor D, Steiner TJ. The Global Burden of Headache. Semin Neurol 2018;38(2): 182–90.
3. Vos T, Flaxman AD, Naghavi M, et al. Years lived with disability (YLDs) for 1160 sequelae of 289 diseases and injuries 1990-2010: a systematic analysis for the Global Burden of Disease Study 2010. Lancet 2012;380(9859):2163–96.
4. GBD 2016 Disease and Injury Incidence and Prevalence Collaborators. Global, regional, and national incidence, prevalence, and years lived with disability for 328 diseases and injuries for 195 countries, 1990-2016: a systematic analysis for the Global Burden of Disease Study 2016. Lancet 2017; 390(10100):1211–59.

5. Burch R, Rizzoli P, Loder E. The prevalence and impact of migraine and severe headache in the United States: figures and trends from government health studies. Headache 2018;58(4):496–505.
6. GBD 2016 Headache Collaborators. Global, regional, and national burden of migraine and tension-type headache, 1990-2016: a systematic analysis for the Global Burden of Disease Study 2016. Lancet Neurol 2018;17(11):954–76.
7. Fuensalida-Novo S, Palacios-Ceña M, Fernández-Muñoz JJ, et al. The burden of headache is associated to pain interference, depression and headache duration in chronic tension type headache: a 1-year longitudinal study. J Headache Pain 2017;18(1):119.
8. Crystal SC, Robbins MS. Epidemiology of tension-type headache. Curr Pain Headache Rep 2010;14(6):449–54.
9. Schwartz BS, Stewart WF, Simon D, et al. Epidemiology of tension-type headache. JAMA 1998;279(5):381–3.
10. Fumal A, Schoenen J. Tension-type headache: current research and clinical management. Lancet Neurol 2008;7(1):70–83.
11. Waldie KE, Poulton R. Physical and psychological correlates of primary headache in young adulthood: a 26 year longitudinal study. J Neurol Neurosurg Psychiatry 2002;72(1):86–92.
12. Jensen RH. Tension-type headache - the normal and most prevalent headache. Headache 2018;58(2):339–45.
13. Creamer A, Ioannidis S, Wilhelm T, et al. Headache in an HIV positive patient: diagnostic challenges and approach to treatment. Clin Med (Lond) 2016; 16(6):548–50.
14. Krasenbaum LJ. A Review of HIV and headache: a cross-sectional study. Headache 2017;57(10):1631–2.
15. Sampaio Rocha-Filho PA, Torres RCS, Ramos Montarroyos U. HIV and Headache: A Cross-Sectional Study. Headache 2017;57(10):1545–50.
16. Dewan MC, Rattani A, Gupta S, et al. Estimating the global incidence of traumatic brain injury. J Neurosurg 2018;1–18.
17. Seifert TD, Evans RW. Posttraumatic headache: a review. Curr Pain Headache Rep 2010;14(4):292–8.
18. Ashina H, Porreca F, Anderson T, et al. Post-traumatic headache: epidemiology and pathophysiological insights. Nat Rev Neurol 2019;15(10):607–17.
19. Chen PK, Wang SJ. Medication overuse and medication overuse headache: risk factors, comorbidities, associated burdens and nonpharmacologic and pharmacologic treatment approaches. Curr Pain Headache Rep 2019;23(8):60.
20. Torres-Ferrus M, Vila-Sala C, Quintana M, et al. Headache, comorbidities and lifestyle in an adolescent population (The TEENs Study). Cephalalgia 2019; 39(1):91–9.
21. Nieswand V, Richter M, Berner R, et al. The prevalence of headache in German pupils of different ages and school types. Cephalalgia 2019;39(8):1030–40.
22. Nieswand V, Richter M, Gossrau G. Epidemiology of headache in children and adolescents-another type of pandemia. Curr Pain Headache Rep 2020; 24(10):62.
23. Balottin U, Fusar Poli P, Termine C, et al. Psychopathological symptoms in child and adolescent migraine and tension-type headache: a meta-analysis. Cephalalgia 2013;33(2):112–22.
24. Blaauw BA, Dyb G, Hagen K, et al. The relationship of anxiety, depression and behavioral problems with recurrent headache in late adolescence - a Young-HUNT follow-up study. J Headache Pain 2015;16:10.

25. Faedda N, Cerutti R, Verdecchia P, et al. Behavioral management of headache in children and adolescents. J Headache Pain 2016;17(1):80.
26. Jesus TS, Landry MD, Hoenig H. Global Need for Physical Rehabilitation: Systematic Analysis from the Global Burden of Disease Study 2017. Int J Environ Res Public Health 2019;16(6):980.
27. Bevilaqua-Grossi D, Gonçalves MC, Carvalho GF, et al. Additional effects of a physical therapy protocol on headache frequency, pressure pain threshold, and improvement perception in patients with migraine and associated neck pain: a randomized controlled trial. Arch Phys Med Rehabil 2016;97(6):866–74.
28. Garrigos-Pedron M, La Touche R, Navarro-Desentre P, et al. Effects of a physical therapy protocol in patients with chronic migraine and temporomandibular disorders: a randomized, single-blinded, clinical trial. J Oral Facial Pain Headache 2018;32(2):137–50.
29. Harris P, Loveman E, Clegg A, et al. Systematic review of cognitive behavioural therapy for the management of headaches and migraines in adults. Br J Pain 2015;9(4):213–24.
30. Lee HJ, Lee JH, Cho EY, et al. Efficacy of psychological treatment for headache disorder: a systematic review and meta-analysis. J Headache Pain 2019; 20(1):17.
31. Probyn K, Bowers H, Caldwell F, et al. Prognostic factors for chronic headache: A systematic review. Neurology 2017;89(3):291–301.
32. Probyn K, Bowers H, Mistry D, et al. Non-pharmacological self-management for people living with migraine or tension-type headache: a systematic review including analysis of intervention components. BMJ Open 2017;7(8):e016670.
33. Day MA, Thorn BE. Mindfulness-based cognitive therapy for headache pain: An evaluation of the long-term maintenance of effects. Complement Ther Med 2017;33:94–8.
34. Linde K, Allais G, Brinkhaus B, et al. Acupuncture for the prevention of tension-type headache. Cochrane Database Syst Rev 2016;(4):CD007587.
35. Linde K, Allais G, Brinkhaus B, et al. Acupuncture for the prevention of episodic migraine. Cochrane Database Syst Rev 2016;(6):CD001218.
36. Wachholtz AB, Malone CD, Pargament KI. Effect of Different Meditation Types on Migraine Headache Medication Use. Behav Med 2017;43(1):1–8.
37. Faedda N, Natalucci G, Baglioni V, et al. Behavioral therapies in headache: focus on mindfulness and cognitive behavioral therapy in children and adolescents. Expert Rev Neurother 2019;19(12):1219–28.
38. Brandes JL. Global trends in migraine care: results from the MAZE survey. CNS Drugs 2002;16 Suppl 1(Suppl 1):13–8.
39. World Health Organization. Atlas of headache Disorders and Resources in the world: 2011. Geneva (Switzerland): WHO; 2011.
40. John D, Ram D, Sundarmurthy H, et al. Study of Barrier to Help Seeking and its Relationships with Disability in Patients with Headache. J Clin Diagn Res 2016; 10(10):VC01–5.
41. Dodick DW, Loder EW, Manack Adams A, et al. Assessing barriers to chronic migraine consultation, diagnosis, and treatment: results from the chronic migraine epidemiology and outcomes (CaMEO) Study. Headache 2016;56(5): 821–34.
42. Lipton RB, Serrano D, Holland S, et al. Barriers to the diagnosis and treatment of migraine: effects of sex, income, and headache features. Headache 2013;53(1): 81–92.

43. Gibbs TS, Fleischer AB, Feldman SR, et al. Health care utilization in patients with migraine: demographics and patterns of care in the ambulatory setting. Headache 2003;43(4):330–5.
44. Lipton RB, Scher AI, Steiner TJ, et al. Patterns of health care utilization for migraine in England and in the United States. Neurology 2003;60(3):441–8.
45. Matsuzawa Y, Lee YSC, Fraser F, et al. Barriers to behavioral treatment adherence for headache: an examination of attitudes, beliefs, and psychiatric factors. Headache 2019;59(1):19–31.
46. Minen MT, Azarchi S, Sobolev R, et al. Factors related to migraine patients' decisions to initiate behavioral migraine treatment following a headache specialist's recommendation: a prospective observational study. Pain Med 2018; 19(11):2274–82.
47. Muller KI, Alstadhaug KB, Bekkelund SI. A randomized trial of telemedicine efficacy and safety for nonacute headaches. Neurology 2017;89(2):153–62.
48. Muller KI, Alstadhaug KB, Bekkelund SI. Headache patients' satisfaction with telemedicine: a 12-month follow-up randomized non-inferiority trial. Eur J Neurol 2017;24(6):807–15.
49. Muller KI, Alstadhaug KB, Bekkelund SI. Telemedicine in the management of non-acute headaches: A prospective, open-labelled non-inferiority, randomised clinical trial. Cephalalgia 2017;37(9):855–63.
50. Muller KI, Alstadhaug KB, Bekkelund SI. Acceptability, feasibility, and cost of telemedicine for nonacute headaches: a randomized study comparing video and traditional consultations. J Med Internet Res 2016;18(5):e140.
51. Qubty W, Patniyot I, Gelfand A. Telemedicine in a pediatric headache clinic: A prospective survey. Neurology 2018;90(19):e1702–5.
52. Hollander JE, Carr BG. Virtually perfect? telemedicine for Covid-19. N Engl J Med 2020;382(18):1679–81.
53. Smith AC, Thomas E, Snoswell CL, et al. Telehealth for global emergencies: Implications for coronavirus disease 2019 (COVID-19). J Telemed Telecare 2020; 26(5):309–13.
54. Smith S, Doarn CR, Krupinski EA, et al. Changes in perception of various telehealth topics before and after a patient-centered outcomes research institute telehealth research dissemination conference. Telemed J E Health 2020;26(6): 827–34.
55. Snoswell CL, Caffery LJ, Haydon HM, et al. Telehealth uptake in general practice as a result of the coronavirus (COVID-19) pandemic. Aust Health Rev 2020;44(5):737–40.
56. Wosik J, Fudim M, Cameron B, et al. Telehealth transformation: COVID-19 and the rise of virtual care. J Am Med Inform Assoc 2020;27(6):957–62.
57. Wamsley CE, Kramer A, Kenkel JM, et al. Trends and challenges of telehealth in an academic institution: the unforeseen benefits of the COVID-19 Global Pandemic. Aesthet Surg J 2020;41(1):109–18.
58. Roy B, Nowak RJ, Roda R, et al. Teleneurology during the COVID-19 pandemic: A step forward in modernizing medical care. J Neurol Sci 2020;414:116930.
59. Koonin LM, Hoots B, Tsang CA, et al. Trends in the Use of Telehealth During the Emergence of the COVID-19 Pandemic - United States, January-March 2020. MMWR Morb Mortal Wkly Rep 2020;69(43):1595–9.
60. McGeary DD, McGeary CA, Gatchel RJ, et al. Assessment of research quality of telehealth trials in pain management: a meta-analysis. Pain Pract 2013;13(5): 422–31.

61. Tassorelli C, Tramontano M, Berlangieri M, et al. Assessing and treating primary headaches and cranio-facial pain in patients undergoing rehabilitation for neurological diseases. J Headache Pain 2017;18(1):99.
62. Cote P, Yu H, Shearer HM, et al. Non-pharmacological management of persistent headaches associated with neck pain: A clinical practice guideline from the Ontario protocol for traffic injury management (OPTIMa) collaboration. Eur J Pain 2019;23(6):1051–70.
63. Reischl S, Dabbagh A, MacDermid JC. Appraisal of Clinical Practice Guideline: OPTIMa revised recommendations for non-pharmacological management of persistent headaches associated with neck pain. J Physiother 2020;66(3):201.
64. Williams KA. Headache management in a Veteran population: First considerations. J Am Assoc Nurse Pract 2020;32(11):758–63.
65. Tauben DJ, Langford DJ, Sturgeon JA, et al. Optimizing telehealth pain care after COVID-19. Pain 2020;161(11):2437–45.
66. Seng EK, Prieto P, Boucher G, et al. Anxiety, incentives, and adherence to self-monitoring on a mobile health platform: a naturalistic longitudinal cohort study in people with headache. Headache 2018;58(10):1541–55.
67. Stubberud A, Linde M. Digital technology and mobile health in behavioral migraine therapy: a narrative review. Curr Pain Headache Rep 2018;22(10):66.
68. Mosadeghi-Nik M, Askari MS, Fatehi F. Mobile health (mHealth) for headache disorders: A review of the evidence base. J Telemed Telecare 2016;22(8):472–7.
69. Hundert AS, Huguet A, McGrath PJ, et al. Commercially available mobile phone headache diary apps: a systematic review. JMIR Mhealth Uhealth 2014; 2(3):e36.
70. van de Graaf DL, Schoonman GG, Habibović M, et al. Towards eHealth to support the health journey of headache patients: a scoping review. J Neurol 2020. https://doi.org/10.1007/s00415-020-09981-3.
71. Pereira-Monteiro J, Wysocka-Bakowska MM, Katsarava Z, et al. Guidelines for telematic second opinion consultation on headaches in Europe: on behalf of the European Headache Federation (EHF). J Headache Pain 2010;11(4):345–8.
72. Craig J, Chua R, Russell C, et al. A cohort study of early neurological consultation by telemedicine on the care of neurological inpatients. J Neurol Neurosurg Psychiatry 2004;75(7):1031–5.
73. American Headache S. The American Headache Society position statement on integrating new migraine treatments into clinical practice. Headache 2019; 59(1):1–18.
74. McLean A, Becker WJ, Vujadinovic Z. Making a new-patient headache education session more patient-centered: what participants want to know. Disabil Rehabil 2020;42(10):1462–73.
75. Valja A, Tenhunen H, Harno H, et al. From tertiary to primary care - understanding context in the transfer of digital headache service pathway. Stud Health Technol Inform 2019;262:304–7.
76. Diener HC, Holle D, Solbach K, et al. Medication-overuse headache: risk factors, pathophysiology and management. Nat Rev Neurol 2016;12(10):575–83.
77. Lipton RB. Risk factors for and management of medication-overuse headache. Continuum (Minneap Minn) 2015;21(4 Headache):1118–31.
78. Andrasik F. Behavioral treatment approaches to chronic headache. Neurol Sci 2003;24(Suppl 2):S80–5.
79. Kropp P, Meyer B, Meyer W, et al. An update on behavioral treatments in migraine - current knowledge and future options. Expert Rev Neurother 2017; 17(11):1059–68.

80. Minen MT, Torous J, Raynowska J, et al. Electronic behavioral interventions for headache: a systematic review. J Headache Pain 2016;17:51.

81. Moman RN, Dvorkin J, Pollard EM, et al. A systematic review and meta-analysis of unguided electronic and mobile health technologies for chronic pain-is it time to start prescribing electronic health applications? Pain Med 2019;20(11):2238–55.

82. Pfeifer AC, Uddin R, Schröder-Pfeifer P, et al. Mobile application-based interventions for chronic pain patients: a systematic review and meta-analysis of effectiveness. J Clin Med 2020;9(11):3557.

83. Lau SC, Bhattacharjya S, Fong MW, et al. Effectiveness of theory-based digital self-management interventions for improving depression, anxiety, fatigue and self-efficacy in people with neurological disorders: A systematic review and meta-analysis. J Telemed Telecare 2020. https://doi.org/10.1177/1357633X20955122. 1357633X20955122.

84. Perlini C, Donisi V, Del Piccolo L. From research to clinical practice: a systematic review of the implementation of psychological interventions for chronic headache in adults. BMC Health Serv Res 2020;20(1):459.

85. Klausen SH, Rønde G, Tornøe B, et al. Nonpharmacological interventions addressing pain, sleep, and quality of life in children and adolescents with primary headache: a systematic review. J Pain Res 2019;12:3437–59.

86. Jiang W, Li 0, Wei N, et al. Effectiveness of physical therapy on the suboccipital area of patients with tension-type headache: A meta-analysis of randomized controlled trials. Medicine (Baltimore) 2019;98(19):e15487.

87. Alvarez-Melcon AC, Valero-Alcaide R, Atín-Arratibel MA, et al. Effects of physical therapy and relaxation techniques on the parameters of pain in university students with tension-type headache: A randomised controlled clinical trial. Neurologia 2018;33(4):233–43.

88. Durban NR. President's message. Orthop Phys Ther Pract 2020;32(3):177–9.

89. Levy CE, Silverman E, Jia H, et al. Effects of physical therapy delivery via home video telerehabilitation on functional and health-related quality of life outcomes. J Rehabil Res Dev 2015;52(3):361–70.

90. Bell A. Telehealth: What's Next. APTA Magazine 2020;12–5.

91. Adams J, Barbery G, Lui CW. Complementary and alternative medicine use for headache and migraine: a critical review of the literature. Headache 2013;53(3):459–73.

92. Anheyer D, Klose P, Lauche R, et al. Yoga for treating headaches: a systematic review and meta-analysis. J Gen Intern Med 2020;35(3):846–54.

93. Zhang Y, Dennis JA, Leach MJ, et al. Complementary and alternative medicine use among US adults with headache or migraine: results from the 2012 national health interview survey. Headache 2017;57(8):1228–42.

94. Jasti N, Bhargav H, George S, et al. Tele-yoga for stress management: Need of the hour during the COVID-19 pandemic and beyond? Asian J Psychiatr 2020;54:102334.

95. Mathersul DC, Mahoney LA, Bayley PJ. Tele-yoga for chronic pain: current status and future directions. Glob Adv Health Med 2018;7. 2164956118766011.

96. Bayley L, McDermott K, Donesky D, et al. Appropriateness and acceptability of a Tele-Yoga intervention for people with heart failure and chronic obstructive pulmonary disease: qualitative findings from a controlled pilot study. BMC Complement Altern Med 2015;15:21.

97. Schulz-Heik RJ, Meyer H, Mahoney L, et al. Results from a clinical yoga program for veterans: yoga via telehealth provides comparable satisfaction and health improvements to in-person yoga. BMC Complement Altern Med 2017;17(1):198.
98. Wells C, Malins S, Clarke S, et al. Using smart-messaging to enhance mindfulness-based cognitive therapy for cancer patients: A mixed methods proof of concept evaluation. Psychooncology 2020;29(1):212–9.
99. Niles BL, Vujanovic AA, Silberbogen AK, et al. Changes in mindfulness following a mindfulness telehealth intervention. Mindfulness 2013;4(4):301–10.
100. Earles J, Folen RA, James LC. Biofeedback using telemedicine: clinical applications and case illustrations. Behav Med 2001;27(2):77–82.
101. Folen RA, James LC, Earles JE, et al. Biofeedback via telehealth: a new frontier for applied psychophysiology. Appl Psychophysiol Biofeedback 2001;26(3):195–204.
102. Morcos MW, Teeter MG, Somerville LE, et al. Correlation between hip osteoarthritis and the level of physical activity as measured by wearable technology and patient-reported questionnaires. J Orthop 2020;20:236–9.
103. Dowling AV, Eberly V, Maneekobkunwong S, et al. Telehealth monitor to measure physical activity and pressure relief maneuver performance in wheelchair users. Assist Technol 2017;29(4):202–9.
104. DeWorsop D, Creatura G, Bluez G, et al. Feasibility and success of cell-phone assisted remote observation of medication adherence (CAROMA) in clinical trials. Drug Alcohol Depend 2016;163:24–30.
105. Steinkamp JM, Goldblatt N, Borodovsky JT, et al. Technological interventions for medication adherence in adult mental health and substance use disorders: a systematic review. JMIR Ment Health 2019;6(3):e12493.
106. Tolley JA, Michel MA, Williams AE, et al. Peer support in the treatment of chronic pain in adolescents: a review of the literature and available resources. Children (Basel) 2020;7(9):129.
107. Barney A, Buckelew S, Mesheriakova V, et al. The COVID-19 pandemic and rapid implementation of adolescent and young adult telemedicine: challenges and opportunities for innovation. J Adolesc Health 2020;67(2):164–71.
108. Minen MT, Stieglitz EJ, Sciortino R, et al. Privacy issues in smartphone applications: an analysis of headache/migraine applications. Headache 2018;58(7):1014–27.
109. Wojciechowski MI. New technology: Keeping it Ethical, keeping it legal. PT in Motion 2019;11(10):30-9.
110. Begasse de Dhaem O, Bernstein C. Headache virtual visit toolbox: the transition from bedside manners to webside manners. Headache 2020;60(8):1743–6.
111. Tenforde AS, Hefner JE, Kodish-Wachs JE, et al. Telehealth in physical medicine and rehabilitation: a narrative review. PM R 2017;9(5S):S51–8.
112. Strowd RE, Strauss L, Graham R, et al. Rapid implementation of outpatient teleneurology in rural Appalachia: Barriers and disparities. Neurology 2020.

Tele-Integrative Medicine to Support Rehabilitative Care

Rashmi S. Mullur, MD[a],*, Seetal Preet Kaur Cheema, MD[b],
Ryan Edward Alano, MD, MPH[c], Lynn Elizabeth Chang, DO, MS[c]

KEYWORDS

- Telemedicine • Integrative medicine • Complementary and integrative health
- Holistic medicine

KEY POINTS

- Complementary and integrative health (CIH) modalities, including yoga, tai chi, mindfulness meditation, hypnosis, self-massage, and acupressure, are simple therapeutic techniques for managing chronic pain with little to no negative effects, and can be easily incorporated into telemedicine care with great potential benefit.
- CIH modalities as a component of a multidisciplinary patient-centered whole health care model are effective in decreasing opioid use and improving overall well-being, as seen for veteran patients at the (Veterans Affairs) VA Healthcare System.
- Although evidence is present that many CIH modalities delivered via telemedicine are effective, studies are small and varied, and there is a need for further research with larger sample sizes and greater pain populations.
- Future direction of incorporating wellness care into telemedicine will need the collaboration of providers from multiple disciplines, ease and low cost of technology, and simple education tools for delivery to providers and patients.

INTRODUCTION

Physical medicine and rehabilitation aim to enhance and restore functional ability and quality of life to people with physical impairments or disabilities, many of whom suffer from chronic pain conditions. Multidisciplinary care including complementary and integrative modalities has beneficial therapeutic value in the care of chronic pain patients. The terms integrative health and integrative medicine refer to a holistic approach to healing that focuses on the biopsychosocial and spiritual wellness of

[a] Department of Medicine, VA Greater Los Angeles Healthcare System, David Geffen School of Medicine at UCLA, 11301 Wilshire Boulevard, Mail Code 111-D, Los Angeles, CA 90073, USA;
[b] Department of Anesthesia (212), VA Greater Los Angeles Healthcare System, 11301 Wilshire Boulevard, Los Angeles, CA 90073, USA; [c] Department of Physical Medicine and Rehabilitation (1415), VA Greater Los Angeles Healthcare System, 1301 Wilshire Boulevard, Los Angeles, CA 90073, USA
* Corresponding author.
E-mail address: rmullur@mednet.ucla.edu

Phys Med Rehabil Clin N Am 32 (2021) 393–403
https://doi.org/10.1016/j.pmr.2020.12.006

each individual, and believes that health is more than just the absence of disease. An integrative medical approach incorporates complementary and integrative health (CIH) therapies into standard medical care and is not considered an alternative to traditional treatment approaches.

For the purpose of this article, the authors will focus on CIH modalities with evidence to support their use in the management of chronic pain and stress including yoga, tai chi, mindfulness meditation, hypnosis, massage, and acupressure. Incorporation of CIH modalities into medical care is an effective strategy to manage chronic pain, and the Veterans Affairs (VA) health care system has been leading efforts in this area. In examining the medical records of more than half a million veterans with musculoskeletal pain, VA researchers found that 27% of veterans were using at least one of these CIH approaches. Additionally, those who did use at least 1 approach reported slightly less pain and had slightly lower health care costs than those who did not use any of the CIH approaches.[1]

Over the past decade, as the use of CIH approaches has continued to grow within the United States, the development of digital health technology and virtual care platforms has modernized how patients access medical care. The delivery of integrative medicine via telehealth platforms provides a novel approach to whole-person care. Telehealth not only increases patients' access to care, but it also limits the burden of travel on patients, which can be critical for those requiring rehabilitative care who may also struggle with limited mobility. Additionally, the ability to virtually care for a patient within his or her own home allows providers tremendous insight into the patient's environment, which is instrumental in providing holistic care. Moreover, many yoga and mind-body programs are available through live-streaming and mobile applications, which increase access to CIH therapies. Finally, remote monitoring technology and mobile health applications are also emerging as novel ways to promote integrative health. This article will review the data supporting the use of established CIH therapies and discuss the feasibility of incorporating these approaches into telehealth-based rehabilitative care.

THE US DEPARTMENT OF VETERANS AFFAIRS: WHOLE-HEALTH AND TELEHEALTH EXPANSION

Facing a large population of patients with chronic pain, opioid use, post-traumatic stress disorder (PTSD), and complex medical disease, in the early 2010s, the VA began to transition from a primarily reactive, disease-focused, physician-centered care model to a personalized, proactive, patient-driven approach that prioritizes the veteran and his or her values to create a personalized strategy to optimize health, healing, and well-being. The VA established Whole-Health System of Care as an "approach to healthcare that empowers and equips people to take charge of their health and well-being and live their life to the fullest."[2] This integrated system of care emphasizes the individual patient working collaboratively with a team of health care providers and using various treatment modalities, blending self-care, conventional care, and complementary approaches (including yoga, tai chi, chiropractic care, massage, meditation, biofeedback, guided imagery, hypnosis, and acupuncture). This program, available nationally, is currently used by 31% of veterans suffering from chronic pain. Preliminary data from a recent report by Bokhour and colleagues[2] demonstrate opioid use among whole-health users decreased by 38%, compared with an 11% decrease among those not subscribing to this approach to care. Outpatient pharmacy costs were lower for those veterans with mental health conditions who used whole-health services (3.5% annual increase compared with 12.5%). Moreover, improvements in health and well-being thus far have been shown to last for up to 6 months, with promising future benefit.

During this same period, the VA had already begun to adopt telehealth services to increase health care access to its large population of veteran users who live in rural areas. The VA encompasses the nation's largest health care system, with more than 152 hospitals and 1100 ambulatory locations. However, most of those patients live in rural areas with no access to a VA facility, and the agency recognized that use of telehealth provides a feasible option to extend care to all veterans. As a result, the agency prioritized the use of telemedicine across the country creating models of virtual care including tele-mental health care, tele-primary care, and tele-subspecialty care. Early reports on the VA's telehealth expansion remained overwhelmingly positive, with evidence to support cost savings from televisits, decreased hospitalization rates, and high veteran satisfaction with the program.[3]

The use of telehealth-based strategies has become a key focus of the VA to manage a multimorbid population, who often require multidisciplinary care. In 2018, as part of the VA Roadmap for Managing Pain,[4] 1 key strategy recommended that VA hospitals also consider establishing telehealth-based programs to utilize nonpharmacological pain care modalities, which several facilities across the nation accomplished. As a result of this confluence of innovation in both integrative health and telehealth, the VA not only has a population that is eager and interested in receiving CIH therapies, but also has established the infrastructure and investment required to deliver these services virtually.

TELEHEALTH IMPLEMENTATION CONSIDERATIONS

The COVID-19 pandemic has accelerated the use of telemedicine and telehealth across the globe, and it has become evident that telehealth-based care will remain vital for several vulnerable groups. During the early months of the COVID-19 pandemic, the VA was able to leverage its telehealth infrastructure to vastly increase telemedicine use for mental health, primary care, and subspecialty care.[5] With the infrastructure in place to deliver most services virtually, the VA was able to offer several CIH services, including group yoga, meditation, and tai chi classes, via virtual platforms throughout the pandemic. Although it is clear that virtual delivery of CIH programs is feasible, it is important to recognize that the system wide implementation of virtual care achieved by the VA may be difficult to reproduce in private settings.

There are several limitations and barriers to the use of telemedicine to deliver CIH therapies. First, the digital divide creates potential disparities in access to telemedicine for those with limited Internet access, which impacts people living in rural areas, older adults, and those with diverse socioeconomic backgrounds. In a cross-sectional study of Medicare beneficiaries, 26% of participants lacked digital access in their home, and this proportion was greater among those with lower socioeconomic status, with age over 85 years, and within communities of color.[6] Additionally, telehealth literacy remains a concern; older adults may have difficulty accessing telemedicine services because of inexperience with technology or physical disabilities. Finally, reimbursement for telemedicine varies greatly by health insurance coverage and by state regulation. For most CIH therapies, telemedicine coverage is lacking. App-based programs and group classes offer an option for patients without insurance access, but out-of-pocket costs may be a deterrent to use.

Despite these challenges, delivery of CIH approaches via telemedicine platforms remains a viable, sustainable long-term option to improve care and decrease opioid use. The delivery of yoga and tai chi programs is relatively easy to translate to the virtual space, and there is evidence that patients find these comparable to in-person classes.[7]

Furthermore, the use of mobile applications is already a popular method for patients to access mindfulness meditation programs,[8] and use of these programs has grown since the pandemic. Similarly, the practice of hypnosis translates easily into the virtual space. There is emerging evidence to support the application of modified and self-guided CIH services such as acupressure and self-massage, also via telehealth.

MOVEMENT THERAPIES: YOGA AND TAI CHI

Movement therapies, like yoga and tai chi, can be beneficial for promoting the healing and overall well-being of chronic pain patients. Yoga refers to the physical, mental, and spiritual practices originating from ancient India. Tai chi is a mind-body movement practice based on the principles of traditional Chinese medicine.[9] Both movement modalities focus on linking the breath with movement and intention to promote and foster healing. Yoga and tai chi are recommended nationally as a first-line treatment for low back pain.[10] Of note, when incorporating mind-body approaches as therapeutic approach, it is important to differentiate these practices from group wellness classes. Therapeutic mind-body medicine requires that instructors have advanced training and expertise in caring for patients with chronic pain, those with differing physical abilities, and complex psychological histories.

Yoga is among the top 10 CIH approaches used by adults in the United States, with many reporting that they practiced yoga to promote general wellness, reduce stress, and improve chronic pain.[11] There are a variety of different yoga styles that have emerged through the ages, including Ashtanga, Bikram, Vinyasa, Hatha, Iyengar, Kundalini, and Yin Yoga. Each of these styles may focus on the physical postures (asanas), breathing techniques (pranayama), and meditation practices to a various degree.[12] It is important to note that clinical studies of yoga as a therapeutic modality may differ from community-based yoga classes for wellness. Research into the clinical benefits of modern yoga practice confirms that the greatest benefit from yoga comes from a practice that includes all 3 components to promote healing and whole health.[13,14] Yoga is thought to improve the physiologic, behavioral, and psychological factors that contribute to chronic pain.[15] In several large reviews and meta-analyses, yoga has been shown to improve back pain, back-related function, and chronic pain.[16] More recently, movement-based therapies, such as yoga and tai chi, are thought to improve an individual's response to pain by modulating the nervous system and pain signaling.[17] In fact, Villemure and colleagues[18] looked at brain MRIs of practitioners proficient in yoga using voxel-based morphometry, and demonstrated an increase in gray matter in the insular cortex, which correlates to pain tolerance.

Like yoga, there are various forms of tai chi, but in Western culture, it is commonly taught as a series of slow, controlled, low-impact movements combined with focused breath work, allowing the practitioner to achieve greater awareness, inner peace, and well-being. This meditative movement is intended to strengthen and stretch the body, and enhance blood flow, proprioception, and balance.[19,20] Tai chi is strongly recommended by the American College of Rheumatology because of its low impact and has consistent positive benefit for patients overall, specifically with benefit for patients suffering from pain caused by knee or hip osteoarthritis.[21] A 2016 systematic review demonstrated that tai chi may positively influence chronic pain among those suffering from low back pain and osteoarthritis if practiced for at least 6 weeks.[22] Additionally, tai chi has also been shown to have beneficial effects on balance and fall prevention compared with conventional exercise or physical therapy.[9]

Both of these movement modalities can easily be incorporated into telehealth as group classes, allowing for decreased cost to the individual, as well as the opportunity to engage in a social group activity. Online yoga and tai chi may eliminate barriers to receiving traditional face-to-face health interventions, such as transportation and time constraints, and many of these classes can be easily found online through many purchasable offerings, as well as through mobile applications. The data for telehealth delivery of these CIH modalities are emerging. A study comparing in-person yoga classes versus telehealth yoga classes revealed similar improvements in back pain, anxiety, and depression, and participants were equally satisfied with either method of delivery.[23] Online therapeutic yoga and tai chi programs may also promote whole health in that both the patient and caregiver can participate and benefit from these modalities.[24]

MINDFULNESS MEDITATION

Mindfulness meditation, or *Vipassana*, translated from Pali to mean "insight," is an ancient Buddhist practice, and, although many different forms and definitions exist, a central aspect of the practice is the intention to be more aware and engaged in the present moment.[25] Two components can be differentiated: the self-regulation of attention so that it is maintained on immediate experiences (thereby allowing for increased recognition of mental events in the present moment) and adopting a particular orientation toward experiences in the present moment (an orientation that is characterized by curiosity, openness, and acceptance). Jon Kabat-Zinn is often credited with popularizing mindfulness in the United States by establishing a mindfulness-based stress reduction (MBSR) program for treating chronic disease, which created institutional capacity for using mindfulness approaches in clinical settings. Although evaluations of a large number and variety of mindfulness interventions have been published, there is only limited agreement on how to define mindfulness interventions, and formats and components vary across interventions.

Mindfulness meditation encompasses practices including breathing exercises and guided imagery techniques that allow the practitioner to focus on the present moment with curiosity and openness.[25] By practicing mindfulness meditation, one focuses on the here and now, with the aim of making one more content in life. Mixed evidence exists for this modality in terms of pain management; however, its benefit lies in the fact that it improves several other components of chronic pain, including improvement in feelings of wellness, and symptoms of depression and chronic stress.[25] Although initial studies did not show subjective decrease in pain intensity among patients with chronic pain, this modality may improve pain acceptance, which in turn may influence subjective experience of pain.[26] Additionally, a large meta-analysis of 38 randomized controlled trials found that mindfulness improved pain symptoms, depression symptoms, and quality of life.[27]

Mindfulness meditation is easily incorporated into virtual care. Several mobile applications offer free trial subscriptions and online courses that are well suited to home-based practice. There is emerging evidence supporting the efficacy of telehealth-based mindfulness interventions on pain, depression, and stress in both patients and caregivers.[28,29] Additionally, reports from Korea reveal that telemedicine-based mindfulness meditation practices were feasible and effective in improving mental health and wellness for patients and caregivers during the COVID-19 pandemic.[30]

HYPNOSIS

Hypnosis falls within the philosophy of mind-body medicine as a simple modality for improving emotional and physical well-being. Clinical hypnosis is a learnable coping skill that is generally safe for individuals of all ages, including children and geriatric patients. Although there is no singular definition, this modality can be defined as "the cultivation of the imagination in an altered state of consciousness (awareness and alertness) within a focused state (with or without physical relaxation), in which an individual is selectively focused, absorbed, and concentrating upon a particular idea or image aimed at improving mental or physical health."[31]

Research has shown evidence that hypnosis can provide safe, beneficial pain reduction for various conditions, including low back pain, migraines, fibromyalgia, multiple sclerosis, and labor pain.[32–36] In a meta-analysis of studies performed by Thompson and colleagues[37] in 2019, significant findings revealed a 42% reduction in pain intensity with high suggestible intervention, and 29% reduction with medium suggestible, revealing further that the specifics of technique may play a role in effective benefit and warrants further study. Hypnotherapy has also been shown to improve emotional health by reducing anxiety and depression.[38] Integrating hypnosis into breast cancer care has benefit for breast cancer-related symptoms, with sparse but promising evidence.[39] Pediatric patients can also benefit from distraction and hypnosis for reducing needle-related pain and distress, as shown with efficacy in systematic reviews.[40] Although more high-quality data are needed with studies over general pain populations, this simple tool has minimal to no negative consequences and significant potential benefit as an adjunct to the overall treatment plan of care.

Clinically, the delivery of hypnosis outside of traditional in-person care is challenging. Prior studies suggest that audiotaped hypnosis and asynchronous delivery methods are more effective than no treatment at all, but less effective than the presence of a live hypnotherapist.[41] Development of virtual-reality (VR) technology offers a viable option to improve remotely delivered hypnosis, but base investment in VR can be cost-prohibitive for many. Despite this challenge, a recent meta-analysis by Rousseaux and colleagues[42] suggest that VR hypnosis provides short-term significant decreases in pain intensity, pain unpleasantness, time spent thinking about pain, and opioid use.

ACUPRESSURE

Acupuncture is a well-known CIH modality developed over 3000 years ago, focusing on the flow of energy, known as *qi* or *chi*, in the body.[43] It is believed that acupuncture stimulates the flow of energy along meridians (networks or channels of energy pathways), and disease and pain result from the blockage of energy flow.[44] Activating or unblocking these meridians through stimulation of specific acupuncture points can restore balance, promote healing, and alleviate pain.[45] Acupuncture affects the modulation of molecules related to analgesia within the brain, spinal cord, and peripheral nervous system, including opioid peptides, cAMP and glutamate, adenosine, dopamine, norepinephrine, serotonin, and endocannabinoids. Acupuncture also affects the immune system, as evidenced by upregulation of immune markers including interleukin and nerve growth factors. Functional MRI studies have shown that acupuncture enhances connectivity between different areas of the brain, promoting neuroplasticity; this whole-brain integration helps with pain modulation.[46,47]

Acupressure refers to the stimulation of points along meridians using manual pressure rather than needles. This technique is a noninvasive, relatively inexpensive intervention with no known adverse effects, and can be a useful modality for patients who are needle-phobic or cannot tolerate a more invasive treatment option.[48] Moreover, this therapeutic technique can be administered at any time, place, or situation. Patients can perform acupressure on themselves, or it can be given to them by their caregivers, with a minimal requirement of technical knowledge.[49,50] Clinically, this promising treatment can be easily and quickly taught, allowing patients to improve their own health.

The data surrounding acupressure is promising. In a study of patients with chronic low back pain, self-administered acupressure with a wooden tool (acu-ki), pencil tip eraser, or fingertip decreased pain 35% to 36% compared with baseline.[51] However, in a study of older patients with osteoarthritis, self-administered acupressure improved pain scale ratings, but there was no difference between the acupressure and the sham-acupressure group.[52] Although this finding seems to imply that acupressure is ineffective, it is likely more accurate that sham-acupressure may not act as a negative control, a finding is that is consistent with prior reports of sham acupuncture.[53] Finally, acupressure can be taught through telemedicine sessions as well as through mobile applications. In a study of patients with dysmenorrhea, app-based self-acupressure decreased pain intensity, number of days with pain, and use of pain medications.[54]

SELF-MASSAGE

Self-massage is the application of various massage strokes to the body's soft tissue for therapeutic purposes, such as soothing tired hands and feet or easing tension headaches. As self-massage research is in its infancy, there are limited data to support its therapeutic value. Historically, however, self-massage has been employed as an integral modality for the treatment and management of many chronic medical conditions. For example, massage therapies can be helpful for managing lymphedema. Specific study of applying self-massage for osteoarthritis of the knee showed significant benefit for patients' pain, stiffness, or functional limitations, with between-group analyses of pain indices,[55] while there was no significant difference in range of motion. Further research has shown decrease in visual analogue scale (VAS) and functional scales for patients practicing self-massage with ginger oil for osteoarthritis of the knee with up to 5 weeks of treatment, compared with nonpractitioners.[56] Additionally, in a randomized controlled trial of patients with fibromyalgia, the use of a self-myofascial release program showed significant benefit in emotional and physical well-being, as shown with Fibromyalgia Impact Questionnaire (FIQ-S) Score, including improvement in days per week feeling good, pain intensity, fatigue, stiffness, and depression/sadness, and range of motion variables.[57]

Overall, self-massage requires additional study, but systematic reviews of this CIH modality reveal that it is feasible and effective in certain populations.[58] Although more high-quality studies are needed on specific techniques and application to various conditions, this simple, learnable tool with few effects can be taught via telemedicine and easily implemented virtually.

SUMMARY

CIH modalities are of great therapeutic value in the multidisciplinary-based rehabilitation of patients with chronic pain and complex disease. This whole-person based approach to health is well established in large health systems such as the VA, and has been shown to improve patient satisfaction, decrease opioid use, and reduce health care expenditure. The telehealth delivery of many CIH programs is feasible and provides an opportunity to increase access for patients with multimorbid disease. It is important to remember that telehealth delivery of such programs requires both patient education and buy-in, as well as investment in telehealth infrastructure for long-term sustainability. Additional research is warranted to evaluate these telehealth CIH programs in larger, more diverse populations, and novel technologies such as virtual reality (VR)-based programs and personal wearable devices represent a new frontier in tele-integrative medicine.

CLINICS CARE POINTS

- CIH approaches are well established tools to improve patients' pain, fatigue, stress, and overall well-being when added to a comprehensive rehabilitation program.
- The delivery of many CIH approaches translates well into the virtual care space, but data on the efficacy of these programs are limited.
- Reimbursement for many virtual CIH programs depends on private insurance coverage, as well as state and federal telemedicine regulations.
- Tele-integrative medicine requires that patients have telehealth literacy and access to digital equipment to facilitate care.
- Online group wellness classes offer a nice option to incorporate mind-body movement modalities such as tai chi and yoga into patient care, but it is important to distinguish virtual group wellness classes from mind-body therapeutic programs that are centered around the whole health of the individual.
- Digital applications and online courses offer a feasible option to incorporate mindfulness-based approaches into clinical care.
- The future of tele-integrative medicine is evolving to incorporate newer technology such as VR and remote health monitoring.

DISCLOSURE

The authors have nothing to disclose.

REFERENCES

1. Peterson K, Anderson J, Ferguson L, et al. Evidence brief: the comparative effectiveness of selected complementary and integrative health (CIH) interventions for preventing or reducing opioid use in adults with chronic neck, low back, and large joint pain. 2016. Available at: https://www.ncbi.nlm.nih.gov/books/NBK409241/. Accessed November 3, 2020.
2. Bokhour BG, Hyde JK, Zeliadt S, et al. Whole health system of care evaluation: a progress report on outcomes of the WHS pilot at 18 flagship sites. Veterans Health Administration, Center for Evaluating Patient-Centered Care in VA (EPCC-VA). 2020. Available at: https://www.va.gov/WHOLEHEALTH/docs/EPCCWholeHealthSystemofCareEvaluation-2020-02-18FINAL_508.pdf. Accessed November 3, 2020.
3. Becker's Hospital Review. 7 key findings on VA telehealth services outcomes. 2014. Available at: https://www.beckershospitalreview.com/healthcare-information-technology/7-key-findings-on-va-telehealth-services-outcomes.html. Accessed November 6, 2020.
4. US Department of Veterans Affairs. VHA pain management: PACT roadmap for managing pain. 2018. Available at: https://www.va.gov/PAINMANAGEMENT/Providers/index.asp. Accessed November 3, 2020.
5. Heyworth L, Kirsh S, Zulman D, et al. Expanding access through virtual care: the VA's early experience with Covid-19. NEJM Catalyst 2020;11. https://doi.org/10.1056/CAT.20.0327.

6. Roberts ET, Mehrotra A. Assessment of disparities in digital access among Medicare beneficiaries and implications for telemedicine. JAMA Intern Med 2020; 180(10):1386–9.

7. Mathersul DC, Mahoney LA, Bayley PJ. Tele-yoga for chronic pain: current status and future directions. Glob Adv Health Med 2018;7. https://doi.org/10.1177/2164956118766011.

8. Champion L, Economides M, Chandler C. The efficacy of a brief app-based mindfulness intervention on psychosocial outcomes in healthy adults: a pilot randomised controlled trial. PLoS One 2018;13(12):e0209482.

9. Hempel S, Taylor SL, Solloway MR, et al. Evidence map of tai chi. 2014. Available at: https://www.ncbi.nlm.nih.gov/books/NBK253200/. Accessed November 3, 2020.

10. Qaseem A, Wilt TJ, McLean RM, et al. Noninvasive treatments for acute, subacute, and chronic low back pain: A clinical practice guideline from the American college of physicians. Ann Intern Med 2017;166(7):514–30.

11. Clarke TC, Barnes PM, Black LI, et al. Use of yoga, meditation, and chiropractors among U.S. adults aged 18 and over, NCHS Data Brief. 2018. Available at: https://pubmed.ncbi.nlm.nih.gov/30475686/. Accessed November 5, 2020.

12. Cramer H, Lauche R, Langhorst J, et al. Is one yoga style better than another? A systematic review of associations of yoga style and conclusions in randomized yoga trials. Complement Ther Med 2016;25:178–87.

13. Wren AA, Wright MA, Carson JW, et al. Yoga for persistent pain: new findings and directions for an ancient practice. Pain 2011;152(3):477–80.

14. Daubenmier J, Mehling W, Price C, et al. OA14.02. Exploration of body awareness and pain and emotion regulation among yoga and meditation practitioners: Does type of mind-body practice matter? BMC Complement Altern Med 2012; 12(Suppl 1):O54.

15. Wieland LS, Skoetz N, Pilkington K, et al. Yoga treatment for chronic non-specific low back pain. Cochrane Database Syst Rev 2017;(1):CD010671.

16. Coeytaux RR, McDuffie J, Goode A, et al. Evidence map of yoga for high-impact conditions affecting veterans 2014. Available at: https://pubmed.ncbi.nlm.nih.gov/25254284/. Accessed November 5, 2020.

17. Phuphanich ME, Droessler J, Altman L, et al. Movement-based therapies in rehabilitation. Phys Med Rehabil Clin N Am 2020;31(4):577–91.

18. Villemure C, Ceko M, Cotton VA, et al. Insular cortex mediates increased pain tolerance in yoga practitioners. Cereb Cortex 2014;24(10):2732–40.

19. Jahnke R, Larkey L, Rogers C, et al. A comprehensive review of health benefits of qigong and tai chi. Am J Health Promot 2010;24(6):e1–25.

20. Qin J, Zhang Y, Wu L, et al. Effect of tai chi alone or as additional therapy on low back pain: Systematic review and meta-analysis of randomized controlled trials. Medicine (Baltimore) 2019;98(37):e17099.

21. Kolasinski SL, Neogi T, Hochberg MC, et al. 2019 American College of Rheumatology/Arthritis Foundation guideline for the management of osteoarthritis of the hand, hip, and knee. Arthritis Rheumatol 2020;72(2):220–33.

22. Kong LJ, Lauche R, Klose P, et al. Tai chi for chronic pain conditions: a systematic review and meta-analysis of randomized controlled trials. Sci Rep 2016;6:25325.

23. Schulz-Heik RJ, Meyer H, Mahoney L, et al. Results from a clinical yoga program for veterans: yoga via telehealth provides comparable satisfaction and health improvements to in-person yoga. BMC Complement Altern Med 2017;17(1):198.

24. Martin AC, Candow D. Effects of online yoga and tai chi on physical health outcome measures of adult informal caregivers. Int J Yoga 2019;12(1):37–44.

25. Hempel S, Taylor SL, Marshall NJ, et al. Evidence map of mindfulness. 2014. Available at: https://pubmed.ncbi.nlm.nih.gov/25577939/. Accessed November 3, 2020.
26. Lachance CC, McCormack S. Mindfulness training and yoga for the management of chronic non-malignant pain: a review of clinical effectiveness and cost-effectiveness. Canadian Agency for Drugs and Technologies in Health. 2019. Available at: http://www.ncbi.nlm.nih.gov/books/NBK549581/. Accessed November 3, 2020.
27. Hilton L, Hempel S, Ewing BA, et al. Mindfulness meditation for chronic pain: systematic review and meta-analysis. Ann Behav Med 2017;51(2):199–213.
28. Tkatch R, Bazarko D, Musich S, et al. A pilot online mindfulness intervention to decrease caregiver burden and improve psychological well-being. J Evid Based Complement Altern Med 2017;22(4):736–43.
29. Sesel AL, Sharpe L, Beadnall HN, et al. The evaluation of an online mindfulness program for people with multiple sclerosis: study protocol. BMC Neurol 2019; 19(1):129.
30. Kwon CY, Kwak HY, Kim JW. Using mind-body modalities via telemedicine during the COVID-19 crisis: Cases in the Republic of Korea. Int J Environ Res Public Health 2020;17(12):4477.
31. Sawni A, Breuner CC. Clinical hypnosis: an effective mind–body modality for adolescents with behavioral and physical complaints. Children 2017;4(4):19.
32. Rizzo RRN, Medeiros FC, Pires LG, et al. Hypnosis enhances the effects of pain education in patients with chronic nonspecific low back pain: a randomized controlled trial. J Pain 2018;19(10):1103.e1-e9.
33. Flynn N. Systematic review of the effectiveness of hypnosis for the management of headache. Int J Clin Exp Hypn 2018;66(4):343–52.
34. Zech N, Hansen E, Bernardy K, et al. Efficacy, acceptability and safety of guided imagery/hypnosis in fibromyalgia - a systematic review and meta-analysis of randomized controlled trials. Eur J Pain 2017;21(2):217–27.
35. Hosseinzadegan F, Radfar M, Shafiee-Kandjani AR, et al. Efficacy of self-hypnosis in pain management in female patients with multiple sclerosis. Int J Clin Exp Hypn 2017;65(1):86–97.
36. Madden K, Middleton P, Cyna AM, et al. Hypnosis for pain management during labour and childbirth. Cochrane Database Syst Rev 2012;(11):CD009356.
37. Thompson T, Terhune DB, Oram C, et al. The effectiveness of hypnosis for pain relief: A systematic review and meta-analysis of 85 controlled experimental trials. Neurosci Biobehav Rev 2019;99:298–310.
38. Ardigo S, Herrmann FR, Moret V, et al. Hypnosis can reduce pain in hospitalized older patients: a randomized controlled study. BMC Geriatr 2016;16:14.
39. Cramer H, Lauche R, Paul A, et al. Hypnosis in breast cancer care: a systematic review of randomized controlled trials. Integr Cancer Ther 2015;14(1):5–15.
40. Birnie KA, Noel M, Parker JA, et al. Systematic review and meta-analysis of distraction and hypnosis for needle-related pain and distress in children and adolescents. J Pediatr Psychol 2014;39(8):783–808.
41. Askay SW, Patterson DR, Sharar SR. Virtual reality hypnosis. Contemp Hypn 2009;26(1):40–7.
42. Rousseaux F, Bicego A, Ledoux D, et al. Hypnosis associated with 3D immersive virtual reality technology in the management of pain: a review of the literature. J Pain Res 2020;13:1129–38.
43. Zhuang Y, Xing J, Li J, et al. History of acupuncture research. Int Rev Neurobiol 2013;111:1–23.

44. Ernst E, White AR. Acupuncture for back pain: a meta-analysis of randomized controlled trials. Arch Intern Med 1998;158(20):2235–41.
45. Hempel S, Taylor SL, Solloway MR, et al. Evidence Map of Acupuncture. 2014. Available at: https://pubmed.ncbi.nlm.nih.gov/24575449/. Accessed November 5, 2020.
46. Han JS, Terenius L. Neurochemical basis of acupuncture analgesia. Annu Rev Pharmacol Toxicol 1982;22:193–220.
47. Yin C, Buchheit TE, Park JJ. Acupuncture for chronic pain: an update and critical overview. Curr Opin Anaesthesiol 2017;30(5):583–92.
48. Jones E, Isom S, Kemper KJ, et al. Acupressure for chemotherapy-associated nausea and vomiting in children. J Soc Integr Oncol 2008;6(4):141–5.
49. Tiwari A, Lao L, Wang AX-M, et al. Self-administered acupressure for symptom management among Chinese family caregivers with caregiver stress: a randomized, wait-list controlled trial. BMC Complement Altern Med 2016;16(1):424.
50. Lee EJ, Frazier SK. The efficacy of acupressure for symptom management: a systematic review. J Pain Symptom Manage 2011;42(4):589–603.
51. Murphy SL, Harris RE, Keshavarzi NR, et al. Self-administered acupressure for chronic low back pain: a randomized controlled pilot trial. Pain Med 2019;20(12):2588–97.
52. Li LW, Harris RE, Tsodikov A, et al. Self-acupressure for older adults with symptomatic knee osteoarthritis: a randomized controlled trial. Arthritis Care Res (Hoboken) 2018;70(2):221–9.
53. Richter HT. Acupuncture studies: are they done with sham or scam? Int J Complement Alt Med 2016;3(1):00060.
54. Blödt S, Pach D, von Eisenhart-Rothe S, et al. Effectiveness of app-based self-acupressure for women with menstrual pain compared to usual care: a randomized pragmatic trial. Am J Obstet Gynecol 2018;218(2):227.e1-e9.
55. Atkins DV, Eichler DA. The effects of self-massage on osteoarthritis of the knee: a randomized, controlled trial. Int J Ther Massage Bodywork 2013;6(1):4–14.
56. Tosun B, Unal N, Yigit D, et al. Effects of self-knee massage with ginger oil in patients with osteoarthritis: an experimental study. Res Theory Nurs Pract 2017;31(4):379–92.
57. Ceca D, Elvira L, Guzmán JF, et al. Benefits of a self-myofascial release program on health-related quality of life in people with fibromyalgia: a randomized controlled trial. J Sports Med Phys Fitness 2017;57(7–8):993–1002.
58. Miake-Lye IM, Mak S, Lee J, et al. Massage for pain: an evidence map. J Altern Complement Med 2019;25(5):475–502.

Telehealth in Rehabilitation Psychology and Neuropsychology

Mary J. Wells, PhD[a],*, Paul Dukarm, PhD, ABPP-CN[a], Ana Mills, PsyD[b]

KEYWORDS

• Telepsychology • Teleneuropsychology • telehealth • Rehabilitation • COVID-19

KEY POINTS

- Although telepsychology had been in use for many years with good clinical and research outcomes, the demand for safety during the COVID-19 pandemic accelerated the implementation of telehealth platforms and solidified their value in providing rehabilitation psychology care.
- Successful use of telepsychology for rehabilitation care requires close communication between administrative staff, patients, caregivers, and providers, including education, skills training, developing efficient workflows, on-the-spot problem solving, and back-up plans to ensure the safety of all involved.
- Developing clear guidelines and screening processes is essential for identifying problems with patient access, technology capability, and clinical appropriateness, particularly for high-risk populations, such as patients with substance abuse and suicidality.
- Teleneuropsychological evaluation offers an innovative and feasible alternative to traditional in-person examination, although remote in-home evaluations are limited in the scope of testing and diagnostic conclusions.
- Continued use of telepsychology will be predicated on the development of sustainable billing and coding practices that reflect the complex aspects of rehabilitation psychology and neuropsychology care.

Major health crises often set the stage for needed reform in medicine and social services by illuminating underlying structural problems that have previously existed but gone largely unaddressed. These catastrophic events offer a unique opportunity to examine barriers to health care provision and enact necessary change for the betterment of patient care. The COVID-19 (coronavirus) pandemic has served as one such reckoning. Both nationally and internationally, one of the key pandemic responses was to postpone elective procedures and services in order to limit the spread of infection.

[a] Department of Physical Medicine and Rehabilitation, Virginia Commonwealth University Health System, PO Box 980677, Richmond, VA 23298, USA; [b] Department of Physical Medicine and Rehabilitation, Virginia Commonwealth University, PO Box 980206, Richmond, VA 23298-0206, USA
* Corresponding author.
E-mail address: mary.wells@vcuhealth.org

Phys Med Rehabil Clin N Am 32 (2021) 405–418
https://doi.org/10.1016/j.pmr.2020.12.009
1047-9651/21/© 2020 Elsevier Inc. All rights reserved.
pmr.theclinics.com

Although necessary and beneficial, this dramatic shift also exposed many problems in the US health care system, including limited access to affordable care, exacerbated impact on underserved populations, lack of insurance coverage because of widespread unemployment, deficits in technology infrastructure, cost inflation, and antiquated payment structures.[1] These challenges are substantial and no more apparent than in the field of behavioral health care.

Past studies of epidemics such as the Ebola virus have shown that the prevalence of mental health concerns exceeds the prevalence of infection.[2] In addition, the mental health implications can last longer and have a more pervasive impact on the population. Preliminary data from the COVID-19 pandemic indicate a similar trend, with an exacerbation of symptoms in individuals with pre-existing psychiatric conditions and the development of significant stress in individuals with no premorbid psychiatric history.[3,4]

The COVID-19 pandemic has also brought into stark relief the disparity between demand and supply in behavioral health care. Epidemiologic studies confirm that in any given year 25% of the American population may experience mental illness, with a lifetime occurrence as high as 57%.[5] Yet, there are demonstrated shortages of behavioral health professionals in many areas of the United States. As of 2018, over 115 million people lived in designated health professional shortage areas, in which the ratio of professionals to residents was less than 1 professional per 30,000 population.[6] Shortages are more likely in rural regions because of lack of infrastructure, funding, and provider supply. This service gap increased dramatically during the pandemic, as many providers closed in-person services. Given the increase in demand for behavioral health services, telepsychology is one means by which the safety and wellbeing of patients and providers can be ensured, while maintaining the necessary safety precautions to limit infection transmission.

TELEPSYCHOLOGY SERVICE

Telepsychology has been in existence for many years prior to the onset of the COVID-19 pandemic. Beginning as early as the mid-1970s, behavioral health professionals began utilizing phone-based telehealth to address the needs of underserved populations. With the development of computers, smart phones, and user-friendly video platforms, telehealth options have expanded dramatically. The US Department of Defense and the US Department of Veterans Affairs (VA) became leaders in telehealth clinics for various health care services.[6] Embedded in the development of videoconferencing technology was a surge to disseminate telehealth services to rural and other underserved patients.

Notwithstanding these advances, implementation of telehealth in behavioral health care remained limited until recently because of multiple barriers, including reimbursement, security concerns, and limited provider competency. Medicare and other commercial payers were reluctant to offer reimbursement at a comparable rate for telehealth services. There were also concerns about confidentiality and the ability of both patient and clinician to ensure safety and privacy.[7–9]

Research indicates that telepsychology is supported both from a financial and treatment efficacy perspective. The cost of telepsychology services has been found to be equivalent to in-person care.[10] Multiple studies have shown that video-and phone-based telehealth service provision is comparable to in-person treatment of a variety of conditions, including depression,[11] PTSD,[12,13] anxiety,[14] and mild cognitive impairment.[15]

In the field of rehabilitation, a meta-analysis of telephone-based counseling for individuals with newly acquired disability found improved quality of life 12 months later for adult patients receiving telephone based counseling after stroke and spinal cord injury.[16] Telepsychology has also been found to be effective with children and families. One study of children with moderate to severe TBI and their families found that tele-psychology was rated as equal or superior to in-person interventions.[17] Cited benefits included increased family motivation, ease of scheduling, attendance, decreased stigma, equivalent therapeutic alliance, progression, and homework completion. Challenges included increased environmental distractions, limited non-verbal cues, and technology disruptions.

Evidence also supports the delivery of cognitive rehabilitation by telehealth for a variety of rehabilitation populations. Telehealth cognitive rehabilitation has been successfully used for combat veterans diagnosed with mild TBI.[18] A randomized controlled trial indicated that telehealth rehabilitation was effective for older adults with cognitive impairments and dementia, provided that modifications are made for requiring patients or caregivers to manipulate materials.[19] Myers and colleagues[9] found that a telehealth psychoeducation-based cognitive rehabilitation program for survivors of breast cancer was associated with adequate program adherence, participant satisfaction, and improved self-report of cognitive functioning.

TELENEUROPSYCHOLOGY SERVICE

Extension of health services into rural and underserved areas has been the primary goal of telepsychology services. Remote video-based neuropsychological assessment (teleneuropsychology) has been shown to enhance service access and reduce health care costs for both the provider and patient. Teleneuropsychology has also been shown to demonstrate high patient satisfaction and consumer acceptability.[20] Additional benefits of teleneuropsychology evaluation include clarification of diagnosis, detection of either unrecognized or unmet mental health needs, delivery of psychological intervention targeting affective disturbance, caregiver education and support, and neurobehavioral wellness strategies designed to optimize healthy living.

Historically, teleneuropsychology utilized a remote in-person model, in which the patient is seen at a location remote to the provider and testing at the remote site is facilitated by a health care assistant who conducts in-person physical and neuropsychological examination procedures with the patient under the supervision of the provider. Barton and colleagues[21] described the delivery of videoconferencing as a component of their memory disorders clinic at the San Francisco VA Medical Center. Illustration of their approach emphasizes the need for a health care assistant at the designated remote location. Several other studies have demonstrated the feasibility and validity of conducting teleneuropsychology evaluations over video conferencing.[22–26]

In the advent of restrictions imposed on in-person clinical services during the COVID-19 pandemic, perhaps no other facet of clinical psychology has been as negatively affected as the neuropsychology service. In many hospitals, clinics, and private practices, the gold-standard of in-person evaluation was suspended to allow for development of safety procedures. Providers shifted to remote in-home evaluations, in which the patient is assessed in his or her unsecured home environment and the neuropsychologist is either at home or at his or her office. Remote in-home evaluations provide unique limitations, including control of the patient environment, security of tests administered, and availability of qualitative data.

Many neuropsychological tests do not transfer well from in-person examination to in-home video examination. Therefore, the breadth of tests traditionally available to the neuropsychologist is narrower, and the neuropsychologist acquires fewer neuro-cognitive data from which to infer brain dysfunction. Provided there is adequate audio quality on the provider and recipient device, tests in the auditory domain are more suitable for in-home video examination. These include auditory tasks of basic language, attention, learning and memory, and fluid reasoning. Tests that require the patient to physically handle manipulatives create the greatest challenge to test transfer. Screen sharing capability has reduced this problem considerably, but test security issues remain and should be considered prior to such delivery.

Brearly and colleagues[27] conducted a systematic meta-analysis to determine the effect of videoconference-mediated administration on neuropsychological tests, and differences in scores between videoconference-mediated versus on-site administration. Their analyses demonstrated that there was no clear trend toward inferior scores when tests were delivered through remote videoconference. Disruptions in the technology by means of loss of connectivity or audio showed no clear influence on score variability. Moreover, small effects were observed on tests deemed robust to videoconferencing administration because of their lack of timing and repetition. Verbal tasks such as list learning, digit span, and verbal associative fluency were not affected by videoconference administration. Other tests such as clock drawing and the Mini Mental State Exam showed extensive variability between studies, limiting the ability to determine their effect. It was hypothesized that sources of influence outside of videoconferencing were likely to be driving the distribution of scores across settings.

SPECIAL CONSIDERATIONS WHEN STARTING TELEPSYCHOLOGY SERVICES
Referral Question

With new patients, the nature of the referral question generally drives the modality of the initial consultation. For patients referred exclusively for rehabilitation psychotherapy service, the initial intake can usually be completed virtually. Video is preferred, as completing an initial intake without visual cues may result in less than optimal ability to obtain essential information. Referrals for legal purposes or medical care prescreening are much more challenging to complete via telehealth. Many if not most clinicians require an in-person assessment given the high stakes nature of such evaluations, such as psychological assessments for bariatric surgery and implantable pain devices, or neuropsychological evaluations for epilepsy or deep brain stimulation for Parkinson disease.

Provider Competency

All rehabilitation psychology providers utilizing telehealth platforms should possess the basic competencies required for adequate telepractice, including understanding of clinical, technical, ethical, and legal issues. Continuing education is available through key organizations, including the Inter Organizational Practice Committee, the American Psychological Association, and others.[28–32]

In cognitive evaluation, an important distinction should be made in the labeling of examination services. Block and Johnson-Greene[33] provide a clarification between cognitive screening, cognitive testing, and neuropsychological assessment. These practices are often incorrectly used interchangeably, whereas the distinction is critical for determining who conducts the remote evaluation and what is being done. Although telehealth cognitive screening and abbreviated testing can be conducted by medical and other rehabilitation providers, neuropsychological assessment should be the sole domain of the clinical neuropsychologist (**Table 1**).

Table 1
Classification system for cognitive evaluation services

Level of Evaluation	Complexity	Specialty	Training	Scope	Examples
Cognitive screening	Low – no contextual information and scores interpreted in isolation	Licensed and trained health care providers (physicians, physician assistants, SLPs, registered nurses, nurse practitioners, psychologists, neuropsychologists)	Low – entry level licensed health care providers	Narrow – cursory; emphasis on global cognitive functioning	MMSE, MoCA, CLOX, Min-Cog
Cognitive testing	Medium – normative adjustments made; little contextual information	Non-neuropsychologists, speech pathologists, other licensed health care providers working in neurology or rehabilitation settings where cognition is an issue	Medium – familiarity with principles of neurocognition and neuropsychology based on formalized education or training in neuropsychology	Circumscribed cognitive domains in absence of deeper probing and other contextual factors	DRS-2, RBANS; WAIS/WISC; WMS
Neuropsychological assessment	High – demographic adjustments; qualitative contextual information	Clinical neuropsychologist	High – specialized internship and 2 years of fellowship training in clinical neuropsychology according to Houston criteria	Comprehensive – integration of cognitive, emotional, behavioral domains in setting of contextual factors	Fixed or flexible batteries including psychological and neuropsychological measures; qualitative neurobehavioral observations

Adapted from Block CK, Johnson-Greene D, Pliskin N, Boake C. Discriminating cognitive screening and cognitive testing from neuropsychological assessment: implications for professional practice. Clin Neuropsychol. 2017;31(3):487–500. https://doi.org/10.1080/13854046.2016.1267803; with permission.

Patient Accessibility

Although research and anecdotal evidence suggest that most patients transition reasonably well to video-based telepsychology, certain populations are likely to have greater difficulty, including older patients and patients with limited technology familiarity or Internet access. With patients who have less reliable Internet access, the telephone is a necessary back up option. The American Psychological Association (APA) Committee on Aging identified several barriers to successful telehealth with older adults.[31] Although 7 in 10 older adults have access to computers, only 11% were comfortable with the telehealth platforms currently available. Older adults may also present with sensory, motor, or cognitive issues that impede their ability to utilize a telehealth platform, especially with audio-only telehealth options. These barriers to care can be lowered by recruiting caregivers and providing front-end training and support in advance of clinical appointments. The APA Office & Technology Checklist for Telepsychology Services is a useful guide for screening patients for potential remote-based services[28] (**Table 2**).

Informed Consent

Informed consent for any psychology service should be obtained at initial contact when feasible. Initial consent should be obtained in writing, with either a signed form or indication via email or telehealth platform. Providers should discuss privacy, security, and limits of telehealth platforms including loss of service, back up options, and data cost for video platforms.[28] With each encounter, a verbal consent to the telehealth platform is recommended and should be documented in each encounter note.

Consenting individuals to psychological assessments such as teleneuropsychology evaluation requires an additional level of care. The IOPC[15] has devised foundational elements to informed consent, and these include, but are not limited to

- Standard test administration will be modified, and this may affect results in ways that are so far unknown, thereby reducing confidence in diagnostic conclusions and recommendations for treatment.
- Involvement of a third-party in the evaluation (eg, caregiver, guardian, parent, and facilitator) may add additional validity concerns.
- Error may be compounded when assessment procedures are used with people who come from culturally and linguistically diverse populations, require an interpreter, or have limited experience or comfort with the technology.
- There will be a loss of some qualitative data usually obtained during an in-person examination, and this loss may reduce the richness of the clinical data and further limit conclusions and recommendations.

Interstate Practice

With the mobility provided by telehealth services, rehabilitation providers and patients may either purposely or inadvertently be located across state boundaries. States vary in the specific regulations on telepsychology services and provisions for out-of-state clinicians, which can limit services across state lines. Providers should be familiar with the regulations in their state of practice, as well as other state regulations if their patient resides across state lines.

In order to reduce this service barrier, the APA has worked with state licensing boards to provide cross-state licensing processes and practices with the launch of the Psychology Interjurisdictional Compact (PSYPACT). Formed in February 2015 by the Association of State and Provincial Psychology Boards (ASPPB), PSYPACT was created to facilitate interstate telepsychology and temporary in-person

Table 2	
American Psychological Association Office & Technology Checklist for Telepsychology Services	
Screening	• Screen patient's cognitive status. • Assess for adequate technology/comfort level. • Evaluate privacy and safety. • Determine necessity for guardian or caregiver.
Technology	• Is the psychologist's technology platform consistent with HIPAA-(Health Insurance Portability and Accountability Act) complaint practice? • Is there a business associate agreement with the vendor? • Confirm adequate internet connectivity • Confirm secure Internet connection. • Confirm that security protection software is up to date. • Establish log-in protocol.
Set-up	• Ensure private location. • Ensure adequate lighting. • Ensure good camera positioning. • Ensure adequate picture and audio quality. • Maintain eye contact and articulate clearly.
Before the session	• Discuss risks and benefits with the patient. • Get signed informed consent (electronic signatures are sufficient). • Discuss backup plan when technological problems arise. • Discuss billing. • If evaluating a minor, determine where the adult guardian will be.
Beginning of virtual session	• Verify patient identity. • Verify the patient in view of the camera. • Confirm location and phone number where the patient can be reached. • Review importance of privacy at both locations. • Confirm that the evaluation is not being recorded. • Turn off all applications and notifications on smart device or computer. Ask the patient to do the same. • Conduct evaluation or intervention as with an in-person session.

Data from American Psychological Association. Office and technology checklist for telepsychology services. March 2020. Accessed 09/20/2020.

psychology services. As of May 2020, PSYPACT legislation has been enacted in 14 states: Arizona, Colorado, Delaware, Georgia, Illinois, Missouri, Nebraska, Nevada, New Hampshire, Oklahoma, Pennsylvania, Texas, Utah, and Virginia.

Group Psychotherapy

Group psychotherapy via telehealth requires unique considerations. All patients should be screened individually, either in person or via video format, prior to initiation of the group. The purpose and goals of group treatment should be made explicit, and consent to this form of treatment should be obtained prior to enrollment. Patients must verbally consent to their email information being available to other group members to allow access to the video platform. Patients should also be encouraged to access via computer if at all possible as it allows them to see all the members simultaneously, which is more challenging on cell phone platforms generally.

Risk Management

Although there is substantial literature supporting the use of telehealth with a wide variety of patient populations and treatment modalities,[34] historically these studies have not included high-risk patients, such as those with severe mental illness or suicidal behavior. The limited evidence suggests that telepsychology can be used appropriately with high acuity populations, such as individuals experiencing interpersonal abuse, suicidality, and other emergent situations.[35,36] Telehealth platforms have been found to enhance patient satisfaction and safety with collaborative development of safety plans.[37,38] There is also evidence that telepsychology services can reduce repeat hospitalization rates and increase treatment adherence.[39,40]

Practice guidelines for managing suicidality via telehealth have been published by multiple government and professional organizations, including the APA, the joint task force of the American Psychiatric Association and American Telemedicine Association (Practice Guidelines),[41] the VA, and the US Department of Defense.[42,43] Guidelines recommend careful screening to determine appropriateness of telehealth platforms, identifying emergency contact and nearby resources, and assessing cognitive capacity, history of cooperation, substance and psychiatric history, and history of violence or self-destructive behavior. Providers should routinely confirm the location of the patient at each visit, to allow for rapid access to emergency services in the event of a crisis. High acuity patients should have a patient-specific emergency plan. Incorporating family members in the care plan can facilitate safety.

Coding and Billing

Historically, the paucity of reimbursement by insurance providers has proven a barrier to provision of telepsychology services. Prompted by the demand for services during the COVID-19 pandemic, as of May 2020 the Centers for Medicare and Medicaid Services (CMS) approved all psychology and neuropsychology codes for video telepsychology.[15] Billing coverage continues to vary state-by-state, and it is unclear to what extent expanded coverage for telepsychology services will remain once the COVID-19 pandemic resolves. State-specific billing code coverage can also be accessed through the IOPC Web site. Interested readers are referred to https://iopc.squarespace.com/state-by-state-teleneuropsychology-resources. The APA also provides data on the specific CPT codes and billing recommendations for telepsychology services.[29]

ADAPTATION TO TELEPSYCHOLOGY DURING COVID-19

Several recently published research articles confirm that the greatest barriers to use of telehealth services before the pandemic were clinicians themselves, who felt uncomfortable with virtual platforms and lacked adequate training to use telehealth platforms effectively.[44] Additionally, psychologists demonstrated a negative bias against telehealth platforms despite many years of research supporting the claim that telepsychology is no less effective than in-person treatment with a wide variety of patient populations and conditions.[45]

The transition to telepsychology during the COVID-19 pandemic has been remarkable. A study completed in August 2020 looked at telehealth service provision by a cross-section of 2600 psychologists around the country.[46] It found that before the pandemic, 7% of psychological services were rendered virtually, whereas telepsychology increased twelvefold to 85% during the pandemic. Psychologists were optimistic that they could continue to provide about one-third of their care in a virtual format even after pandemic restrictions were lifted.

In June 2020, a case example was published of the rapid transition to telehealth in a primary care psychology service.[47] Within a 2-week window, the service moved to an entirely virtual format. Facilitating factors included a pre-existing telepsychology platform and policies related to an existing research project. Challenges included limited clinic capacity for telehealth service, decreased referral volume, scheduling and electronic health record access from remote sites, technology disruption, and patient preference.

A CASE EXAMPLE OF RAPID TRANSITION TO TELEPSYCHOLOGY SERVICE

VCU Health is a large Level 1 trauma center and academic medical center located in Richmond, Virginia. The health system serves a diverse patient population uniquely characterized by a high volume of urban and rural residents. Of the 840,000 plus outpatient clinic visits in 2019, only a fraction were provided by telehealth. As of early March 2020, all rehabilitation psychology and neuropsychology services in the Department of Physical Medicine & Rehabilitation (PM&R) were provided in-person, with no established platform for telepsychology services.

On March 12, 2020, the health system elected to reduce and redefine ambulatory services in order to limit COVID-19 transmission. In-person ambulatory services were reduced to 20% of normal volume, and widespread telehealth was implemented. By April 2020, consistent with other sectors of VCU ambulatory care, 90% of VCU PM&R psychological services were provided virtually. Throughout the shelter-in-place months of April, May, and June, 80% to 90% of all services were rendered virtually by video platform or telephone. With the establishment of safety procedures for in-person services and stabilization of infection rates, in-person psychology services increased gradually through the summertime (**Fig. 1**).

This case example illustrates that rehabilitation psychology services care can be maintained even with an abrupt transition to telehealth service. Without an established telepsychology platform, the rapid transition from in-person to virtual services required agility by providers, patients, and administrators. During the emergent ramp-down phase, providers maintained close contact with patients by phone or available videoconferencing technology such as FaceTime. A formal triage system was developed to identify patients who would be best served by telepsychology,

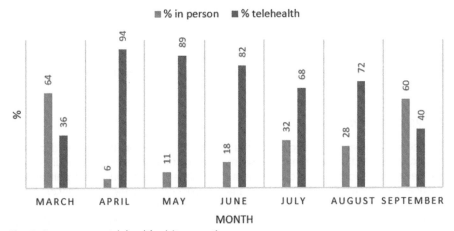

Fig. 1. In person vs. telehealth visits over time.

which required extensive training of providers and support staff. Communication between staff, providers, and patients was integral, with office staff playing a critical role in information dissemination. Patients were provided with education on using the telehealth platform in advance of their first appointment and were provided with a backup option should the first platform fail. Multiple HIPAA-compliant video telehealth platforms were trialed, including Zoom, Doximity, and Connect Well. Due to easier facilitation of group psychotherapy, Zoom was implemented for all rehabilitation telepsychology services. With the exception of comprehensive neuropsychological evaluations, all psychological services were able to be provided via telehealth, including

- Neurobehavioral status examination
- Psychiatric diagnostic interview
- Treatment consultation
- Abbreviated neuropsychological assessment
- Psychological assessment
- Group psychotherapy
- Cognitive behavioral therapy
- Acceptance and commitment therapy
- Affect processing therapy
- Motivational interviewing
- Relaxation training
- Lifestyle change and management
- Psychoeducation

Patient feedback suggests that although not optimal, telepsychology services provide a safe option for continued services when in-person rehabilitation services are not feasible. Many patients find it more convenient to be able to be seen in their homes. For some rehabilitation patients, the telehealth is the only means for access because of transportation limitations and other barriers to care. As one patient observed, "it would not be possible for me to attend in person sessions even if (the therapist) were allowed to do so. Also, it has been a blessing to be able to still have interaction with (the therapist) and the members of the group on a regular basis. Even with the occasional technical glitches, being able hear from and talk to the others in the group is better than not communicating at all." Other patients have reported less than optimal experiences, owing to issues of confidentiality, intimacy, and familiarity. As observed by another patient, telehealth "has been wonderful, because we have been able to keep up within our group with most issues for group members. On the down side,-...not having a place to meet, to get out of the house and see each other, have a place to go that is private, has made personal sharing harder and feedback more stilted. Not to mention the camaraderie that is essential to group is missing, the personal touch of eye to eye, direct feedback is gone."

FUTURE DIRECTIONS

The use of telehealth in response to the COVID-19 pandemic has resulted in dramatic changes in the way rehabilitation psychologists and neuropsychologists provide services. Guidelines for clinical care, risk management, maintaining an ethical practice, test security, and billing have been published on numerous practice organization Web sites and training webinars. Prior research indicates that telepsychology can be used to successfully provide psychotherapy and cognitive rehabilitation services to various rehabilitation patients, including SCI, TBI, stroke, and dementia.

Moving forward, continued efforts to ensure adequate insurance reimbursement for these types of services will be essential. In the field of psychology, most billed services are timed, and the need for compatible payment for timed services will need to be taken into account to ensure fair reimbursement. The current temporary provisions suspending requirement of in-person service provision and HIPPA-compliant platforms will need to be replaced with more permanent solutions for coding and billing.

Studies have also demonstrated the feasibility and validity of administering neuropsychological evaluations via videoconferencing. More work is needed to demonstrate the validity of conducting teleneuropsychology in uncontrolled patient settings and developing methods for the remote use of manipulatives for motor and visuospatial assessment. Using traditional nineteenth century evaluation methods in remote evaluations is difficult, which further serves as motivation for the evolution of orthodox and novel technologies[12] The goal of the Disruptive Technologies Initiative of the American Academy of Clinical Neuropsychology is to embrace novel methods in engineering, computer programming, and biotechnology so that the next generation of neuropsychologists is at the forefront of informing rather than reacting to technological innovations and health care crises.[13] Further lobbying for continuing reimbursement of remote neuropsychological services will potentially serve to redefine the way in which a typical neuropsychological evaluation is conducted.

It is too early to tell if the rapid transition to telepsychology will be sustained over time. Uncertainty remains regarding whether the reimbursement of telehealth services will be reversed or integrated into broader health care reform.[1] Although there are limitations to telepsychology, there are also clear advantages that were identified during the COVID-19 pandemic, including supporting continuity of care, facilitating service access, and maintaining patient and provider safety. The case study of the VCU Health PM&R psychology service illustrates that rapid and dramatic changes can be successfully executed when transitioning to telehealth. Additional research and clinical care evaluation are being conducted daily, and there is good reason for optimism regarding the future role of telehealth in the provision of rehabilitation psychology and neuropsychology care.

CLINICS CARE POINTS

- The specific referral question is a major determining factor in assessing appropriate use of telehealth for both initial assessment and follow-up treatment.

- Providers require tailored training in the technical use of the telehealth platforms and how to conduct an assessment via video, including an appreciation of limits to data collection and diagnostic accuracy.

- Informed consent for use of the telehealth format must be obtained at initial consultation and for each subsequent treatment session. Written consent should be obtained through some form of electronic documentation.

- Careful screening of high-risk patient populations is imperative, with clear documentation of risk assessment and clarification that use of telehealth platforms may need to be altered or discontinued based on ongoing risk assessment and changes in clinical presentation.

- Group psychotherapy can be provided via telehealth platforms that allow for multiple participants. Patients being considered for group psychotherapy service provision will require individual assessment prior to initiation of this form of treatment.

- Remote neuropsychological testing presents unique challenges and may result in reduction in diagnostic confidence and validity by introducing additional error variance.

- Reliance on validated measures and adhering to established guidelines when conducting a remote assessment are strongly recommended.
- At present, the Centers for Medicare and Medicaid have suspended most prior limits for telepsychology billing, but this is likely to change in the near future. Attention to ongoing changes is essential in order to maintain compliance.

REFERENCES

1. Bashshur R, Doarn CR, Frenk JM, et al. Telemedicine and the COVID-19 pandemic, lessons for the future. Telemed E-health 2020;26(5):571–3.
2. Reardon S. Ebola's mental-health wounds linger in Africa: health-care workers struggle to help people who have been traumatized by the epidemic. Nature 2015;519(7541):13–5. Available at: https://go.gale.com/ps/i.do?p=AONE&sw=w&issn=00280836&v=2.1&it=r&id=GALE%7CA404276279&sid=googleScholar&linkaccess=fulltext. Accessed November 6, 2020.
3. Brooks SK, Webster RK, Smith LE, et al. The psychological impact of quarantine and how to reduce it: rapid review of the evidence. Lancet 2020;395(10227):912–20.
4. Shigemura J, Ursano RJ, Morganstein JC, et al. Public responses to the novel 2019 coronavirus (2019-nCoV) in Japan: mental health consequences and target populations. Psychiatry Clin Neurosci 2020;74(4):281–2.
5. Weil TP. Insufficient Dollars and Qualified Personnel to Meet United States Mental Health Needs. J Nerv Ment Dis 2015;203(4):233–40.
6. Mental Health and Substance Use State Fact Sheets | KFF. Available at: https://www.kff.org/statedata/mental-health-and-substance-use-state-fact-sheets/. Accessed November 6, 2020.
7. Antoniotti NM, Drude KP, Rowe N. Private payer telehealth reimbursement in the United States. Telemed E-health 2014;20(6):539–43.
8. Cowan KE, McKean AJ, Gentry MT, et al. Barriers to use of telepsychiatry: clinicians as gatekeepers. Mayo Clin Proc 2019;94(12):2510–23.
9. Myers JS, Cook-Wiens G, Baynes R, et al. Emerging from the haze: a multicenter, controlled pilot study of a multidimensional, psychoeducation-based cognitive rehabilitation intervention for breast cancer survivors delivered with telehealth conferencing. Arch Phys Med Rehabil 2020;101(6):948–59.
10. Egede LE, Gebregziabher M, Walker RJ, et al. Trajectory of cost overtime after psychotherapy for depression in older veterans via telemedicine. J Affect Disord 2017;207:157–62.
11. Egede LE, Acierno R, Knapp RG, et al. Psychotherapy for depression in older veterans via telemedicine: effect on quality of life, satisfaction, treatment credibility, and service delivery perception. J Clin Psychiatry 2016;77(12):1704–11.
12. Bolton AJ, Dorstyn DS. Telepsychology for posttraumatic stress disorder: a systematic review. J Telemed Telecare 2015;21(5):254–67.
13. Moring JC, Dondanville KA, Fina BA, et al. Cognitive processing therapy for posttraumatic stress disorder via telehealth: practical considerations during the COVID-19 pandemic. J Trauma Stress 2020;33(4):371–9.
14. Varker T, Brand RM, Ward J, et al. Efficacy of synchronous telepsychology interventions for people with anxiety, depression, posttraumatic stress disorder, and adjustment disorder: a rapid evidence assessment. Psychol Serv 2018. https://doi.org/10.1037/ser0000239.

15. Cotelli M, Manenti R, Brambilla M, et al. Cognitive telerehabilitation in mild cognitive impairment, Alzheimer's disease and frontotemporal dementia: a systematic review. J Telemed Telecare 2019;25(2):67–79.

16. Dorstyn DS, Mathias JL, Denson LA. Psychosocial outcomes of telephone-based counseling for adults with an acquired physical disability: a meta-analysis. Rehabil Psychol 2011;56(1):1–14.

17. Wade SL, Moscato EL, Raj SP, et al. Clinician perspectives delivering telehealth interventions to children/families impacted by pediatric traumatic brain injury. Rehabil Psychol 2019;64(3):298–306.

18. Riegler L, Wade SL, Narad M, et al. POWER-A telehealth rehabilitation program for veterans: feasibility and preliminary efficacy. Perspect ASHA Spec Interes Groups 2017;2(18):3–14.

19. Burton RL, O'Connell ME. Telehealth rehabilitation for cognitive impairment: randomized controlled feasibility trial. JMIR Res Protoc 2018;7(2):e43.

20. Parikh M, Grosch MC, Graham LL, et al. The clinical neuropsychologist consumer acceptability of brief videoconference-based neuropsychological assessment in older individuals with and without cognitive impairment. Taylor Fr 2013;27(5):808–17.

21. Barton C, Morris R, Rothlind J, et al. Video-telemedicine in a memory disorders clinic: evaluation and management of rural elders with cognitive impairment. Telemed E-health 2011;17(10):789–93.

22. Loh PK, Ramesh P, Maher S, et al. Can patients with dementia be assessed at a distance? The use of Telehealth and standardised assessments. Intern Med J 2004;34(5):239–42.

23. Cullum CM, Weiner MF, Gehrmann HR, et al. Feasibility of telecognitive assessment in dementia. Assessment. 2006;13(4):385–90. Available at: journals.sagepub.com.

24. Munro Cullum C, Hynan LS, Grosch M, et al. Teleneuropsychology: Evidence for video teleconference-based neuropsychological assessment. J Int Neuropsychol Soc 2014;20(10):1028–33.

25. Grosch MC, Weiner MF, Hynan LS, et al. Video teleconference-based neurocognitive screening in geropsychiatry. Psychiatry Res 2015;225(3):734–5.

26. Wadsworth H. JG-G-A of C, 2016 undefined. Remote neuropsychological assessment in rural American Indians with and without cognitive impairment. Available at: academic.oup.com https://academic.oup.com/acn/article-abstract/31/5/420/2726825. Accessed October 31, 2020.

27. Brearly TW, Shura RD, Martindale SL, et al. Neuropsychological test administration by videoconference: a systematic review and meta-analysis. Neuropsychol Rev 2017;27(2):174–86.

28. Office and technology checklist for telepsychological services. Available at: https://www.apa.org/practice/programs/dmhi/research-information/telepsychological-services-checklist. Accessed November 6, 2020.

29. Telepsychology best practice 101 series. Available at: https://apa.content.online/catalog/product.xhtml?eid=15132. Accessed November 6, 2020.

30. A neuropsychology telemedicine clinic - PubMed. Available at: https://pubmed.ncbi.nlm.nih.gov/11370198/. Accessed November 6, 2020.

31. Guidelines for the practice of telepsychology. Available at: https://www.apa.org/practice/guidelines/telepsychology. Accessed November 6, 2020.

32. Guidelines for the practice of telepsychology. Am Psychol 2013;68(9):791–800.

33. Block CK, Johnson-Greene D, Pliskin N, et al. The clinical neuropsychologist discriminating cognitive screening and cognitive testing from neuropsychological assessment: implications for professional practice. Taylor Fr 2016;31(3):487–500.
34. Hubley S, Lynch SB, Schneck C, et al. Review of key telepsychiatry outcomes. World J Psychiatry 2016;6(2):269.
35. Sorvaniemi M, Ojanen E, Santamäki O. Telepsychiatry in emergency consultations: a follow-up study of sixty patients. Telemed E-health 2005;11(4):439–41.
36. Thomas CR, Miller G, Hartshorn JC, et al. Telepsychiatry program for rural victims of domestic violence. Telemed E-health 2005;11(5):567–73.
37. Godleski L, Nieves JE, Darkins A, et al. VA telemental health: suicide assessment. Behav Sci Law 2008;26(3):271–86.
38. Pruitt LD, Luxton DD, Shore P. Additional clinical benefits of home-based telemental health treatments. Prof Psychol Res Pract 2014;45(5):340–6.
39. Godleski L, Cervone D, Vogel D, et al. Home telemental health implementation and outcomes using electronic messaging. J Telemed Telecare 2012;18(1):17–9.
40. D'souza R. Improving treatment adherence and longitudinal outcomes in patients with a serious mental illness by using telemedicine. J Telemed Telecare 2002; 8(2_suppl):113–5.
41. Wright JH, Caudill R. Remote treatment delivery in response to the COVID-19 Pandemic. Psychother Psychosom 2020;89(3):130–2.
42. McGinn M, Roussev M. ES-PC of, 2019 undefined. Recommendations for using clinical video telehealth with patients at high risk for suicide. Available at: psycnet.apa.org https://psycnet.apa.org/record/2019-65479-011. Accessed November 1, 2020.
43. Sall J, Brenner L, Bell AMM, et al. Assessment and management of patients at risk for suicide: synopsis of the 2019 U.S. Department of Veterans Affairs and U.S. Department of Defense Clinical Practice Guidelines. Ann Intern Med 2019; 171(5):343–53.
44. Perle JG, Burt J, Higgins WJ. Psychologist and physician interest in telehealth training and referral for mental health services: an exploratory study. J Technol Hum Serv 2014;32(3):158–85.
45. Perry K, Gold S, Shearer EM. Identifying and addressing mental health providers' perceived barriers to clinical video telehealth utilization. J Clin Psychol 2020; 76(6):1125–34.
46. Pierce BS, Perrin PB, Tyler CM, et al. The COVID-19 telepsychology revolution: a national study of pandemic-based changes in U.S. mental health care delivery. Am Psychol 2020. https://doi.org/10.1037/amp0000722.
47. Perrin PB, Rybarczyk BD, Pierce BS, et al. Rapid telepsychology deployment during the COVID-19 pandemic: a special issue commentary and lessons from primary care psychology training. J Clin Psychol 2020;76(6):1173–85.

Virtual Physical Therapy and Telerehabilitation

Mark A. Havran, DPT[a,b,]*, Douglas E. Bidelspach, MPT[c]

KEYWORDS

- Telehealth • Telerehabilitation • Virtual physical therapy • Tele-physical therapy

KEY POINTS

- Virtual physical therapy (PT) has been demonstrated to be an effective service to be provided through telerehabilitation, showing improvements in function as an additional mode of evaluation and treatment.
- Recent reimbursement changes due to the pandemic are leading to innovative ways to further enhance this type of service.
- Virtual PT can be used to perform types of evaluation and treatment that addresses functional declines related to musculoskeletal, cardiovascular, pulmonary, neurologic, and integumentary system disorders.
- Service delivery incorporates durable medical equipment, home evaluations, and follow-up treatments that may include caregivers and other interdisciplinary team members.
- There are many options for services to be provided that enhance the patient experience.

BACKGROUND/HISTORY

The COVID 19 pandemic in 2020 led to an increased emphasis on telemedicine and telerehabilitation across health care worldwide. Telehealth services can be traced back to the Civil War in how supplies, casualties, and probable medical consultations were used.[1] Over time, the importance and utilization of telehealth has evolved. The American Physical Therapy Association (APTA) supports telehealth to help mitigate rising health care costs, address the disparity in accessibility to services, and leverage existing staff where workforce shortages exist.[2] Telerehabilitation provided by physical therapy, also known as virtual physical therapy, has grown significantly within the federal sector. The expansion of the US Army Medical Command telehealth now spans over 50 countries, across 19 time zones and at least 22 different medical services.[3] Similarly, the US Veterans Health Administration has significantly increased

[a] Department of Veterans Affairs, Des Moines, IA, USA; [b] Rehabilitation and Extended Care (117CLC) VA Central Iowa HCS, 3600 30th Street, Des Moines, IA 50310, USA; [c] Department of Veterans Affairs, 1700 South Lincoln Avenue, Lebanon, PA 17042, USA
* Corresponding author. Rehabilitation and Extended Care (117CLC) VA Central Iowa HCS, 3600 30th Street, Des Moines, IA 50310.
E-mail address: Mark.Havran@va.gov

Phys Med Rehabil Clin N Am 32 (2021) 419–428
https://doi.org/10.1016/j.pmr.2020.12.005
1047-9651/21/Published by Elsevier Inc.
pmr.theclinics.com

telehealth programming and projected over 300% increase in the number of unique veterans receiving clinical video telehealth for PT services in fiscal year 2020.

Virtual PT provides convenient, high-quality services with similar benefits to other health care services provided. Benefits from virtual PT can be described as

- Provide access to PT services at a place of the patient's preference, better serving those who may be isolated geographically, minimizing travel distance, and allowing for more timely responses for care
- Allow the addition of other health care advocates to participate
- Enhance follow-up to care and incur less societal cost[4,5]

Traditionally, payment for services rendered was a hindrance in providing virtual PT services. This has changed rapidly in response to the COVID-19 public health emergency. In April 2020, CMS expanded their list of eligible virtual care providers to include rehabilitation therapists providing payment for two-way, real-time interactive telehealth services that are furnished remotely by PTs. These telehealth services include e-visits, virtual check-ins, remote evaluation of recorded video or images, and telephone assessment and management services. These telehealth services may also be covered by commercial payers. For all payers, physical therapists need to first determine if state practice act enables them to legally provide services.

Telehealth services that are being covered for virtual PT will be described.[6]

Two-Way, Real-Time Interactive Communication

This form of telehealth entails real-time 2-way interaction between the provider and patient or caregiver using audio and video communication technology. Eligible services are reported using the same current procedural terminology (CPT) codes that describe in-person services.

E-Visit

An e-visit is a patient-initiated online assessment and management service for an established patient that is furnished using an online patient portal, not in real time.

Virtual Check-In

Virtual check-ins are brief, real-time remote communication services for an established patient.

Remote Evaluation of Recorded Video or Images

Reviewing a prerecorded video or image that an established patient has submitted is considered a remote evaluation of recorded video or images. This is another example of asynchronous technology used by physical therapists. This asynchronous video or image review by a physical therapist may be paired with a real-time follow-up discussion with the patient, or communicated through texting, e-mail, and an electronic health record's patient portal (**Fig. 1**).

Telephone Assessment and Management Services

Telephone assessment and management services are initiated by the patient or, for a child, the parent, or guardian and involves a real-time discussion with the physical therapist over the telephone.

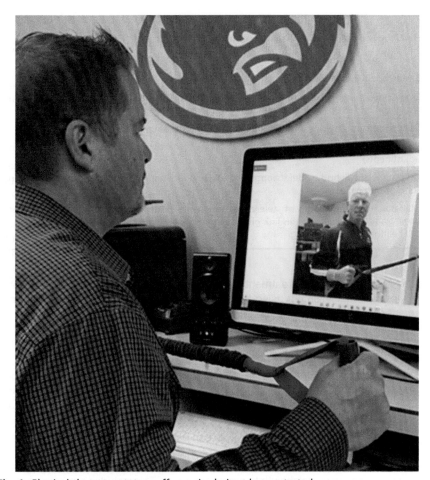

Fig. 1. Physical therapy rotator cuff exercise being demonstrated.

CURRENT EVIDENCE

In patient-centered care, there must be a strong rapport and therapeutic alliance that exist to not only achieve buy in, but also trust.[7,8] Telerehabilitation has been demonstrated to have a high alliance,[9] with high ratings of satisfaction for virtual PT for all patient-centered outcome metrics (93.7%–99%), and value in future telehealth visits (86.8%).[10]

Systematic reviews of virtual PT have shown it to have good concurrent validity for pain, edema, range of motion, strength, balance, gait, functional outcomes, special orthopedic tests, neurodynamic tests, and scar assessment.[11] Diagnosing upper and lower extremity primary pathoanatomical diagnoses has been demonstrated. These conditions have shown increased functional improvement for gait, transfers, and other instrumental activities of daily living when using virtual PT.[12–24]

Furthermore, virtual PT has been shown to decrease pain and disability for patients with chronic neck pain. The enhanced ability for home exercise program follow-up and adherence may have led to the improved outcomes.[25] Agreement between virtual PT and face-to-face assessments for the low back demonstrated a 68.1% agreement

---

Box 1
Technology considerations for tele-physical therapy

- Learn how to use the technology
- Ensure adequate bandwidth
- Does system and software comply with HIPAA (Health Insurance Portability and Accountability Act of 1996) requirements for privacy and security?
- Does patient or caregiver understand how to use technology?
- Determine best surroundings (ie, quiet location, lighting, camera angle, and background adjustments)
- Utilization of a hybrid model if appropriate-face to face and virtual PT visits in combination for best outcomes
- Marketing of utilization of telerehabilitation to patients, referring providers, and community organizations; this link gives some helpful resources: https://www.telehealthresourcecenter.org/

---

was found when applying a treatment-based classification. The results suggest that a telerehabilitation assessment using the modified TBC system may be able to direct treatment of patients with acute and subacute low back pain (LBP).[26,27]

Additionally, virtual PT has been demonstrated to improve functional status with disease processes such as: Parkinson disease,[28] cerebral vascular accident,[29] cardiopulmonary,[30] oncology programs and fall prevention programs.[31–35]

Virtual PT initial preparation involves several steps.

- Examine your state's PT licensure law and corresponding licensure board regulations/rules to determine whether telehealth is addressed in your state practice act. In addition, be aware of any requirements for those who might manage patients remotely across state lines. This can be found at the APTA list of state actions permitting physical therapists to provide virtual PT at: www.apta.org.
- Review each payer's policy regarding eligibility on payment for furnishing, implementing, and using telehealth to provide services. This includes ensuring compliance with practice billing and documentation requirements.

Box 2
Key factors in providing tele-physical therapy visits

- Evaluation and treatment; he standard of care for practicing telehealth is the same as that of in-person physical therapist services
- Informed consent ensures that the patient is informed, understands, and is comfortable with treatment via telehealth; the Center for Connected Health Policy provides a report on telehealth laws and policies, and informed consent: https://www.cchpca.org/
- Emergency contact Information is available
- Explain technology
- Explain that questions can be asked at any point by patient
- Utilize clinical judgment; it may be determined that you should see the patient face to face if applicable and require some type of hybrid frequency
- Document the location of the patient and others involved in the session, including if a PT assistant or other providers involved (eg, telehealth technician or prosthetist)

Table 1
Physical therapy relevant diagnostic, equipment, and outcome suggestions

Physical Therapy Treatment Diagnostic Groupings	Equipment Considerations	Possible Outcome Measures for Consideration
Musculoskeletal conditions (pre-/postoperative, joint impairment, muscle imbalances, pain management, amputations)	Tape measure, resistance band, ruler, firm chair	Promis 6b Pain Interference, Promis Upper Extremity Short Form 7a, Defense & Veterans Pain Rating Scale (DVPRS), APTA Telehealth PT Services Patient Satisfaction Survey, 5x Sit to Stand, 30 Second Sit to Stand, Lower Extremity Functional Index
Cardiovascular and pulmonary conditions (chronic obstructive pulmonary disease, COVID-19, lymphedema)	Pulse oximeter, blood pressure cuff, supplemental oxygen, lymphedema pump, tape measure	Three Minute Walk Test, Two Minute Step Test, St. George Respiratory Questionnaire, SF36, Gait Speed, pulse oximetry weaning progress, vital signs, One Minute Sit to Stand
Neurologic and chronic progressive debilitating conditions (traumatic brain injury, stroke, SCI, ALS)	Metronome, timer, measuring tape/able to measure distance	5x Sit to Stand, Four Square Step Test, Montreal, ABC Scale, Berg, 10 Minute Walk Test, 6-minute walk
Gait and balance deficits	Tape measure, resistance band, ruler, cones or small obstacles, canes, firm chair with and without arms, pillow or foam, eye chart, metronome, pen/pencil	Berg Balance Test, Dynamic Gait (DGI), Four Square Step Test, Single Limb Stance, One Minute Sit to Stand, Four Stage Balance Test, Timed Up and Go (TUG), L-Test, Functional Reach Test, Vertigo Symptom Scale-short form
Durable medical equipment evaluation, intervention, dispensing, training, follow-up, including wheelchair and other mobility assessment	Tape measure, TENS device, walker, cane, crutches, wheelchair	Promis Physical Function with Mobility Aid-short form, pain rating scale, Berg Balance Test, DGI,Examples of wheelchair assessments and other telerehabilitation programs can be accessed at: https://marketplace.va.gov/practices/telerehab-wheeled-mobility-clinic-to-cnh

(continued on next page)

Table 1 (continued)		
Physical Therapy Treatment Diagnostic Groupings	**Equipment Considerations**	**Possible Outcome Measures for Consideration**
Oncology, integumentary, and women's health and pelvic health	Wound care supplies, home biofeedback unit	Pelvic Floor Distress Inventory (PFDI-20), Pelvic Floor Impact Questionnaire (PFIQ-7), Chronic Prostatitis Symptoms Index (CPSI)
Caregiver and family needs/ concerns including cognitive impairments	Access to areas	Geriatric Depression Scale, Patient Health Questionnaire (PHQ-9), MoCA, Brief Test for Adult Cognition
Home and/or work environmental evaluation	Tape measure	Example of how to perform a home safety evaluation can be accessed at: http://www.rstce.pitt.edu/varha/

- Check with your malpractice insurance carrier for any coverage policies specific to telehealth prior to providing physical therapy services. A helpful article titled Telemedicine: Risk Management Issues, Strategies and Resources can be found by Healthcare Providers Service Organization at: http://www.hpso.com/risk-education/individuals/articles/Risk-Management-Considerations-in-Telehealth-and-Telemedicine.
- Prepare policies and procedures before your start, including consent, protected health information protection, and a medical emergency plan to incorporate in overall process.
- Track outcomes (**Box 1**)

VIRTUAL PHYSICAL THERAPY COMMUNICATION TIPS

The Academy of Communication in Healthcare describes telehealth communication: quick tips that can be used in building trust and confidence while getting buy in. This focuses on

- Being present. Think of how you are feeling, with whom you are meeting, and a genuine way to connect.
- Identify the patient's needs. Think of what the other person may expect and notice your own assumptions. Ask open-ended questions to identify the patient's needs.
- Listen. Time and resource limitations tempt people to interrupt. Brief moments of attentive listening allow the other person to feel heard, and often improves understanding of his or her needs and expectations. Try to identify both the content and emotion you hear as you listen.
- Respond. Provide empathy. Summarize what you heard in terms of content and attempt to name and validate the patient's emotion. Offer a short statement of empathy.
- Share information. Provide jargon-free information in small chunks. Ask patients to summarize what they heard to ensure you have been clear (**Box 2**).

More information can be found at: http://www.achonline.org/Telehealth.

Demonstrated Examples of successful physical therapy evaluations and interventions using telerehabilitation include

- Modified musculoskeletal, neurologic, cardiovascular, pulmonary, and/or integumentary system evaluations
- Home exercise program and follow-up
- Group interdisciplinary visits
- Assistive device assessment and training
- Modality and self-care training
- Biopsychosocial chronic pain and spine programming
- Home environmental assessments
- Wheelchair and/or other mobile equipment assessments

The table (**Table 1**) below gives more insight on equipment considerations and possible outcome measures for different diagnostic groupings.

SUMMARY

PT can be effectively applied as part of telerehabilitation. The benefits to the consumer can be measured in timely access, functional improvements, decreased travel time, and other decreased societal costs. Providers are benefitted by applying safety protocols, establishing therapeutic alliances, ability to connect if distance or other factors are a challenge, and the ability to perform follow-up on adherence to any recommendations to sustain functional improvements. Research continues to grow in the area. Continued technological enhancements and further research will create future innovations to further improve patient care in this area. Potentially, the care models and research will lead to successful hybrid models that may encompass a ratio of face-to-face visits and virtual visits depending on clinical presentation. The authors' intent was to demonstrate that virtual physical therapy is a successful telerehabilitation intervention, provide a few key points to make successful, and invoke thought that may lead to additional research, treatment strategies, and create a vision on how to expand. There is certainly room to manage the present, but also an opportunity to create the future in leading innovation for virtual PT.[36]

CLINICS CARE POINTS

- Utilize technology that you and your patient can use
- Ensure a private, quiet area that is not distracting
- Welcome the patient-
  ○ Introduce yourself and establish rapport
  ○ Ensure consent and reinforce the amount of time available
  ○ Explain next steps if for some reason the visit is cut off because of technical issues
- During evaluation and treatment
  ○ Open-ended history of illness-be an active listener
  ○ Avoid interrupting, looking away, or leaning back in chair-be aware of nonverbal communication
  ○ Assess any red or yellow signs that may be emergent or identified throughout session
  ○ Utilize appropriate camera angles in order to perform evaluative and objective tests
  ○ Identify any equipment that the patient may need to enhance evaluation or objective tests to ensure efficient use of time
- Utilize and arrange caregiver or technician as needed for assistance in care or moving technology device for better viewing

- Plan on what type of media to use to demonstrate, educate, and ensure home exercise program is understood by patient or caregiver
- Document session and coordinate scheduling of any follow-up appointments (if indicated)
- Identify if face-to-face or duty to refer is indicated prior to next virtual visit

DISCLOSURE

The authors have nothing to disclose.

REFERENCES

1. Institute of Medicine (US). Committee on Evaluating Clinical Applications of Telemedicine. In: Field MJ, editor. Telemedicine: a guide to assessing telecommunications in health care. Washington, DC: National Academies Press (US); 1996. p. 34-52.
2. American Physical Therapy Association. 2020. Available at: https://www.apta.org/. Accessed October 1, 2020.
3. Poropatich R, Lai E, McVeigh F, et al. The U.S. Army Telemedicine and m-Health Program: making a difference at home and abroad. Telemed J E Health 2013; 19(5):380–6.
4. Chern CC, Chen YJ, Hasoi B. Decistion tree-based classifier in providing telehealthservice. BMC Med Inform Decis Mak 2019;19(1):104–18.
5. Kloek CJJ, vanDongen JM, de Bakker DH, et al. Cost-effectiveness of a blended physiotherapy intervention compared to usual physiotherapy in patients with hip and/or knee osteoarthritis: a cluster randomized controlled trial. BMC Public Health 2018;18(1):1082.
6. Centers for Medicare & Medicaid Services. 2020. Available at: www.medicare.gov. Accessed October 1, 2020.
7. Muller I, Kirby S, Yardley L. The therapeutic relationship in telephone-delivered support for people undertaking rehabilitation: a mixed-methods interaction analysis. Disabil Rehabil 2015;37(12):1060–5.
8. Diener I, Kargela M, Louw A. Listening is therapy: Patient interviewing from a pain science perspective. Physiother Theor Pract 2016;32(5):356–67.
9. Lawford BJ, Bennell KL, Campbell PK, et al. Therapeutic alliance between physiotherapists and patients with knee osteoarthritis consulting via telephone: a longitudinal study. Arthritis Care Res 2019. https://doi.org/10.1002/acr.23890.
10. Tenforde AS, Borgstrom H, Polich G, et al. Outpatient physical, occupational, and speech therapy synchronous telemedicine: a survey study of patient satisfaction with virtual visits during the COVID-19 Pandemic. Am J Phys Med Rehabil 2020; 99(11):977–81.
11. Mani S, Sharma S, Omar B, et al. Validity and reliability of Internet-based physiotherapy assessment for musculoskeletal disorders: a systematic review. J Telemed Telecare 2017;23(3):379–91.
12. Canoso JJ, Saavedra MÁ, Pascual-Ramos V, et al. Musculoskeletal anatomy by self-examination: A learner-centered method for students and practitioners of musculoskeletal medicine. Ann Anat 2020;228:151457.
13. Basteris A, Pedler A, Sterling M. Evaluating the neck position sense error with a standard computer and a webcam. Man Ther 2016;26:231–4.

14. Lade H, McKenzie S, Steele L, et al. Validity and reliability of the assessment and diagnosis of musculoskeletal elbow disorders using telerehabilitation. J Telemed Telecare 2012;18(7):413–8.
15. Worboys T, Brassington M, Ward EC, et al. Delivering occupational therapy hand assessment and treatment sessions via telehealth. J Telemed Telecare 2018; 24(3):185–92.
16. Hoenig HM, Amis K, Edmonds C, et al. Testing fine motor coordination via tele-health: Effects of video characteristics on reliability and validity. J Telemed Tele-care 2018;24(5):365–72.
17. Steele L, Lade H, McKenzie S, et al. Assessment and diagnosis of musculoskel-etal shoulder disorders over the internet. Int J Telemed Appl 2012;2012:945745.
18. Russell T, Truter P, Blumke R, et al. The diagnostic accuracy of telerehabilitation for nonarticular lower-limb musculoskeletal disorders. Telemed J E Health 2010; 16(5):585–94.
19. Richardson BR, Truter P, Blumke R, et al. Physiotherapy assessment and diag-nosis of musculoskeletal disorders of the knee via telerehabilitation. J Telemed Telecare 2017;23(1):88–95.
20. Wong YK, Hui E, Woo J. A community-based exercise programme for older per-sons with knee pain using telemedicine. J Telemed Telecare 2005;11(6):310–5.
21. Azma K, RezaSoltani Z, Rezaeimoghaddam F, et al. Efficacy of tele-rehabilitation compared with office-based physical therapy in patients with knee osteoarthritis: A randomized clinical trial. J Telemed Telecare 2018;24(8):560–5.
22. Pastora-Bernal JM, Martin-Valero R, Baron-Lopez FJ, et al. Evidence of benefit of telerehabilitation after orthopedic surgery: a systematic review. J Med Internet Res 2017;19(4):1–12.
23. Panda S, Bali S, Kirubakaran R, et al. Telerehabilitation and total knee arthro-plasty: A systematic review and meta-analysis of randomised controlled trials. Int J Ther Rehabil 2015;(supplement 22):S6.
24. Agostini M, Moja L, Banzi R, et al. Telerehabilitation and recovery of motor func-tion: a systematic review and meta-analysis. J Telemed Telecare 2015;21(4): 202–13.
25. Gialanella B, Ettori T, Faustini S, et al. Home-based telemedicine in patients with chronic neck pain. Am J Phys Med Rehabil 2017;96(5):327–32.
26. Truter P, Russell T, Fary R. The validity of physical therapy assessment of low back pain via telerehabilitation in a clinical setting. Telemed J E Health 2014; 20(2):161–167..
27. Peterson S, Kuntz C, Roush J. Use of a modified treatment-based classification system for subgrouping patients with low back pain: agreement between telere-habilitation and face-to-face assessments. Physiother Theor Pract 2018. https:// doi.org/10.1080/09593985.2018.1470210.
28. Chen YY, Guan BS, Li ZK, et al. Application of telehealth intervention in Parkin-son's disease: a systematic review and meta-analysis. J Telemed Telecare 2018. https://doi.org/10.1177/1357633X18792805.
29. Rintala A, Paivarinne V, Hakala S, et al. Effectiveness of technology-based dis-tance physical rehabilitation interventions for improving physical functioning in stroke: a systematic review and meta-analysis of randomized controlled trials. Arch Phys Med Rehabil 2019. https://doi.org/10.1016/j.apmr.2018.11.007.
30. Garvey C, Singer JP, Bruun AM, et al. Moving pulmonary rehabilitation into the home: a clinical review. J Cardiopulm Rehabil Prev 2018;38(1):8–16.
31. Finnegan S, Seers K, Bruce J. Long-term follow-up of exercise interventions aimed at preventing falls in older people living in the community: a systematic

review and meta-analysis. Physiotherapy 2018;105(1). https://doi.org/10.1016/j.physio.2018.09.002.

32. Van Egmond MA, van der Schaaf M, Vredeveld T, et al. Effectiveness of physiotherapy with telerehabilitation in surgical patients: a systematic review and meta-analysis. Physiotherapy 2018;104:277–98.

33. Cheville AL, Moynihan T, Herrin J, et al. Effect of collaborative telerehabilitation on functional impairment and pain among patients with advanced-stage cancer: a randomized clinical trial. JAMA Oncol 2019. https://doi.org/10.1001/jamaoncol.2019.0011.

34. Jansen-Kosterink S, Huis in 't Veld R, Hermens H, et al. Telemedicine service and partial replacement of face-to-face physical rehabilitation: the relevance of use. Telemed J E Health 2015;21(10):808–13.

35. Tsai LL, McNamara RJ, Moddel C, et al. Home-based telerehabilitation via real-time videoconferencing improves endurance exercise capacity in patients with COPD: the randomized controlled TeleR study. Respirology 2017;22(4):699–707.

36. Govindarajan V. The three box solution: a strategy for leading innovation. Boston: Harvard Business Review Press; 2016.

Logistics of Rehabilitation Telehealth

Documentation, Reimbursement, and Health Insurance Portability and Accountability Act

Anne H. Chan, DPT, MBA

KEYWORDS

- Telehealth • Rehabilitation • Telehealth documentation • Telehealth billing
- Telehealth coding • Telehealth privacy

KEY POINTS

- As a result of the COVID-19 public health emergency (PHE), the Centers for Medicare & Medicaid Services expanded its telehealth benefit on a temporary and emergency basis.
- Effective March 6, 2020, Medicare began to pay for Medicare telehealth services at the same rate as regular, in-person visits.
- To bill telehealth claims for services delivered during the PHE, providers should include the place of service in which the service would have been furnished if the visit was in person, and providers should add modifier 95 to denote the service took place via telehealth.
- Non–public-facing remote communications like Apple FaceTime®, Zoom®, and Skype® can be used for the delivery of Medicare telehealth services.

INTRODUCTION

The Centers for Medicare & Medicaid Services (CMS) defines telehealth, telemedicine, and related terms as "the exchange of medical information from one site to another through electronic communication to improve a patient's health."[1] Additionally, the Health Resources and Services Administration of the US Department of Health and Human Services (HHS) describes telehealth as "the use of electronic information and telecommunication technologies to support long-distance clinical health care, patient and professional health-related education, public health, and health administration. Technologies include videoconferencing, the internet, store-and-forward imaging, streaming media, and landline and wireless communications."[2]

With the COVID-19 public health emergency (PHE), the CMS expanded its telehealth benefit on a temporary and emergency basis. Effective March 6, 2020,

Department of Physical Medicine and Rehabilitation, Virginia Commonwealth University, 1223 East Marshall Street, PO Box 980677, Richmond, VA 23298, USA
E-mail address: Anne.Chan@vcuhealth.org

Phys Med Rehabil Clin N Am 32 (2021) 429–436
https://doi.org/10.1016/j.pmr.2021.01.006
1047-9651/21/© 2021 Elsevier Inc. All rights reserved.

Medicare began to pay for office, hospital, and other visits furnished via telehealth. Prior to this expansion, Medicare "could only pay for telehealth on a limited basis: when the person receiving the service is in a designated rural area and when they leave their home and go to a clinic, hospital, or certain other types of medical facilities for the service."[1] Furthermore, prior to the COVID-19 PHE telehealth expansion, Medicare was making payments for virtual check-ins, and Medicare Part B was paying for e-visits, which are "non-face-to-face patient-initiated communications through an online patient portal."[1]

Note that guidance from the CMS and other agencies are evolving, and the most current policies can be found on the CMS Web site. Also note that coverage for telehealth varies by payer and by state.

Medicare classifies 3 main types of virtual services that physicians and other health care professionals can provide to Medicare beneficiaries:

1. Medicare telehealth visits: these visits are furnished using telecommunications technology that must be real-time, 2-way interactive, and with audio and visual capabilities. Effective March 6, 2020, and for the duration of the PHE, Medicare will pay for Medicare telehealth services at the same rate as regular, in-person visits. Additional details on Medicare telehealth visits are discussed later.
2. Virtual check-ins: these visits are briefer than Medicare telehealth visits and do not require audio and visual capabilities for real-time communication. Examples include "synchronous discussion over a telephone or exchange of information through video or image."[1] Virtual check-ins are done with established patients, are patient-initiated, and require verbal patient consent.
3. E-visits: using online patient portals, Medicare patients initiate communications with their physicians. These are established patients, and "the Medicare coinsurance and deductible would apply to these services."[1]

MEDICARE TELEHEALTH VISITS: EXPANSIONS DUE TO THE COVID-19 PUBLIC HEALTH EMERGENCY

On March 30, 2020, the CMS issued an Interim Final Rule with Comment Period, which, in addition to its March 17, 2020, announcement, expanded telehealth by waiving its geographic and place of service (POS) restrictions and by adding more flexibility in the use of telehealth. The key elements of this expansion are as follows:

- The Medicare telehealth expansions are effective for March 6, 2020, through the period of the PHE.
- The geographic and POS restrictions are waived, such that Medicare pays for Medicare telehealth visits in patient locations, such as their homes and outside of designated rural areas.
- Medicare telehealth visits must be furnished using telecommunications technology that is real-time, 2-way interactive, and with audio and visual capabilities. An exception to this rule is that "CMS has used its waiver authority to allow, beginning on March 1, 2020, telephone evaluation and management codes and certain counseling behavior health care and educational services, to be furnished as telehealth services using audio-only communications technology (telephones or other audio-only devices)."[3]
- Medicare telehealth visits can be furnished by distant site practitioners from their home during the PHE. The POS code should be reported as the place where the service would have been reported if the service had been provided in person.

- Providers may see both new and established Medicare patients via telehealth.
- Medicare telehealth visits must be reasonable and necessary.
- The types of telehealth services covered by Medicare during the COVID-19 PHE can be found at https://www.cms.gov/Medicare/Medicare-General-Information/Telehealth/Telehealth-Codes.
- The HHS Office of Inspector General (OIG) will not sanction health care providers for reducing or waiving cost-sharing obligations for telehealth services paid for by Medicare. More information can be found at the following:
  - https://oig.hhs.gov/fraud/docs/alertsandbulletins/2020/policy-telehealth-2020.pdf
  - https://www.oig.hhs.gov/fraud/docs/alertsandbulletins/2020/factsheet-telehealth-2020.pdf
  - https://oig.hhs.gov/fraud/docs/alertsandbulletins/2020/telehealth-waiver-faq-2020.pdf
- The CMS has allowed providers to deliver telehealth services across state lines. Providers are subject, however, to the requirements established by the states involved. The following resources are available:
  - Federation of State Medical Boards: this link provides a list of US states and territories that have modified their telehealth requirements in response to the COVID-19 PHE: https://www.fsmb.org/siteassets/advocacy/pdf/states-waiving-licensure-requirements-for-telehealth-in-response-to-covid-19.pdf.
  - Federation of State Medical Boards: this link provides a list of US states and territories that have modified licensure requirements for physicians in response to the COVID-19 PHE: https://www.fsmb.org/siteassets/advocacy/pdf/state-emergency-declarations-licensures-requirementscovid-19.pdf.
  - Federation of State Medical Boards: this link provides a list of US states and territories that have expedited licensure for inactive/retired licensees in response to the COVID-19 PHE: https://www.fsmb.org/siteassets/advocacy/pdf/states-expediting-licensure-for-inactive-retired-licensees-in-response-to-covid19.pdf.
  - The National Telehealth Policy Resource Center: this link provides information by state on changes states have made to remove policy barriers to telehealth in response to the COVID-19 PHE: https://www.cchpca.org/covid-19-related-state-actions.
  - Interstate Medical Licensure Compact (IMLC): the IMLC, created by state medical boards, executives, and administrators, significantly streamlines the licensure process for physicians wanting to practice in multiple states. The intent of the IMLC was to increase access to health care (eg, geographic access and access to specialists), and the benefits to physicians include faster licensure and fewer administrative burdens: https://www.imlcc.org/a-faster-pathway-to-physician-licensure/.
  - Medicare: this link provides information on Medicare's recognition of IMLCs: https://www.cms.gov/files/document/SE20008.pdf.
  - IMLCs also exist for other health care providers:
    - Emergency medical services workers: https://www.emscompact.gov/
    - Nurses: https://www.ncsbn.org/nurse-licensure-compact.htm
    - Physical therapists: http://ptcompact.org/
    - Psychologists: https://psypact.org/page/PracticeUnderPSYPACT
    - Speech language pathologists/therapists: https://aslpcompact.com/
- As a result of the COVID-19 PHE, the Drug Enforcement Administration (DEA) has made the following key changes:

- The DEA has allowed DEA-registered practitioners to prescribe schedule II–V controlled substances via telehealth. The following 3 conditions must be met:
  - "The prescription is issued for a legitimate medical purpose by a practitioner acting in the usual course of his/her professional practice;
  - The telemedicine communication is conducted using an audio-visual, real-time, two-way interactive communication system; and
  - The practitioner is acting in accordance with applicable Federal and State laws."[4]
- The DEA, through the Controlled Substances Act, "allows practitioners to dispense narcotic drugs, including buprenorphine, to individuals with OUD [opioid use disorder] for maintenance or detoxification treatment if the practitioners separately register with DEA as an opioid treatment program."[5]
- The DEA has granted an exception to DEA-registered practitioners, such that DEA-registered practitioners are not required to register with the DEA in additional states where they dispense controlled substances. Further detail is available at https://www.deadiversion.usdoj.gov/GDP/(DEA-DC-018)(DEA067)%20DEA%20state%20reciprocity%20(final)(Signed).pdf.
- The DEA has granted an exception to requirements for paper delivery of an emergency oral prescription. Further detail is available at https://www.deadiversion.usdoj.gov/GDP/(DEA-DC-021)(DEA073)%20Oral%20CII%20for%20regular%20CII%20scirpt%20(Final)%20+Esign%20a.pdf.

MEDICAID COVERAGE FOR TELEHEALTH

Because Medicaid coverage differs by state, the National Telehealth Policy Resource Center has compiled a resource on COVID-19–related state actions: https://www.cchpca.org/covid-19-related-state-actions. The link provides state-by-state information on the allowance of telehealth, changes to geographic restrictions, and coverage for telehealth services.

UNINSURED PATIENTS: FEDERAL COVID-19 REIMBURSEMENTS

Health care providers and health centers can be reimbursed by the federal government for testing and treating uninsured individuals for COVID-19. Claims can be submitted to the Health Resources and Services Administration COVID-19 Uninsured Program Portal (https://coviduninsuredclaim.linkhealth.com/). Claims generally are paid at Medicare rates, upon availability of funding.

MEDICARE BILLING, CODING, AND REIMBURSEMENT

The types of telehealth services covered by Medicare during the COVID-19 PHE can be found at https://www.cms.gov/Medicare/Medicare-General-Information/Telehealth/Telehealth-Codes. Medicare reimburses a telehealth visit at the same fee-for-service-rate as an in-person visit during the PHE. To bill telehealth claims for services delivered during the PHE, providers should include the POS in which the service would have been furnished if the visit were in person, and providers should add modifier 95 in order to denote the service took place via telehealth.

The catastrophe/disaster-related (CR) modifier is not needed when billing for telehealth services. The CMS requires modifiers, however, for Medicare telehealth professional claims for the following 2 scenarios:

- "Furnished as part of a federal telemedicine demonstration project in Alaska and Hawaii using asynchronous (store and forward) technology, use GQ (*Via an asynchronous telecommunications system* when reporting telehealth services) modifier."[6]
- "Furnished for diagnosis and treatment of an acute stroke, use G0 (used to identify Telehealth services furnished for purposes of diagnosis, evaluation, or treatment of symptoms of an acute stroke) modifier."[6]

For office/outpatient evaluation and management (E/M) services furnished via telehealth, level selection can be based on medical decision making or time. Medical decision making refers to the existing definition of "the complexity of establishing a diagnosis and/or selecting a management option, which is determined by considering these factors: the number of possible diagnoses and/or the number of management options that must be considered; the amount and/or complexity of medical records, diagnostic tests, and/or other information that must be obtained, reviewed, and analyzed; [and] the risk of significant complications, morbidity, and/or mortality as well as comorbidities associated with the patient's presenting problem(s), the diagnostic procedure(s), and/or the possible management options."[7] Additional information on time can be found at https://www.aap.org/en-us/professional-resources/practice-transformation/getting-paid/Coding-at-the-AAP/Pages/Using-Time-to-Report-Outpatient-EM-Services.aspx.

Examples of Healthcare Common Procedure Coding System/Current Procedural Terminology codes: Medicare telehealth visits

Service	Healthcare Common Procedure Coding System/ Current Procedural Terminology Code
New patient office/outpatient E&M services	99201 99202 99203 99204 99205
Under new or established patient office/outpatient E&M services	99221 99222 99223 99224 99225
Telehealth consultations, emergency department, or initial inpatient	G0425 G0426 G0427
Follow-up inpatient consultation, furnished via telehealth to beneficiaries in hospitals or skilled nursing facilities	G0406 G0407 G0408

Examples of Healthcare Common Procedure Coding System/Current Procedural Terminology codes: virtual check-ins

Service	Healthcare Common Procedure Coding System/ Current Procedural Terminology Code
Brief virtual check-in (5-10 minutes of medical discussion) with an established patient, not resulting from a service provided within the past 7 days nor leading to a service within the next 24 hours or next available appointment	G2012
Remote evaluation with interpretation of recorded video or images submitted by an established patient, inclusive of follow-up with the patient within 24 business hours, not resulting from a service provided within the past 7 days nor leading to a service within the next 24 hours or next available appointment	G2010

Examples of Healthcare Common Procedure Coding System/Current Procedural Terminology codes: e-visits

Service	Healthcare Common Procedure Coding System/ Current Procedural Terminology Code
Under non–face-to-face on-line digital E/M service	99421 99422 99423
Qualified nonphysician health care professional online assessment and management service, for an established patient, for up to 7 days, cumulative time during the 7 days	G2061 G2062 G2063

- Residents furnishing services at primary care centers may provide an expanded set of services to beneficiaries, including levels 4-5 of an office/outpatient Evaluation and Management (E/M) visit, telephone E/M, care management, and some communication technology-based services
- This expanded set of services at CPT® codes 99204-99205, 99214-99215, 99495-99496, 99421-99423, 99452, and 99441-99443 and HCPCS codes G2010 and G2012

- Teaching physicians may submit claims for these services furnished by residents in the absence of a teaching physician using the GE modifier."[6]

HEALTH INFORMATION PORTABILITY AND ACCOUNTABILITY ACT

During the COVID-19 PHE, the Office for Civil Rights at HHS has issued a Notification of Enforcement Discretion and "will not impose penalties for noncompliance with the regulatory requirements under the HIPAA [Health Insurance Portability and Accountability Act of 1996] Rules against covered health care providers in connection with the good faith provision of telehealth."[8] Non–public-facing remote communications like Apple FaceTime®, Zoom®, and Skype® can be used. Public-facing applications like Facebook Live®, Twitch®, and TikTok® are not allowed to be used.

CLINICS CARE POINTS

- The CMS defines telehealth, telemedicine, and related terms as "the exchange of medical information from one site to another through electronic communication to improve a patient's health."[1]
- Guidance from the CMS and other agencies is evolving, and the most current policies can be found on the CMS Web site.
- Coverage for telehealth varies by payer and by state.
- Providers may see both new and established Medicare patients via telehealth.
- Medicare telehealth visits must be reasonable and necessary.
- The CMS has allowed providers to deliver telehealth services across state lines. Providers are subject, however, to the requirements established by the states involved.
- The DEA has allowed DEA-registered practitioners to prescribe schedule II–V controlled substances via telehealth, with specific required conditions.

DISCLOSURE

The author has nothing to disclose.

REFERENCES

1. Centers for Medicare and Medicaid Services. Medicare telemedicine health care provider fact sheet. 2020. Available at: https://www.cms.gov/newsroom/fact-sheets/medicare-telemedicine-health-care-provider-fact-sheet. Accessed November 3, 2020.
2. U.S. Department of Health and Human Services, Office for Civil Rights. FAQs on telehealth and HIPAA during the COVID-19 nationwide public health emergency. Available at: https://www.hhs.gov/sites/default/files/telehealth-faqs-508.pdf. Accessed November 3, 2020.
3. Centers for Medicare and Medicaid Services. COVID-19 frequently asked questions (FAQs) on Medicare fee-for-service (FFS) billing. 2020. Available at: https://www.cms.gov/files/document/medicare-telehealth-frequently-asked-questions-faqs-31720.pdf. Accessed November 3, 2020.
4. U.S. Department of Justice, Drug Enforcement Administration, Diversion Control Division. COVID-19 information page. Available at: https://deadiversion.usdoj.

gov/coronavirus.html?inf_contact_key=410e6a45f5ef27deb85e6b6a8b284664. Accessed November 4, 2020.

5. U.S. Department of Justice, Drug Enforcement Administration. Use of telephone evaluations to initiate buprenorphine prescribing. 2020. Available at: https://www.deadiversion.usdoj.gov/GDP/(DEA-DC-022)(DEA068)%20DEA%20SAMHSA%20buprenorphine%20telemedicine%20%20(Final)%20+Esign.pdf. Accessed November 4, 2020.

6. Centers for Medicare and Medicaid Services, Medicare Learning Network. Medicare fee-for-service (FFS) response to the public health emergency on the coronavirus (COVID-19). 2020. Available at: https://www.cms.gov/files/document/se20011.pdf. Accessed November 3, 2020.

7. Centers for Medicare and Medicaid Services, Medicare Learning Network. Evaluation and management services guide. 2020. Available at: https://www.cms.gov/outreach-and-education/medicare-learning-network-mln/mlnproducts/downloads/eval-mgmt-serv-guide-icn006764.pdf. Accessed November 4, 2020.

8. U.S. Department of Health and Human Services, Health Information Privacy. Notification of enforcement discretion for telehealth remote communications during the COVID-19 nationwide public health emergency. 2020. Available at: https://www.hhs.gov/hipaa/for-professionals/special-topics/emergency-preparedness/notification-enforcement-discretion-telehealth/index.html. Accessed November 4, 2020.

Using Biometric Technology for Telehealth and Telerehabilitation

Thiru M. Annaswamy, MD, MA[a],*, Gaurav N. Pradhan, PhD[b],
Keerthana Chakka, BS[c], Ninad Khargonkar, MS[d],
Aleks Borresen, MD[e], Balakrishnan Prabhakaran, PhD[d]

KEYWORDS

- Telehealth • Telerehabilitation • Biometric • Pose estimation • Kinematics
- Electromyography • Wearable sensors • Virtual reality

KEY POINTS

Biometric data in telerehabilitation have utility in:

- Remote physical assessment
- Remote biometric monitoring of patients to assess safety, and/or progress in community-based rehabilitation.
- Biometric data also better engage patients and customize rehabilitation.

INTRODUCTION, BACKGROUND, AND DEFINITIONS

Telerehabilitation can be performed synchronously when the rehabilitation clinician and the patient are interacting with each other in real time, or asynchronously when patient-specific data is transmitted to the clinician and when clinical information and patient education may be transmitted to the patient offline. Most telerehabilitation systems currently used in the practice of physical medicine and rehabilitation use audio and video, but biometric data including vital signs and other physical biometric data are not routinely collected or utilized in the delivery of telerehabilitation. Currently, bio-peripherals, Internet of Things (IoT) and mobile health (mHealth) devices (smartphones)

[a] PM&R Service, Department of PM&R, VA North Texas Health Care System, UT Southwestern Medical Center, 4500, South Lancaster Road, Dallas, TX-75216, USA; [b] Biomedical Informatics, Mayo Clinic College of Medicine, 13400, East Shea Boulevard, Scottsdale, AZ-85259, USA; [c] UT Southwestern Medical School, 5323, Harry Hines Boulevard, Dallas, TX-75390, USA; [d] Department of Computer Science, University of Texas at Dallas, 800, West Campbell Road, Richardson, TX-75080, USA; [e] Department of Physical Medicine and Rehabilitation, University of Alabama at Birmingham, 157 Spain Rehabilitation Center, 1717 6th Avenue South, Birmingham, AL 35249, USA
* Corresponding author.
E-mail address: thiru.annaswamy@va.gov
Twitter: @T_Doc (T.M.A.)

Phys Med Rehabil Clin N Am 32 (2021) 437–449
https://doi.org/10.1016/j.pmr.2020.12.007
1047-9651/21/Published by Elsevier Inc.

can provide physiologic biometric data such as heart rate (HR), blood pressure (BP), temperature, oxygen saturation, electrocardiogram (EKG), oxygen saturation, heart rate (HR) variability, sleep parameters, and similar physiologic measures. The reader is referred to other publications for an overview of applications of such technology in telehealth.[1] In this article, the current state of research and clinical applications of technology that allow collection and analysis of physical and biomechanical biometric data such as electromyography, sensory data (position sense), force, torque, displacement, velocity, tone, range of motion, and motor control are discussed.

Telehealth systems, their features, characteristics, and application to the rehabilitation settings, and how biometric data may be utilized in such systems are summarized in **Table 1**.

This article will be discussing the following clinical uses of biometric data in telerehabilitation and a snapshot of the state of science in this field:

- Capturing and utilizing biometric data for remote physical assessment
- Remote biometric monitoring of patients to assess safety, and/or progress in-home rehabilitation
- Utilizing biometric data to better engage patients and customize their rehabilitation

DISCUSSION
Capturing and Utilizing Biometric Data for Remote Physical Assessment

Synchronous tele-physical assessment using haptics and augmented reality
An immersive augmented reality (AR)-based synchronous telerehabilitation system with haptics (ARTESH) was designed and evaluated for performing remote

Table 1					
Types of telehealth systems and their characteristics					
	Audio and Video	Synchronous/ Asynchronous	Biometrics/ Bioperipherals	Clinician: Patient	Rehabilitation Application
Traditional telehealth	Yes	Asynchronous or synchronous	None	Many:1 or 1:1	• Rural telerehabilitation • Remote consultation • Tele-rounds during COVID-19
eVisits or virtual video visits	Yes	Synchronous	Usually no	1:1	Most common-outpatient rehabilitation clinics: VA Video Connect, EHR-Platform, Teladoc and others
Remote patient monitoring	Usually no	Usually asynchronous	• HR/blood pressure/ pulse oximeter/ thermometer • Virtual reality and wearable sensors	Many:1	• Home therapy • SCI-home monitoring • Remote physical examination

musculoskeletal physical examination.[2] ARTESH used a haptic feedback device and depth sensing red-green-blue-depth (RGB-D) cameras to allow clinicians and patients to interact remotely in real time through audio, video, and touch. The 2 sites were connected via the Internet, and ARTESH's novel features including force rendering and other algorithms to process, compress, decompress and transmit 3-dimensional data in real time allowed real-time interactions to occur without noticeable lag or degradation in quality of immersion or physical assessment experience. Fifteen participants including patients with stroke and shoulder pathology used the system, and rated it as user-friendly and as providing a high quality-of-experience, and compared their physical examination favorably with an in-person assessment performed on the same day.[2]

Comparison of the remote and in-person shoulder examination of passive range-of-motion (PROM), strength and pain revealed greater than 75% agreement of PROM and greater than 80% agreement on strength and pain assessments. PROM and presence or absence of pain were better assessed by the video portion of the synchronous physical assessment, and strength was adequately assessed (on a binary scale of normal or impaired) using the resistance feedback delivered by the haptic device. ARTESH shows promise that synchronous tele-physical assessment is possible using AR and haptic technology.

Asynchronous physical assessment using remote pose estimation

Research is ongoing to evaluate how asynchronous physical assessment can be performed remotely using whole-body kinematics assessment based on RGB-D camera sensors. Reasonably accurate joint angle estimation can be obtained from an RGB-D setup in the context of 4 simple tasks like squatting, stepping, or body tilting.[3] It uses the Kinect sensor to extract the skeleton and a variation of the Kalman filter that tracks the joint centers to quantify acceleration and velocity parameters. A human body biomechanical model is used for reference to enable joint angles and segment lengths to be physically consistent. However, the model parameters need to be estimated from reference data each time a new exercise is to be analyzed.

Another article studied hand telerehabilitation in the context of remote control of a wearable hand exoskeleton.[4] During exercise, the position and movement of the hand joints in a 3-dimensional space were recorded using an RGB-D camera that guided exoskeleton movements remotely while recording interaction forces for the rehabilitation task.

Omnidirectional treadmill systems are effective platforms that allow unrestricted exploration of a virtual environment.[5] Control parameters for an omnidirectional treadmill were estimated through the computation of velocity, acceleration, and orientation vectors of lower body joints guided by skeleton extraction from RGB-D sensors. Further similar research in remote force estimation including use of 3-dimensional rigid body modeling using Lie groups seems promising.[6] Other research papers continue to report potential solutions to the problem of force estimation[7–9] as they enforce physically consistent estimates about the joint angles and body segment lengths. The use of virtual mannequins to evaluate the performance of Kinect-based pose estimation on artificially produced configurations is 1 intriguing option.[10] Kinect was used in a study on remote ergonomic evaluation of upper limbs.[11] Here, the raw data were combined with an upper limb dynamic model to estimate upper limb forces and torques. The estimates were accurate despite some occlusion.

An approach toward the problem of pose estimation relies on a monocular camera rather than a depth sensor.[12–14] However, this is a harder problem to solve because of the absence of depth information. Furthermore, the general lack of rigid body constraints often leads to undesirable poses generated, and there is also a lack of temporal consistency in most of the models. The general pipeline here is first estimating the 2-dimensional pose information and then lifting it to 3 dimensions using a feed-forward neural network.[15,16]

There are several large data sets available for training such pose networks with either single or multiple people in an image like Human3.6 M[17] or PoseTrack.[18] A model to jointly estimate the motion and actuated forces in the course of a human-object interaction has been proposed.[12] Another paper used human motion in isolation (ie, no object interaction) with a higher degree of dynamic motion involved, and crucially this method does not require hand labeling data, unlike other studies.[13] However, it is expensive. Scott[19] presents a deep learning model to directly estimate foot pressure distribution, while in Shimada's model,[14] a global 3-dimensional pose is first inferred and then used in a physics-based pose optimizer.

Electromyography (EMG) signals can also be used to estimate muscle activation. Studies[20,21] have compared torque and force estimates with activation patterns.[8] Future studies are warranted to better estimate pose can combine EMG and Kinect data. EMG might be more accurate, as it does not have the occlusion problem but requires wearing sensors, whereas computer vision methods are contactless but have other limitations (occlusion).

Remote Biometric Monitoring of Patients to Assess Progress in Home Rehabilitation and Safety

Biometric data from electromyography

Dynamic EMG signals collected from limb muscles during movements can provide valuable physiologic and biomechanical information. This information can be effectively used to augment musculoskeletal (caused by injury or degenerative arthritis) or neurologic (eg, stroke or Parkinson disease) rehabilitation programs for patients living in their homes or a community setting. With the advancement in science and telecommunications technologies, analyzing EMG signals and interacting with the results in real-time is now achievable in telerehabilitation platforms. Virtual reality technology (VR) has shifted the paradigm of interactivity and interests of users by immersing them in virtual worlds. Integrating VR with telerehabilitation has potential to increase the fidelity and reach of rehabilitation.

EMG-enhanced motion analysis is increasingly used in biomechanical and clinical research and for diagnosis and treatment planning.[22–24] Similarly, VR systems are being used in rehabilitation programs[25,26] to design and modify exercise programs, to further evaluate patients' performance, and to investigate and rehabilitate cognitive and perceptual impairments. Although dynamic EMG is widely used in traditional rehabilitation, there have been few studies that have evaluated the relationships between VR-based telerehabilitation and changes in muscle performance. Evaluating changes in structural and functional properties of skeletal muscles during and after telerehabilitation is important. Dynamic EMG can be used in remote assessment of patients to

- Predict changes in the properties of muscles based on time in a rehabilitation program and make training exercises immersive and intelligent, increasing interest and active participation
- Quantify and track the performance levels of muscles

VR-based telerehabilitation exercise programs need to be able to integrate analysis and evaluate real-time EMG data based on 4 key areas:

Creating VR-based telerehabilitation exercise activities

Mine association rules embedded in the EMG data streams with the associated time in telerehabilitation program and a predetermined dose of VR-based exercises to predict changes in muscle function

Content-based similarity searching techniques such as clustering models in the collected EMG data streams to reflect similar characteristics and performance variations in exercise/balance tasks for longitudinal monitoring in telerehabilitation

Real-time performance evaluation/score for lower and/or upper body skeletal muscles based on EMG data streams during telerehabilitation

Creating virtual reality-based telerehabilitation exercise activities: designing and conducting experiments. Evaluating changes in muscle performance during telerehabilitation can be achieved by designing virtual environments (VEs) based on rehabilitative exercises. During these exercises, along with the continuous monitoring of dynamic EMG data streams, several attributes can be extracted for the development of the computational predictive models:

- Kinetic parameters describe what the muscles are doing, particularly the timing of their contractions, the amount of force generated, and the energy of the muscle activity (integral absolute value).[27] Inverse dynamics will be used to derive the torque (moment) and force at each joint based on the movement.
- Correlation parameters represent interstream relationships using quantitative attributes such as the onset of lower/upper-limb joint movements and muscle activity or firing pattern.

Mine association rules embedded in the electromyography data streams with the associated time in telerehabilitation program and a predetermined dose of virtual reality-based exercises to predict changes in muscle function. Time series pattern mining (TSPM) finds correlations or dependencies in the same series or in multiple time series. The main interest lies in discovering the structural and temporal relationships hidden inside these data streams. The dependencies or the association rules can be mined to give information on the frequent co-occurrences of the events in multiple EMG data streams for a given activity.[28] In this work, a fast, 2-stage approach is discussed that suits a real-time VR-based telerehabilitation environment. This approach mines high confidence patterns/rules in multiple EMG time series data where the raw time series is also associated with quantitative attributes. For an illustration, a sample rule was discovered that involves 3 EMG streams during a simple exercise, "Raise Arm," And it reads as follows, "While raising the arms, if the flexor muscle (SF) has an onset of approximately (13/120) sec and extensor muscle (SE) has an onset of approximately (10/120) sec after the start of the activity, the onset of gastrocnemius leg muscle (SG) had been activated (9/120) sec before the start of the activity." This rule reveals the fact that, when a person gets ready to raise his or her arms, just a few seconds before, his or her legs are prepared for the action (to compensate for the center of gravity shift), although the legs may or may not be actively seen to be involved in the actual motion.

The major telerehabilitation exercises tracked by EMG activity from arm and leg muscles form multidimensional time series data streams. It is necessary to discover the structural and temporal relationships or dependencies hidden inside and between these streams in relation to the time in telerehabilitation and a predetermined amount of VR-based exercise stimuli. The challenge here is that the searching space increases as more entities are involved in the mining process. As a result, traditional algorithms for association rule mining may suffer from large computational overheads. This challenge can be overcome by extending existing association rule mining approaches to develop a multistage approach that performs multidimensional association rule mining on heterogeneous streams.[28] As the purpose and goal of every exercise are different, one needs to mine strong association rules for each exercise separately. It should be noted that it is crucial to measure the strength of the association rules by measuring the uncertainty of the rules using 3 factors: support, confidence, and interest.[29]

Content-based similarity searching techniques such as clustering models in the collected electromyogram data streams to reflect similar characteristics and performance variations in exercise/balance tasks for longitudinal monitoring in telerehabilitation. A content-based similarity searching technique for classifying whole-body motion is a well-studied research problem.[30–33] Such similarity searching techniques are important for longitudinal monitoring of motions of patients who are enrolled in the telerehabilitation program so that physicians/therapists can monitor their progress or decline or variations in the movements. Because EMG is nonstationary with a weak signal-to-noise ratio, it requires fuzzy clustering model techniques such as Fuzzy c-means (FCM) to perform content-based similarity searching.[31]

In telerehabilitation, evaluating the variations in similar functional movements is a key element to monitor the progress of rehabilitation. To investigate the sources of the differences in similar motions that drive their separation in clustering, there are approaches[30] based on multivariate analysis of variance. For each of the major telerehabilitation exercises (VR-based or non-VR-based), one can track and collect EMG activity from different arm and leg muscles. By utilizing the previously mentioned computational architecture based on FCM clustering, one can develop clustering models for the exercise tasks such that each cluster represents the exercise based on a leg and arm muscular performance. In evaluating the variations in similar exercises, the specific quantitative attributes can be the time in the telerehabilitation program and a predetermined dose of rehabilitative exercises, so that changes in muscular performance can be correlated with the amount and duration of exercises performed. This will inform a predictive model for determining changes in the properties of skeletal muscles as a function of time in telerehabilitation and a predetermined amount of rehabilitative exercise stimulus in the VR system.

Real-time performance evaluation/score for lower and/or upper body skeletal muscles based on electromyogram data streams during telerehabilitation. Telerehabilitation requires an analytical model to integrate multiple body sensor data streams (ie, dynamic EMG from different muscles). This type of model should be able to visualize the performance difference between individuals for a given functional movement and be able to visualize the performance difference between repetitive trials of the same functional movement for the same individual. In this article, a 2-stage multidimensional factor analysis (MFA) model discusses similar properties.[34] The first stage is the intrastructure stage, wherein the separate analysis is performed on the structure of each EMG data stream based on the corresponding extracted quantitative attributes. These structures are termed as global analysis of the corresponding EMG stream, as they analyzed and interpreted the differences between the participants' performances for the individual EMG stream. The second stage is the interstructure stage that integrates the global analyses of all EMG streams to get the interglobal analysis structure termed as compromise structure that represents the aggregate effect of all EMG sensors on legs and arms for a given activity. This led to generating the performance score for the performed functional movement.

Telerehabilitation exercises require the activation of multiple muscle groups. The most common examples are knee extensors/flexors, adductors, gastrocnemius, tibialis anterior, biceps brachii, and triceps brachii. Hence, models like MFA are well-suited in VR-based telerehabilitation programs. This can benefit patients and caregivers to perform and monitor the exercises. This model can take input in the form of the multidimensional streams from all EMG sensors during exercise and other factors such as duration, amount, and type of exercise stimulus, and report a performance score as an outcome. Besides an overall score of performance, factors that can account for the performance of specific muscle activity can be derived. This information will be useful to understand the relationships between the duration of telerehabilitation, the amount of exercises, muscle changes, and performance levels as patients progress in telerehabilitation.

Utilizing Biometric Data to Better Engage Patients and Customize Their Rehabilitation

Research update on biometric kinematic and kinetic data

Traditionally, surface markers are used for kinematic analysis of movement. Then an inverse kinematics process allows for the decomposition of complex limb motions into joint trajectories. A dynamic model can then be used to determine the joint torques required to produce joint motion using physics-based equations. Classic methods extract 2-dimensional data from the video or picture. However, such data can only provide information from projections and are susceptible to illumination changes. The use of inexpensive and robust depth sensors like Kinect help alleviate this problem (using infrared) with low relative cost. Using telerehabilitation, home exercises can be performed and monitored remotely, using motion capture technology such as Kinect, without the need to wear sensors for tracking. In addition, the movements are less constrained and less susceptible to interference without the need for external sensors and a complicated setup.

However, it is difficult to estimate the forces in play in such movements using noninvasive sensors like Kinect.[8,9,35] The procedure involves capturing the motion of a human body using such a sensor or camera to track the different joints and the associated angles between them across time. The force dynamics equations require the computation of angular velocity and acceleration involved in the calculation of forces and torques acting on the joints through the kinematic equations. Inverse dynamic processes, joint angles are estimated from joint positions.[9] These joint angles are crucial to estimate, as the velocities (and acceleration) can be obtained by numerical differentiation.[9] The Kinect camera captures the motion at a sampling rate of 30 fps, and hence the Δt in numerical differentiation can only go as small as one-thirtieth of a second. With the Kinect camera sensor, the following pipeline followed

Obtaining the skeleton that is tracked; this gives the 3-dimensional orientation and position map for a predetermined set of joints
The skeleton provides the 3-dimensional position of each joint in the camera's reference frame, which can also be used to determine angles using vector products

There is some evidence to support that the forces estimated through such a method are comparable to traditional force plate measurements as reported in this study where they compared these 2 methods during a jump and land procedure.[35] However, this study only considered the upward force acting on the body by tracking the displacement of a spine-based position in a rectilinear manner. This is perhaps only a basic starting point in terms of force and torque estimation. Another thesis work compared the Kinect sensor with a CurieNano sensor (which has an inertial measurement unit) for angular velocity and acceleration measurements across a series of experiments involving the arm and head.[36]

Clinical studies on biometric kinematic and kinetic data

Virtual reality systems. Exergaming in a VR environment has recently been used to improve the outcomes of neurologic rehabilitation for patients with stroke. A randomized controlled trial exploring exergaming using Xbox Kinect system for home-based therapy on mobility and physical performance of 20 stroke survivors showed that patients' functional level after therapy and concentration during the therapy sessions improved compared with the control group.[37] During the Xbox Kinect therapy, patients played games such as boxing or soccer in the Kinect Sports Pack. These results show that the Kinect system can provide an immersive and engaging environment for stroke survivors to perform therapeutic exercises, promoting extrinsic motivation and ease of access without a high cost.

Mystic Isle is a Kinect V2-based system that calculates gait parameters to help stroke patients improve their motor function in lower limbs and was recently modified for upper body movements also.[38] It allows users to interact with a virtual environment through full-body, multiplanar movements and tracks 20 different points distinguishing both gross motor (ie, jumping) and fine motor (ie, hand waving) movements. In this study, 30 participants completed 6 trials on the Kinect system. Each of these trials involved various arm and torso movements to successfully complete the game. The signals representing the joint locations were evaluated for spatiotemporal accuracy using a signal-to-noise ratio (SNR). For arm joints, the signal was observed to be at least 5 times greater than the noise; hand joints had the largest SNRs. However, it was noted that spatial accuracy for lower body joints was lower in the Kinect system than the control. Other measured gait parameters such as extent of reach and hand velocity were evaluated for error by comparison to the Vicon system. The percentage error across all 6 trials was less than 5%, and the values obtained from the Kinect were highly correlated with the Vicon system. These findings support the use of such systems for remote, home-based rehabilitation because of its quality and ease of use.

A study on evaluating joint range of motion (ROM) in patients with hemophilia showed that the Kinect V2 system provides a low-cost, accessible alternative to measuring joint function compared with traditional exercise therapy.[39]

The VERITAS system, a virtual rehabilitation program for patients who have undergone total knee arthroplasty (TKA), consists of a digitally simulated instructional avatar, visual and audible instructions, and video connection capabilities for synchronous visits with physical therapists.[40] The system also has 3-dimensional tracking technology that can quantify pose and motion, thus allowing for the transmission of relevant real-time data points to health professionals. To evaluate VERITAS, 306 participants were randomized into a control and a test group. The intervention group participated in a virtual 12-week physical therapy (PT) program using the VERITAS system, in which patients had 1 weekly synchronous remote visit with their provider and completed the rest of the therapy asynchronously. Overall, virtual PT showed no significant difference from conventional PT and was associated with significantly lower billable costs, and most participants found it easy to use and adhere to.

A VE telerehabilitation system consisting of Polhemus sensors worn on the hand and upper arm to track the motion of the upper limb was studied.[41] Data obtained were synchronously transmitted for the PT to have a real-time view and control over the patient's upper extremity, and complemented by video conferencing so that therapy is a social and rich interactive experience. Twelve stroke patients participated in a 6-week program of 1-h synchronous PT-guided sessions consisting of exercises that involve hand-to-body movements, control of hand, transporting hand away from body, and reciprocal movement. Engaging VE scenes were fitted to each exercise. All subjects showed significant and sustained functional gains, showing that VE motor training can enhance upper extremity motor function in stroke patients.

Wearable sensors

Force-based sensors Zhang and colleagues designed a mechanical instrument that connects a physical therapist to a patient to enable real-time monitoring of physical activity.[42] The therapist operated an upper limb master device while the patient wore an exoskeleton slave device that received sensory input from the master device. Because patients with severe impairments have limited motor function, therapists often need to directly assist their patients with certain movements. With the use of these paired telerehabilitation devices, the therapist can provide partial assistive force remotely. The therapist's master device is thus able to both provide sensory input to the patient and can monitor motion. A prototype of this device was constructed using a motor that provides torque based on weight and an elastic element (SEA) that aids with shock tolerance and stability control. The force-sensing element of the master device measures the detection of the elastic elements in the instrument. On the patient's side, the exoskeleton slave device consists of a motor, a drive pulley, and a torque limiter to ensure that the patient's movements are safe. To evaluate the prototype, multiple experiments were performed to test the output and to calculate the relationship between the deflection of the SEA elements and the amount of sensed force. The root mean squared error of this experiment was 0.004198, which is a relatively low rate of error. The master device was comfortable and easy to wear, and the motion from the therapist's side was effectively transmitted to the patient side.

A kinetic, force-sensing instrument that can monitor lower limb function in environments outside of the laboratory was studied.[43] Such a device could be potentially used for remote rehabilitation. The study explored a wearable shoe insert technology that contained load-sensing elements and motion tracking devices, each containing an accelerometer, a gyroscope, and a magnetometer. The combination of different sensors allows real-time monitoring of dynamic movements and static measures. The devices are constructed with readout electronics and data storage capabilities, allowing for asynchronous transmission and processing of the collected biometric data. The device was evaluated by subjects wearing the insole while walking on different terrains outside of a laboratory environment. The results were evaluated against data collected by subjects walking on force-plated treadmills. This exploratory study obtained gait parameters that are accurate and responsive to different types of movement. Future fully powered trials can evaluate its clinical implementation.

Speed-based sensors A study explored a new method of tracking freezing of gait (FoG) symptoms in patients with Parkinson disease through the use of support vector machines (SVMs) and a tri-axial accelerometer[44] worn at the waist. Twenty-one participants performed 2 tests while wearing the accelerometer in their homes. The data collected from the accelerometer were analyzed and processed through SVM, a machine learning technique that can classify whether a pattern of movement is representative of FoG or not. Using SVM, the model showed a sensitivity of 88.1% and a specificity of 80.1% in accurately detecting FoG types of motion. Personalized SVM models, in which the data processing and classifier methodologies are adjusted to each individual patient, can outperform generic SVM models.

eFisioTrack, a virtual PT system, allows for providers to synchronously monitor patients as they work through their rehabilitation exercises.[45] eFisioTrack uses a modified Wii Remote gamepad that contains an accelerometer that collects values of linear acceleration. The system contains online and offline connectivity modes so that data can be efficiently stored and transmitted to the therapist. To use the eFisioTrack system remotely, the patient first performs a customized movement. The resulting sequence of acceleration values collected from the Wii Remote gamepad is processed by being compared to a prerecorded master standard for each movement. The comparison allows the therapist to evaluate if the patient's movement and repetitions are correctly performed. This system was evaluated in 10 volunteers who participated in a short rehabilitation plan. Testers deliberately performed half of the exercises erroneously to see how the system would respond. The system's average accuracy recognition rate was 99.9%. A participant survey showed that the system was perceived to be accessible and appropriate.

Other sensor-based systems Another study evaluated a hybrid synchronous and asynchronous telerehabilitation program that uses biometric sensors to enhance the process of in-home rehabilitation for TKA-patients.[46] Using 2 connected platforms, the patients performed knee exercises at home while wearing 2 SimpleLink SensorTag sensors on the operated leg, with sensors on the thigh and shin. Patients' progress was tracked by processing the acquired motion data and evaluating the knee angle calculated from the sensors. In the asynchronous mode, data synchronization occurred once Internet connection was available. In the synchronous mode, real-time data synchronization occurs. Preliminary tests of the system revealed high levels of user satisfaction.

Another study evaluated an interactive virtual telerehabilitation (IVT) that tracked biometric data as patients perform exercises after TKA using WAGYRO wireless sensors (2 gyroscopes and a 3-axis accelerometer) that calculate patient's movement trajectories.[47] The system also contained interactive software with a 3-dimensional instructional avatar and a Web portal that allows therapists to record data and modify the rehabilitation exercises over the course of the therapy. Participants who had undergone TKA were randomized into a control and intervention group in a comparative trial. In most exercises, there were no significant differences between the IVT and control groups, showing that IVT-based rehabilitation is not inferior to traditional therapy; however, in quadriceps strength, the IVT group achieved a greater increase compared with the control group. Overall, the results of this study showed that IVT including biometric monitoring was equally effective as conventional therapy, while offering the benefits of accessibility, cost, and the comfort of going through exercises at one's own home.

SUMMARY

Ongoing research and clinical studies suggest that using biometric data, telerehabilitation can be enhanced to perform a more thorough and nuanced remote physical assessment; remotely monitor patients to assess their safety, and progress in home or community-based rehabilitation; and better engage patients to improve their adherence to and participation in their rehabilitation programs thereby driving better outcomes.

CLINICS CARE POINTS

- Synchronous tele-physical assessment using haptics and AR is possible, and a pilot study revealed high concordance between remote and in-person physical examination findings. However, this requires availability of a haptic device and reliable, high-speed, Internet connectivity.

- Asynchronous physical assessment incorporating remote pose estimation principles using contactless cameras such as Kinect and/or EMG-sensor derived data is an intriguing option that requires further study before clinical implementation.
- Remote monitoring and evaluating progress in kinematics and kinetics of movement during telerehabilitation have been studied using biometric sensors such as EMG and other wearable and noncontact sensors based on force and speed. Using such biometric information, type, dosage, and duration of telerehabilitive exercises can be potentially altered over time.
- Telerehabilitation using VR and virtual environments has demonstrated clinical utility and outcome improvement in various rehabilitation populations including stroke, Parkinson disease, knee replacement, degenerative joint disease, and other chronic, disabling conditions.

DISCLOSURE

No commercial or financial conflicts of interest is reported by any authors of this article. Some of the work reported in this article did receive outside support.

REFERENCES

1. Celler BG, Sparks RS. Home telemonitoring of vital signs—technical challenges and future directions. IEEE J Biomed Health Inform 2014;19(1):82–91.
2. Borresen A, Wolfe C, Lin C-K, et al. Usability of an immersive augmented reality based telerehabilitation system with haptics (Artesh) for synchronous remote musculoskeletal examination. Int J Telerehabil 2019;11(1):23.
3. Colombel J, Bonnet V, Daney D, et al. Physically consistent whole-body kinematics assessment based on an RGB-D sensor. Application to simple rehabilitation exercises. Sensors 2020;20(10):2848.
4. Airò Farulla G, Pianu D, Cempini M, et al. Vision-based pose estimation for robot-mediated hand telerehabilitation. Sensors 2016;16(2):208.
5. Ekram MAU. Measurement of control parameters for omnidirectional treadmills using RGBD camera. Masters Dissertation, Ingram School of Engineering - Texas State University; 2017. Available at: https://digital.library.txstate.edu/handle/10877/7722.
6. Brubaker MA, Sigal L, Fleet DJ. Physics-based human motion modeling for people tracking: a short tutorial. Rochester, NY): Image; 2009. p. 1–48.
7. Brubaker MA, Sigal L, Fleet DJ. Estimating contact dynamics. Paper presented at: 2009 IEEE 12th International Conference on Computer Vision. Kyoto, September 29 - October 02, 2009.
8. Matthew RP, Seko S, Bailey J, et al. Estimating sit-to-stand dynamics using a single depth camera. IEEE J Biomed Health Inform 2019;23(6):2592–602.
9. Matthew RP, Seko S, Bajcsy R, et al. Kinematic and kinetic validation of an improved depth camera motion assessment system using rigid bodies. IEEE J Biomed Health Inform 2018;23(4):1784–93.
10. Plantard P, Auvinet E, Pierres A-SL, et al. Pose estimation with a kinect for ergonomic studies: evaluation of the accuracy using a virtual mannequin. Sensors 2015;15(1):1785–803.
11. Plantard P, Muller A, Pontonnier C, et al. Inverse dynamics based on occlusion-resistant Kinect data: is it useable for ergonomics? Int J Ind Ergon 2017;61:71–80.
12. Li Z, Sedlar J, Carpentier J, Laptev I, et al. Estimating 3D motion and forces of person-object interactions from monocular video. Paper presented at: Proceedings

of the IEEE Conference on Computer Vision and Pattern Recognition. Long Beach, June 16 - 20, 2019.

13. Rempe D, Guibas LJ, Hertzmann A, et al. Contact and human dynamics from monocular video. Presented at: European Conference on Computer Vision. Springer, August 23-28, 2020.

14. Shimada S, Golyanik V, Xu W, et al. PhysCap: physically plausible monocular 3D motion capture in real time. ACM Transactions on Graphics (TOG) 39.6 2020;1–16.

15. Habibie I, Xu W, Mehta D, et al. In the wild human pose estimation using explicit 2D features and intermediate 3D representations. Paper presented at: Proceedings of the IEEE Conference on Computer Vision and Pattern Recognition. Long Beach, June 16 - 20, 2019.

16. Martinez J, Hossain R, Romero J, et al. A simple yet effective baseline for 3d human pose estimation. Paper presented at: Proceedings of the IEEE International Conference on Computer Vision. Venice, October 22 - 29, 2017.

17. Ionescu C, Papava D, Olaru V, et al. Human3. 6m: large scale datasets and predictive methods for 3d human sensing in natural environments. IEEE Trans Pattern Anal Mach Intell 2013;36(7):1325–39.

18. Andriluka M, Iqbal U, Insafutdinov E, et al. Posetrack: A benchmark for human pose estimation and tracking. Paper presented at: Proceedings of the IEEE Conference on Computer Vision and Pattern Recognition. Salt Lake City, June 18 - 22, 2018.

19. Scott J, Ravichandran B, Funk C, et al. From image to stability: learning dynamics from human pose. Presented at: European Conference on Computer Vision. Springer, August 23-28, 2020.

20. Clancy EA, Bida O, Rancourt D. Influence of advanced electromyogram (EMG) amplitude processors on EMG-to-torque estimation during constant-posture, force-varying contractions. J Biomech 2006;39(14):2690–8.

21. Lloyd DG, Besier TF. An EMG-driven musculoskeletal model to estimate muscle forces and knee joint moments in vivo. J Biomech 2003;36(6):765–76.

22. Kadaba MP, Ramakrishnan H, Wootten M. Measurement of lower extremity kinematics during level walking. J Orthop Res 1990;8(3):383–92.

23. Perry J, Davids JR. Gait analysis: normal and pathological function. J Pediatr Orthop 1992;12(6):815.

24. Winter D. Concerning the scientific basis for the diagnosis of pathological gait and for rehabilitation protocols. Physiother Can 1985;37(4):245–52.

25. Lewis JA, Deutsch JE, Burdea G. Usability of the remote console for virtual reality telerehabilitation: formative evaluation. Cyberpsychol Behav 2006;9(2):142–7.

26. Trepagnier C. Virtual environments for the investigation and rehabilitation of cognitive and perceptual impairments. NeuroRehabilitation 1999;12:63–72.

27. Zardoshti-Kermani M, Wheeler BC, Badie K, et al. EMG feature evaluation for movement control of upper extremity prostheses. IEEE Trans Rehabil Eng 1995;3(4):324–33.

28. Pradhan GN, Prabhakaran B. Association rule mining in multiple, multidimensional time series medical data. J Healthc Inform Res 2017;1(1):92–118.

29. Zhang C, Zhang S. Association rule mining: models and algorithms. 1st edition. Germany: Springer-Verlag Berlin Heidelberg; 2002.

30. Pradhan GN, Prabhakaran B. Evaluating the effect of local variations in visually-similar motions on the clustering of body sensor features. Proceedings of the 2009 Sixth International Workshop on Wearable and Implantable Body Sensor Networks. Berkeley, June 3 - 5, 2009.

31. Pradhan GN, Prabhakaran B. Clustering of human motions based on feature-level fusion of multiple body sensor data. Proceedings of the 1st ACM International Health Informatics Symposium. Arlington, November 10-11, 2010.

32. Li C, Pradhan G, Zheng S-Q, et al. Indexing of variable length multi-attribute motion data. Paper presented at: Proceedings of the 2nd ACM international workshop on Multimedia databases. Arlington, November 13, 2004.

33. Li C, Zheng SQ, Prabhakaran B. Segmentation and recognition of motion streams by similarity search. ACM Transactions on Multimedia Computing, Communications, and Applications (TOMM) 2007;3(3):16-es.

34. Pradhan GN, Prabhakaran B. Analyzing and visualizing jump performance using wireless body sensors. ACM Trans Embed Comput Syst 2012;11(S2). Article 47.

35. Gaddam SPR, Chippa MK, Sastry S, et al. Estimating forces during exercise activity using non-invasive Kinect camera. Paper presented at: 2015 International Conference on Computational Science and Computational Intelligence (CSCI). Las Vegas, December 7–9, 2015.

36. Yuan Q. The performance of the depth camera in capturing human body motion for biomechanical analysis. Masters Dissertation, School of Engineering Sciences in Chemistry Biotechnology and Health - KTH Royal Institute of Technology; 2018. (URN: urn:nbn:se:kth:diva-235944)

37. Park D-S, Lee D-G, Lee K, et al. Effects of virtual reality training using Xbox Kinect on motor function in stroke survivors: a preliminary study. J Stroke Cerebrovasc Dis 2017;26(10):2313–9.

38. Ma M, Proffitt R, Skubic M. Validation of a Kinect V2 based rehabilitation game. PLoS One 2018;13(8):e0202338.

39. Mateo F, Carrasco JJ, Aguilar-Rodríguez M, et al. Assessment of Kinect V2 for elbow range of motion estimation in people with haemophilia using an angle correction model. Haemophilia 2019;25(3):e165–73.

40. Bettger JP, Green CL, Holmes DN, et al. Effects of virtual exercise rehabilitation in-home therapy compared with traditional care after total knee arthroplasty: VERITAS, a randomized controlled trial. J Bone Joint Surg Am 2020;102(2):101–9.

41. Holden MK, Dyar TA, Dayan-Cimadoro L. Telerehabilitation using a virtual environment improves upper extremity function in patients with stroke. IEEE Trans Neural Syst Rehabil Eng 2007;15(1):36–42.

42. Zhang S, Guo S, Gao B, et al. Design of a novel telerehabilitation system with a force-sensing mechanism. Sensors 2015;15(5):11511–27.

43. Lacirignola J, Weston C, Byrd K, et al. Instrumented footwear inserts: a new tool for measuring forces and biomechanical state changes during dynamic movements. Paper presented at: 2017 IEEE 14th International Conference on Wearable and Implantable Body Sensor Networks (BSN). Eindhoven, May 9 - 12, 2017.

44. Rodríguez-Martín D, Samà A, Pérez-López C, et al. Home detection of freezing of gait using support vector machines through a single waist-worn triaxial accelerometer. PLoS One 2017;12(2):e0171764.

45. Ruiz-Fernandez D, Marín-Alonso O, Soriano-Paya A, et al. eFisioTrack: a telerehabilitation environment based on motion recognition using accelerometry. ScientificWorldJournal 2014;2014:495391.

46. Naeemabadi M, Dinesen B, Andersen OK, et al. Developing a telerehabilitation programme for postoperative recovery from knee surgery: specifications and requirements. BMJ Health Care Inform 2019;26(1):e000022.

47. Piqueras M, Marco E, Coll M, et al. Effectiveness of an interactive virtual telerehabilitation system in patients after total knee arthroplasty: a randomized controlled trial. J Rehabil Med 2013;45(4):392–6.

Innovative Approaches to Delivering Telehealth

Mary E. Matsumoto, MD[a,b,*], Grace C. Wilske, OTR/L[a], Rebecca Tapia, MD[c,d]

KEYWORDS

- Telerehabilitation • Telehealth • Technology • Locations of care

KEY POINTS

- Approaches to telerehabilitation differ based on patient needs and access to technology, clinical judgment of provider, ongoing advances in technology, and existing infrastructure.
- Telerehabilitation is delivered across multiple settings and in multiple formats.
- Delivering care to different locations and through use of different technologies can help overcome barriers, improve delivery of care, and customize care to the patient's needs.
- Use of telerehabilitation can bridge the gap to provide care when conditions prevent face-to-face care, whether that be rural location or global pandemic.
- Increased adoption of telerehabilitation during the COVID-19 pandemic has forced rapid innovation with potential to expand access, improve interdisciplinary collaboration, and customize patient-centered evaluations to an unprecedented degree.

Telerehabilitation is an evolving modality for the delivery of rehabilitation care. It allows for innovative approaches for delivery of care in different locations and using different technology based on the patient's needs, clinical judgment of the provider, access to technology, and existing infrastructure of the health care system. Technology continues to evolve to expand the scope of care that can be provided over telerehabilitation, particularly to home. The COVID-19 pandemic has led to accelerated adoption of telerehabilitation with potential to expand access, improve interdisciplinary collaboration, and customize patient-centered care to an unprecedented degree.

INTRODUCTION

Telerehabilitation is the remote delivery of rehabilitation services via telecommunications technologies including the telephone, the Internet, and videoconference communication. In recent years, the delivery of rehabilitation services through telehealth has

a Department of Physical Medicine and Rehabilitation, Minneapolis VA Health Care System, 1 Veterans Drive, Mail Stop 117, Minneapolis, MN 55417, USA; b Department of Rehabilitation Medicine, University of Minnesota, Minneapolis, MN, USA; c South Texas Veterans Healthcare System, 7400 Merton Minter Boulevard, San Antonio, TX 78229, USA; d Department of Rehabilitation Medicine, UT Health San Antonio, San Antonio, TX, USA
* Corresponding author. Department of Physical Medicine and Rehabilitation, Minneapolis VA Health Care System, 1 Veterans Drive, Mail Stop 117, Minneapolis, MN 55417.
E-mail address: Mary.Matsumoto@va.gov

Phys Med Rehabil Clin N Am 32 (2021) 451–465
https://doi.org/10.1016/j.pmr.2020.12.008
1047-9651/21/Published by Elsevier Inc.
pmr.theclinics.com

increased.[1] In addition to increased provision of services via telehealth, the scope of services provided through this modality has also expanded with advances in technology.[2] Patients now have more access to connect using the Internet or Wi-Fi and their own personal devices, such as smart phones, tablets, or computers.[3,4] Most recently, the novel coronavirus pandemic (COVID-19) has led to the rapid adoption of telehealth in efforts to minimize exposures for patients and health care workers.[5,6]

Telerehabilitation has seen increased adoption for many reasons. Some benefits are decreased travel time and time away from work or home; increased access to specialty care, especially for patients in rural areas; improved continuity of care; and decreased cost.[2,7,8] Several studies show high patient satisfaction with telerehabilitation.[9-11] In populations with mobility impairments, such as spinal cord injury, multiple sclerosis, or amyotrophic lateral sclerosis, it has the advantage of easier access to care: avoiding transportation barriers, facilitating caregiver or family participation, and allowing for evaluation of the patient in their home environment.[12-14] From a systems and practice perspective, it also has certain advantages, such as decreasing overhead, allowing specialists to cover a larger geographic area without adding travel time, and increasing flexibility for coverage during provider absence.

Drawbacks to telerehabilitation from a clinical perspective are limitations in physical examination and technical challenges.[9,10] Administrative barriers to the use of telehealth have traditionally been payment and regulatory structures, state licensing, credentialing, and data protection.[2] Since the start of the COVID-19 pandemic, some of these have been removed with Centers for Medicare & Medicaid Services expanding reimbursement for telehealth services and permitting use of everyday communication technologies.[15,16]

Through innovative delivery of rehabilitation services, telerehabilitation provides a tool that was previously not available to meet health care challenges, expand access, improve interdisciplinary collaboration, and customize patient-centered evaluations to an unprecedented degree. Furthermore, creative approaches and new technologies can also be used to mitigate some of the traditional challenges of telemedicine. This article focuses on two approaches that can be used in the delivery of telehealth to customize care to the patient's needs. The first is the location where care is delivered over telehealth. The second is the use of different technologies.

LOCATIONS AND COMMUNITY PARTNERSHIPS

One tool provided by telerehabilitation is the ability to see the patient in a variety of locations. Previously, a clinic visit could only occur in the clinic or by the provider traveling to the patient's home. Through the use of telerehabilitation, a provider can see a patient at a hospital, at a clinic, at a community location, or in the home, whatever location is most appropriate based on the most convenient location for the patient, the goals of the visit, and the technology available to connect.

This can help improve access for populations for whom this is a challenge, such as rural patients, patients with mobility issues, and institutionalized patients. It also allows specialists to see patients over a greater geographic area than could otherwise be accomplished.

Choice of location can also help to minimize barriers to telerehabilitation. For instance, if a patient is not be able to connect because of lack of Internet or a device, conducting the visit at a nearby community location may provide resources to overcome this barrier. If a physical examination is needed, the visit can be conducted at a location with a skilled provider, such as a nurse or a therapist to assist with this.

Home

One of the most critical benefits of video telehealth in the physical medicine and rehabilitation (PM&R) continuum is the ability to assess the patient in their native home environment. There are several components of the virtual modality that can add to the evaluation and assessment and inform the eventual treatment plan.

Visual inspection of environment

The wholistic picture of a patient comes to life when interfacing with them in their home setting. This interaction can answer questions in far greater detail than collecting a verbal history in the clinic setting. Is the area organized or chaotic? What does their pill box or medication management look like? Does the area seem safe and clean? How is the lighting? If they use durable medical equipment, such as a rollator, do they have it nearby if indicated for safety or is it over in the corner? Are there any functionally relevant tasks that could be viewed through telehealth to inform the treatment plan or evaluate response to intervention, such as navigating a tight doorway with the new wheelchair or pulling open a kitchen drawer after treatment of upper extremity spasticity? A full home evaluation can be conducted via telehealth technology (discussed later). The information gathered is inherently customized and relevant because the patient is being seen in the environment in which they spend the most time with the most relevant challenges or barriers in daily life.

Interpersonal interactions and caregiver participation

One of the more surprising benefits of telehealth technology is the opportunity to witness real-time interpersonal interactions, which is particularly helpful for patient populations with communication or behavioral disorders. This can happen organically, such as watching a patient interact with their spouse, caregiver, or child during the visit. This could also be a specific function of the examination in which the patient is asked to advocate for their needs in some way, such as explaining to a caregiver what they need retrieved from an upstairs bathroom. There are also instances where a caregiver would not be able to attend a clinic visit because of obligations, such as work or childcare, making a virtual visit a better option for them to actively participate. A systematic review of the use of telehealth to provide support and training to caregivers of persons with traumatic brain injury showed positive findings in terms of feasibility, user satisfaction, and preliminary explorations of effectiveness.[17]

Other considerations

When evaluating a patient in clinic, especially those with mobility or neurologic deficits who are not driving independently, there is potential for interference in the presentation related solely to the transportation effort expended to get from home to clinic. The fatigue related to transportation arrangements, car transfers, extended duration seated in the vehicle, and arriving at the correct clinic location at the correct time is burdensome and contributes to a less accurate picture of how the patient is experiencing their day-to-day life in their home or local community. For example, a 2015 study showed significantly higher energy expenditure for overground walking in stroke patients compared with healthy control subjects.[18] This is in addition to the potential cost savings of travel, improved customer satisfaction, and most importantly improved access for the patient, not to mention the space and resource savings for the physical clinic location. Telehealth services into the home quickly became a critical lifeline for care during the COVID-19 pandemic with the emphasis on reducing community contacts and travel.[19] It allowed patients to continue to receive needed care and prevent complications, as discussed in a pilot study of an exercise program delivered over telehealth to older adults living at home to alleviate the negative effects of quarantine and social distancing and to prevent functional decline.[20] The same potential benefit could be applied in other natural disasters, such as extreme weather, or physical barriers to care including road construction or lack of safe and affordable transportation.[21] Overall, developing avenues for patients to receive virtual care in the home improves access for populations that may already face multiple barriers to care.

Groups

There are many areas where rehabilitation services are more appropriate to be conducted in a group setting, such as support groups, exercise groups, and education classes. Group care can also be delivered over telehealth; interestingly, the first documented use of telehealth was to provide group therapy in 1959.[22] Recent studies have suggested similar outcomes and high participant satisfaction for video teleconference groups compared with in-person.[23,24] Another promising application for delivery of rehabilitation services via group telehealth is in complimentary and integrative health approaches, such as tai chi and yoga.[25] Allowing a virtual option may make groups or classes more accessible to patients, and in the instance of caregivers who provide 24/7 in-home care this may be the only option available to them to receive support. The configuration and administration of group care varies greatly between platforms, but in most instances, it is beneficial to have the flexibility to selectively mute or unmute participants to ensure that the communication is understandable and not chaotic. An important consideration for the group setting is to evaluate impact on patient privacy and have policies, procedures, and consents in place for participants to fully understand the process.

Outpatient

Virtual connections between clinics is helpful to expand access to specialty care for several reasons. It can allow a patient to connect virtually to a specialist at a tertiary care center without having to travel there, which is particularly beneficial in populations with disabilities, such as multiple sclerosis and amyotrophic lateral sclerosis.[13,14] The Department of Veterans Affairs (VA) has leveraged this through its Polytrauma and Amputation Systems of Care where traumatic brain injury and amputation rehabilitation specialists at a regional hub are able to evaluate patients at smaller VA facilities where that specialty care may not be available.[22] Moreover, this approach can also allow a specialist to be present virtually to provide training and instruction to a generalist at the remote site, as in the assistive technology protocol described by Schein and coworkers[26] wherein a therapist with expertise in wheelchair and seating joins a remote clinic virtually with a generalist therapist. Virtual care between clinics may also help cover gaps in coverage because of prolonged absence of a provider at one clinic, which can be covered by a provider located at a different clinic.

Outpatient care in rehabilitation often involves multidisciplinary, team-based care. This has traditionally occurred in person; however, there is a role for virtual options to enhance access and communication. Virtual conferencing can help bring together rehabilitation staff at multiple locations and facilitate integration of the patient and caregiver through telehealth. Scholten and colleagues[22] describe an interdisciplinary teleamputee clinic including physician, prosthetist, and physical therapist where different members of the team may be physically present with the patient, whereas others are joining virtually.

From a technology standpoint, it is not unusual for patients in remote or rural settings to not have Internet access stable enough to complete a video visit, so having access at a satellite clinic to receive care from the hub or main clinic helps bridge this gap. In other instances, it is beneficial for a patient to report to their local clinic area to complete the video visit and then also be able to complete parts of the plan, such as imaging or laboratory work, before returning home.

Community Locations

With telerehabilitation, patients can connect in locations in their community such as

- Prosthetist's office
- Therapist's office (ie, physical therapist, occupational therapist, speech language pathologist)
- Nursing home
- Durable medical equipment vendor

There are several benefits to community locations. One is that they often require less travel than to the hospital or clinic. Another is that there may be a skilled facilitator there to assist with the visit and performing the physical examination, such as a nurse, therapist, or prosthetist. Additionally, this can help with coordination of care if the patient is receiving part of their care at that location. For instance, if the physiatrist sees the patient at the physical therapist's office, the therapist can report on progress and is also present to hear any recommendations or changes in plan of care from the physiatrist during the visit. As part of its teleamputation rehabilitation program, the VA Amputation System of Care is doing virtual visits to evaluate a patient in the office of their prosthetist.[22]

Another example is seeing a patient at a nursing home where the nursing home staff can report on how the patient is doing and the physiatrist can more efficiently and reliably communicate the plan of care to them. Forducey and coworkers[27] describe a case where a physical therapist from a metropolitan rehabilitation center connected virtually to a nursing home more than 100 miles away to provide neurodevelopmental treatment for a patient and to mentor staff. Finally, if the patient is not able to connect because of lack of Internet or video device, the facilitator at the community location can assist.

The benefit of using community locations to connect to patients and to bridge the digital divide is evidenced by the ATLAS Project (Accessing Telehealth through Local Area Stations), which was launched by the VA to allow Veterans to connect to medical appointments in locations closer to home while providing Internet access and technology to connect. These locations include Walmart, Phillips, The American Legion, and Veterans of Foreign Wars.[28]

Inpatient

The use of telemedicine for patients in the inpatient location can facilitate care in several ways. One novel use of telerehabilitation in the inpatient setting is to complete home safety evaluations before discharge, which has been shown to decrease falls in those with high risk.[29] This has many benefits for the patient, including preventing delays in discharge, allowing the patient in the hospital to participate in the evaluation, and improving continuity by allowing the treating inpatient therapist to do the evaluation. For the health care system, it also has tremendous advantages in terms of decreasing the travel time of the therapist and thereby increasing productivity. One study found that there was a 50% increase in home visits before discharge with no increase in staffing with the implementation of telehealth home safety evaluations.[30]

Other uses of telerehabilitation in the inpatient setting are to facilitate participation of family and caregivers. One example is with family meetings or care conferences. Sometimes, it is difficult for family members to travel to the hospital to attend these during the workday. Telerehabilitation provides the ability to connect from their home or place of work more conveniently. A recent study of use of telehealth for family conference in palliative care found that they were able to connect successfully and were highly rated by families.[31] It also allows more flexibility and opportunities for family and caregiver education and training. During the current COVID pandemic, telehealth has been key in allowing this care to continue during a time when visitors were restricted from coming to the hospital.

Finally, telerehabilitation provides an opportunity for continuity of care and improved follow-up and transition of care after discharge. A therapist who was seeing a patient in the hospital can do a post-discharge follow-up to see them in the home via telerehabilitation to follow-up on home exercise program or home accessibility and equipment. One study showed decreased falls with implementation of a multidisciplinary telerehabilitation to home program after discharge in older adults.[32]

TECHNOLOGY

In this day in age we are surrounded by technology, which has transformed our day-to-day lives, our homes, our workplaces, and now more than ever, the medical field. Advances in technology have propelled the growth of telehealth, first with the development of videoconferencing technology, then with widespread access to the Internet and smartphones, and now becoming ever more sophisticated with virtual reality and smart home technology. It is being used to deliver care more and more into the home. The advent of the COVID-19 pandemic has led to health care being delivered virtually at an all-time high.[33] Availability and promotion of telehealth services and advancements of technology has played a prominent role in delivering care through telehealth.[34]

Digital Divide

Widespread access to Internet and camera devices have facilitated the adoption of telehealth. However, this access is not universal. Some populations, such as in rural areas and in older patients, still face challenges connecting. Although 90% of Americans have access to Internet and 81% have a smart phone, these numbers decrease to 85% and 71%, respectively, in rural areas.[35] One study showed that older, rural Veterans had less access to Internet and willingness to connect over telehealth.[36]

To bridge this divide, the Federal Communications Commission created the Lifeline program in 1985, which recently was updated in 2016 to help make communications services more affordable for low-income consumers.[37] It provides subscribers a discount on monthly telehealth phone service, broadband Internet service, or bundled voice-broadband packages from participating wireline or wireless providers. The federal government has an equipment loan program within the VA, which provides Veterans with loaner iPads with cellular data to connect to virtual visits when they do not have other means available.[38]

Digital Platforms

To deliver care virtually, each provider needs to use a digital telehealth platform. There are many companies that are developing digital telehealth platforms or private companies that use proprietary software. Some platforms are HIPAA compliant. During the COVID-19 national emergency, covered health care providers may use popular and accessible applications that allow for video calls without risk that the Office for Civil Rights would penalize the provider for noncompliance with HIPAA Rules.[16] A few samples of digital platforms include Doxy.me, thera-LINK, TheraNest, Zoom,

SimplePractice, Vsee, GoToMeeting, UpDox, and eVisit. The federal government uses a technology platform called VA Video Connect. Many entities have persevered in establishing virtual care and those who have had a digital platform structure have been able to more rapidly mobilize care through telehealth.

Electronic Medical Records

Technology improvements have opened the path to enhance features and interactivity for patients while accessing their own medical records within the electronic medical record. Within this type of system, the patient and their caregivers can engage in managing their health care by communicating with their providers, scheduling appointments, and accessing health education through medical libraries. Engaged patients and their caregivers can even access their virtual visits through this portal.

Health Coaching Applications

There are many technology tools that have been developed to provide support, coaching, and accountability in a remote manner. Several apps are designed to have an automated text messaging program that sends updates, reminders, and health information to patients. Patients can choose to interact with the app program and view charts and graphs of health data they submitted. Patients who engage with these apps have endorsed improved follow through with their cares by simply engaging with the program, which can remind them of their appointments, to take their daily weights or to complete their relaxation exercises, for example.[39]

Peripheral Devices

One noted drawback to telerehabilitation in the past was the inability to collect data, such as vital signs during the visit. Technology has evolved to overcome that barrier with the development of peripheral devices, such as pulse oximeter, blood pressure cuff, and scale, which can be provided to the patient at home and transmit data via Bluetooth. Wootton and colleagues[40] present a case study of providing pulmonary rehabilitation to patients with COVID-19 through telehealth to home and using pulse oximetry to monitor heart rate and oxygen saturation during activity. In another study regarding pulmonary rehabilitation, remote measurement of pulse oximetry data during a session was feasible and valid when compared with face-to-face methods.[41] Home-based cardiac rehabilitation uses remote heart rate monitoring.[42]

Wearable Technology

Moving beyond peripheral devices, wearable technology and sensors, such as smart watches, can be worn throughout the day and collect data on specific parameters. Advances in technology have microsized some components that now allow sensors to be small enough to be embedded in equipment to track movements with clinical applications including remote monitoring, mobile health, and expanded health metrics.[43] Therapists can provide feedback to patients when they are meeting their exercise parameters, and give real time feedback during sessions. Some of these sensors are integrated into equipment or robotics to allow for active or passive motions. Wearable technology can be used to collect data regarding the effectiveness of treatment protocols with the potential to transform the field of rehabilitation.

Remote Home Monitoring

Remote home monitoring, which combines the use of peripheral devices, wearable technology, and telehealth visits, has been of growing interest in developing new models of health care delivery, which has only been accelerated by the COVID-19 pandemic.[44] In addition to synchronous and asynchronous virtual care, home telemonitoring has been used widely for a long time. For patients with chronic conditions that need daily monitoring, such as chronic obstructive pulmonary disease, diabetes, and heart failure, it was normal to call in daily to provide updates, such as vitals, weights, and blood sugars to get feedback from a health care professional. With remote home monitoring, this information and more can be sent securely and automatically. Patients may then have telephone or video visits with their providers to discuss their status and any changes to the plan of care, all while never having to leave the home.

Provider Tools

As providers are shifting their practices from in-person to virtual visits, efforts to improve practices keep emerging as creative tools are being developed for delivering care. In working to improve the practice of telerehabilitation wheeled mobility assessment, the simple act of taking measurements has been challenging and unreliable depending who is on the other end with the patient. A novel means of obtaining an objective and reliable measurement is being developed through use of an application. This is an example of how technological innovations can open the door to providing care over telehealth that was formerly not feasible.

Virtual Reality

As technology improves, another tool within rehabilitation has been the use of virtual reality to assist in with multiple diagnoses to aide in treatment and participation.[45–48] With the immersive quality of virtual reality, the patient can have fun and engage in environments to simulate activities that otherwise would require time to set up or be difficult to access, such as cooking activities, street safety, and community outings. Virtual reality can assist in assessing range of motion, posture, balance, coordination, strength, endurance, and even be a great motivator because of the game feel. There already exists a large library of virtual reality applications, each used for different needs. Each activity can be tracked and monitored for progress and improvements over time.

Store and Forward

Although much of virtual care is synchronous, where a provider connects with a patient at the same time, there are opportunities for asynchronous care. Use of store and forward technologies is common in such practices as dermatology and radiology, but it also has a role in rehabilitation care. Patients may take an image or a video and send it to their provider to review. This is valuable if the patient does not have stable Internet access at home to complete a video visit or if they would need assistance to capture certain images that is not available during the visit. For example, a patient could send a video of their gait taken by their spouse who is not home during the day to help with a video visit. Another promising area for store and forward is in home safety evaluations where the patient can send pictures of the house including measurements based on instructions from the provider. This also has the potential to save the provider time.

CASE STUDIES
Case Study: Virtual Inpatient Occupational Therapy Home Evaluation

A 74-year-old woman was admitted to inpatient rehabilitation following a stroke. The treating occupational therapist requested that her spouse provide a 30-second video of her bathroom using a store and forward application. The therapist described the features he wanted to see and asked to have measurements of the doorway and bathtub included. He later reviewed this video with the patient during a subsequent therapy session and the patient provided insight into her routines. The therapist was able to order a tub bench, a toilet frame, and grab bars for the patient based on his assessment of her current function. He described to the spouse how to install them. The spouse took the equipment home before discharge and installed it. He provided a second video via the store and forward application that the therapist reviewed to determine correct installation. After the patient was discharged home, the patient took a video with the assistance of the spouse showing how she was able to transfer onto the toilet and into the tub using the equipment. After reviewing this video, the therapist made the decision that she could also benefit from a toilet riser. He called the patient and her spouse to tell them that he would mail this to them and they should send another video after it was installed so he could make sure that it was working for her.

Using store and forward, a home safety evaluation was able to be completed before discharge to facilitate discharge planning. In the past, obtaining accurate history and home environment information was difficult when patients were admitted in the hospital. Memory, stress, communication, and recalling details have impacted the accuracy of information provided to the health care team by the patient and caregiver.

The introduction of telerehabilitation to optimize care and gather information has been pivotal in delivering efficient, quality care and expediting discharge planning. The clinician can request specific videos of various areas of the home to review later during therapy with the patient. The patient can provide input to her routines or other details that can contribute to equipment recommendations or plans in treatment. It is important to find a caregiver, family member, friend, or neighbor who is able to take the videos or pictures and transmit them and provide education to them on how to take accurate videos that provide the full view of the space with any necessary measurements. Oftentimes, there are delays in care while waiting for this information to find out what equipment is needed or even if the home is feasible for discharge, so it is best to start the process soon after admission. As the clinician is working with the patient on her progress, the vision of the discharge environment is valuable information obtained at the beginning while the discharge placement is determined. This addition of using virtual technology to enhance to care has become a best practice and shared widely across occupational therapy (OT) departments everywhere.

Case Study: Telerehabilitation Wheeled Mobility Evaluation at a Nursing Home

An 84-year-old woman with Alzheimer dementia residing at a nursing home in a rural town was having issues with her positioning in her standard manual wheelchair. She could not tolerate sitting upright for more than 30 minutes. This was leading to falls when she tried to get out of the wheelchair because of discomfort. She was also beginning to develop a sacral pressure wound. The nursing home therapist believed she needed a custom wheelchair and cushion, but was not sure what to order. He contacted the wheelchair clinic at the university hospital. However, this clinic was 3 hours away and the patient would need someone to accompany her to assist with transferring in and out of the van and to assist her with toileting. These barriers were prohibitive to scheduling this in-person appointment. Because of this, a virtual appointment was scheduled with patient and her treating therapist connecting with the team from the wheelchair clinic. The therapist was able to provide information about the patient's function, transfers, and issues with her current wheelchair. Under the instruction of the team at the wheelchair clinic, he was able to do a mat evaluation and take measurements. The physiatrist placed an order for a custom tilt-in-space manual wheelchair and cushion. This was delivered to the patient at the nursing home by a local durable medical equipment vendor. There was also a follow-up virtual appointment with the vendor joining. The team evaluated the patient's position in the wheelchair and transfers into and out of the wheelchair assisted by the therapist. Some adjustments to the wheelchair were requested, which the vendor was able to make during the appointment. Following the delivery of this wheelchair, the patient was able to tolerate sitting in the chair for 3 hours and use the tilt-in-space function for pressure relief with improvement in skin issues. She also did not have further falls. Through doing these appointments over telerehabilitation, the patient saved more than 21 hours and more than 1100 miles of travel, not to mention the cost of travel for her and an attendant.

Providing specialized wheelchair and seating services at nursing homes over telehealth is an innovative practice that involves multiple team players including specialized therapists, third-party vendors to deliver equipment, community therapists at nursing homes, patients, and their family and caregivers. This virtual process can take place over several visits to (1) to assess the patient, (2) trial demo equipment, (3) continued trialing and fitting of equipment, (4) delivery of the equipment, and (5) follow-up visit 3 weeks after delivery and as needed. Training and education for nursing home staff, family, and caregivers is also included in these visits. It has many potential benefits including reducing the time, cost, and burden of travel; evaluating the patient in their home environment; improving education and training for caregivers; and providing improved follow-up. For instance, the patient would likely not have traveled more than 3 hours for an in-person follow-up after the delivery of the wheelchair, but this was done over telerehabilitation with less burden and cost to the patient.

Case Study: Using Telerehabilitation During COVID-19 Pandemic

A 56 year-old previously independent man presented to the emergency room for fatigue and difficulty breathing, was found to be positive for COVID-19, and was admitted to an acute medicine service for supplemental oxygen and monitoring. The patient experienced a deterioration in clinical status on Day 5 of admission and was transferred to the intensive care unit for more aggressive care including intubation. He remained in the intensive care unit care for 8 days until stabilizing and transferring back to the acute medicine service. The patient was discharged home on Hospital Day 19 with recommendations for home health services including physical therapy and OT. He was scheduled for a virtual follow-up appointment with a local PM&R provider on discharge. He was set up with a remote home monitoring system to track daily vital signs given potential for complications.

Video connection was established on the day of appointment and the patient along with his spouse were interviewed by the PM&R provider and case manager. The patient detailed current functional challenges and discussed focus areas being addressed through home health therapy. Education was provided regarding energy conservation and importance of a home exercise program with the goal of gradual strengthening and endurance. To improve continuity of care, the patient agreed to conduct the next follow-up visit during a home health therapy session.

At the next virtual follow-up visit, the PM&R provider and case manager collaborated with the patient and home health therapist regarding progress and challenges encountered in the therapy course. Ambulation was jointly observed by the physician and on-site therapist. Vital signs were monitored during therapy. It was determined that the patient would benefit from a custom ankle-foot orthosis to aid in safe ambulation, so orders were placed with ongoing follow-up established.

Before the use of virtual in-home follow-up services, it is likely that this patient would have reported to a physical clinic location for care that could have exposed him to repeat infection or other complications. The opportunity for collaboration with the home health therapy team would be limited to telephone or written communication. Even outside of a pandemic situation, virtual in-home follow-up visits stands to improve multiple aspects of care including access, continuity, and interdisciplinary communication.

Case Study: Increasing Access to Specialty Care Through Telerehabilitation

A 42-year-old man with history of traumatic right transradial amputation living in rural North Dakota was evaluated in a local amputation rehabilitation clinic over telerehabilitation with a physiatrist specializing in amputation rehabilitation at a regional center, which was more than 650 miles away. Through the use of telerehabilitation, this physiatrist was able to cover amputation rehabilitation clinics within the health system throughout the region including rural areas. During this initial visit, a prosthesis was prescribed to be made at a local prosthetist's office and OT was ordered for evaluation for adaptive equipment and treatment of phantom limb pain using desensitization techniques and mirror therapy.

The patient also lived at a distance of 120 miles from his local clinic and was working full-time. He was able to have therapy visits over telerehabilitation using his personal device to work on residual limb desensitization during his lunch breaks in his private office. He did not have a mirror at work to do mirror therapy, so the therapist provided education about an application that he could download on his smartphone, which would reflect the image of his left hand and forearm on the screen, allowing him to practice mirror therapy during breaks at work.

He was also able to have OT sessions in his home environment working on his activities of daily living. He had difficulty buttoning his shirt, tying his shoes, and cutting food. The appropriate one-handed and adaptive equipment was ordered for him. He was also able to join the Amputee Support Group virtually, which he otherwise would not have been able to participate in because of distance and work schedule.

A follow-up visit was conducted at his local prosthetist's office connecting with the physiatrist and therapist over telerehabilitation. An issue with his harness was identified during the visit and the prosthetist and physiatrist agreed on a change in his prescription to improve his comfort. The local occupational therapist did not have experience in upper extremity prosthetic training, so the occupational therapist at the regional center with this expertise planned to join their initial sessions virtually to assist.

After several in-person sessions, the patient completed his training doing virtual sessions at his home. This allowed him to work on real-life tasks in his home environment, such as working in his workshop and garden. Based on this evaluation, the occupational therapist recommended ordering some activity-specific terminal devices.

During one therapy visit, the patient was having difficulty operating his prosthesis. The prosthetist joined virtually and suggested adjusting one of the straps on his harness, which resolved the issue. This saved him a 2-hour trip to see his prosthetist in-person.

Before the use of telerehabilitation, this patient would have had to choose between traveling to a clinic or hospital that had amputation rehabilitation specialty care and staying there for his initial prosthetic fabrication and training. He would have been separated from his family and had to take time off work. However, through the use of telerehabilitation services, he was able to receive care from an interdisciplinary amputation rehabilitation specialty team in collaboration with this local prosthetist and therapist. He was able to remain at home and continue work. Moreover, he was able to have part of his treatment in his home environment, which helped with providing him with the right equipment and prosthetic componentry, as well as his carryover after training was complete.

SUMMARY

Telerehabilitation is an evolving modality for the delivery of rehabilitation care. It allows for innovative approaches for delivery of care in different locations and using different technology based on the patient's needs, the goals of the visit, clinical judgment of the provider, access to technology, and existing infrastructure of the health care system. Technology continues to evolve to expand the scope of care that can be provided over telerehabilitation, particularly to home. The COVID-19 pandemic has led to accelerated adoption of telerehabilitation; improvements in infrastructure; removal of traditional barriers; and ongoing innovation with potential to expand access, improve interdisciplinary collaboration, and customize patient-centered care to an unprecedented degree.

CLINICS CARE POINTS

- When deciding in what location to see a patient over telehealth, consider what kind of examination is needed and who will be available to assist with the evaluation (ie, if you need to see the patient's gait, will there be someone there to hold the camera?).
- If a patient lacks the technology to connect via telehealth themselves, consider what other options might be available to bridge the digital divide, such as assistance of a family member, caregiver, neighbor, or home health provider or use of a community location.
- Peripheral devices and wearable technology are used to gather physical examination information, such as vital signs that would otherwise not be available in the telehealth format.
- During the COVID-19 pandemic, providing care into the home when possible is the preferred option to reduce exposures for patients and health care workers.

DISCLOSURE

The authors have nothing to disclose.

REFERENCES

1. Cowper-Ripley DC, Jia H, Wang X, et al. Trends in VA telerehabilitation patients and encounters over time and by rurality. Fed Pract 2019;36(3):122–8.
2. Dorsey ER, Topol EJ. State of telehealth. N Engl J Med 2016;375(14):1400.
3. Mobile Fact Sheet. Available at: https://www.pewresearch.org/internet/fact-sheet/mobile/. Accessed November 15, 2020.
4. Internet/Broadband Fact Sheet. Available at: https://www.pewresearch.org/internet/fact-sheet/internet-broadband/. Accessed November 15, 2020.
5. VA Video Connect Visits Increase 1,000% During COVID-19 Pandemic. VA Office of Connected Care. Available at: https://connectedcare.va.gov/whats-new/

technology/va-video-connect-visits-increase-1000-during-covid-19-pandemic. Accessed November 29, 2020.

6. Mann DM, Chen J, Chunara R, et al. COVID-19 transforms health care through telemedicine: evidence from the field. J Am Med Inform Assoc 2020;27(7): 1132–5.

7. Russo JE, McCool RR, Davies L. VA telemedicine: an analysis of cost and time savings. Telemed J E Health 2016;22(3):209–15.

8. Ihrig C. Travel cost savings and practicality for low-vision telerehabilitation. Telemed J E Health 2019;25(7):649–54.

9. Tenforde AS, Iaccarino MA, Borgstrom H, et al. Telemedicine during COVID-19 for outpatient sports and musculoskeletal medicine physicians. PM R 2020; 12(9):926–32.

10. Tenforde AS, Borgstrom H, Polich G, et al. Outpatient physical, occupational, and speech therapy synchronous telemedicine: a survey study of patient satisfaction with virtual visits during the COVID-19 pandemic. Am J Phys Med Rehabil 2020; 99(11):977–81.

11. Castaneda G. Examining patient and caregiver telehealth satisfaction in the Veterans Health Administration. ATA 2020 Telehealth Virtual Conference & Expo; June 22-26, 2020.

12. Galea M, Tumminia J, Garback LM. Telerehabilitation in spinal cord injury persons: a novel approach. Telemed J E Health 2006;12(2):160–2.

13. Hatzakis M Jr, Haselkorn J, Williams R, et al. Telemedicine and the delivery of health services to veterans with multiple sclerosis. J Rehabil Res Dev 2003; 40(3):265–82.

14. Selkirk SM, Washington MO, McClellan F, et al. Delivering tertiary centre specialty care to ALS patients via telemedicine: a retrospective cohort analysis. Amyotroph Lateral Scler Frontotemporal Degener 2017;18(5–6):324–32.

15. Policy changes during the COVID-19 Public Health Emergency Health Resources and Services Administration. Available at: https://www.telehealth.hhs.gov/ providers/policy-changes-during-the-covid-19-public-health-emergency/. Accessed November 14, 2020.

16. Notification of Enforcement Discretion for Telehealth Remote Communications During the COVID-19 Nationwide Public Health Emergency. U.S. Department of Health and Human Services. Available at: https://www.hhs.gov/hipaa/for-professionals/special-topics/emergency-preparedness/notification-enforcement-discretion-telehealth/index.html. Accessed November 14, 2020.

17. Rietdijk R, Togher L, Power E. Supporting family members of people with traumatic brain injury using telehealth: a systematic review. J Rehabil Med 2012; 44(11):913–21.

18. Kramer S, Johnson L, Bernhardt J, et al. Energy expenditure and cost during walking after stroke: a systematic review. Arch Phys Med Rehabil 2016;97(4): 619–32.e1.

19. Hollander JE, Carr BG. Virtually perfect? Telemedicine for Covid-19. N Engl J Med 2020;382(18):1679–81.

20. Middleton A, Simpson KN, Bettger JP, et al. COVID-19 pandemic and beyond: considerations and costs of telehealth exercise programs for older adults with functional impairments living at home-lessons learned from a pilot case study. Phys Ther 2020;100(8):1278–88.

21. Lurie N, Carr BG. The role of telehealth in the medical response to disasters. JAMA Intern Med 2018;178(6):745–6.

22. Scholten J, Poorman C, Culver L, et al. Department of Veterans Affairs polytrauma telerehabilitation: twenty-first century care. Phys Med Rehabil Clin N Am 2019; 30(1):207–15.

23. Gentry MT, Lapid MI, Clark MM, et al. Evidence for telehealth group-based treatment: a systematic review. J Telemed Telecare 2019;25(6):327–42.

24. Quinn R, Park S, Theodoros D, et al. Delivering group speech maintenance therapy via telerehabilitation to people with Parkinson's disease: a pilot study. Int J Speech Lang Pathol 2019;21(4):385–94.

25. Whitehead AM, Kligler B. Innovations in care: complementary and integrative health in the Veterans Health Administration whole health system. Med Care 2020;58(Suppl 2 9S):S78–9.

26. Schein RM, Schmeler MR, Brienza D, et al. Development of a service delivery protocol used for remote wheelchair consultation via telerehabilitation. Telemed J E Health 2008;14(9):932–8.

27. Forducey PG, Ruwe WD, Dawson SJ, et al. Using telerehabilitation to promote TBI recovery and transfer of knowledge. NeuroRehabilitation 2003;18(2):103–11.

28. VA and ATLAS. VA Office of Connected Care. Available at: https://connectedcare. va.gov/partners/atlas. Accessed November 15, 2020.

29. Cumming RG, Thomas M, Szonyi G, et al. Home visits by an occupational therapist for assessment and modification of environmental hazards: a randomized trial of falls prevention. J Am Geriatr Soc 1999;47(12):1397–402.

30. Nix J, Comans T. Home quick - occupational therapy home visits using mhealth, to facilitate discharge from acute admission back to the community. Int J Telerehabil 2017;9(1):47–54.

31. Kuntz JG, Kavalieratos D, Esper GJ, et al. Feasibility and acceptability of inpatient palliative care E-family meetings during COVID-19 pandemic. J Pain Symptom Manage 2020;60(3):e28–32.

32. Bernocchi P, Giordano A, Pintavalle G, et al. Feasibility and clinical efficacy of a multidisciplinary home-telehealth program to prevent falls in older adults: a randomized controlled trial. J Am Med Dir Assoc 2019;20(3):340–6.

33. Koonin LM, Hoots B, Tsang CA, et al. Trends in the use of telehealth during the emergence of the COVID-19 pandemic—United States, January-March 2020. MMWR Morb Mortal Wkly Rep 2020;69(43):1595–9.

34. Scott BK, Miller GT, Fonda SJ, et al. Advanced digital health technologies for COVID-19 and future emergencies. Telemed J E Health 2020;26(10):1226–33.

35. Kichloo A, Albosta M, Dettloff K, et al. Telemedicine, the current COVID-19 pandemic and the future: a narrative review and perspectives moving forward in the USA. Fam Med Community Health 2020;8(3). https://doi.org/10.1136/fmch-2020-000530.

36. Padala KP, Wilson KB, Gauss CH, et al. VA video connect for clinical care in older adults in a rural state during the COVID-19 pandemic: cross-sectional study. J Med Internet Res 2020;22(9):e21561.

37. Lifeline Support for Affordable Communications. Available at: https://www.fcc.gov/lifeline-consumers. Accessed November 21, 2020.

38. VA expands Veteran access to telehealth with iPad services. . VA Office of Connected Care. Available at: https://www.va.gov/opa/pressrel/pressrelease.cfm?id=5521. Accessed 27, 2020.

39. Willey S, Walsh JK. Outcomes of a mobile health coaching platform: 12-week results of a single-arm longitudinal study. JMIR Mhealth Uhealth 2016;4(1):e3.

40. Wootton SL, King M, Alison JA, et al. COVID-19 rehabilitation delivered via a tele-health pulmonary rehabilitation model: a case series. Respirol Case Rep 2020; 8(8):e00669.

41. Tang J, Mandrusiak A, Russell T. The feasibility and validity of a remote pulse ox-imetry system for pulmonary rehabilitation: a pilot study. Int J Telemed Appl 2012; 2012:798791.

42. Batalik L, Dosbaba F, Hartman M, et al. Benefits and effectiveness of using a wrist heart rate monitor as a telerehabilitation device in cardiac patients: a randomized controlled trial. Medicine (Baltimore) 2020;99(11):e19556.

43. Porciuncula F, Roto AV, Kumar D, et al. Wearable movement sensors for rehabil-itation: a focused review of technological and clinical advances. PM R 2018;10(9 Suppl 2):S220–32.

44. Roblyer D. Perspective on the increasing role of optical wearables and remote patient monitoring in the COVID-19 era and beyond. J Biomed Opt 2020; 25(10). https://doi.org/10.1117/1.JBO.25.10.102703.

45. de Araujo AVL, Neiva JFO, Monteiro CBM, et al. Efficacy of virtual reality rehabil-itation after spinal cord injury: a systematic review. Biomed Res Int 2019;2019: 7106951.

46. Gandolfi M, Geroin C, Dimitrova E, et al. Virtual reality telerehabilitation for postural instability in Parkinson's disease: a multicenter, single-blind, random-ized, controlled trial. Biomed Res Int 2017;2017:7962826.

47. Gutierrez RO, Galan Del Rio F, Cano de la Cuerda R, et al. A telerehabilitation pro-gram by virtual reality-video games improves balance and postural control in multiple sclerosis patients. NeuroRehabilitation 2013;33(4):545–54.

48. Putrino D. Telerehabilitation and emerging virtual reality approaches to stroke rehabilitation. Curr Opin Neurol 2014;27(6):631–6.

Moving?

Make sure your subscription moves with you!

To notify us of your new address, find your **Clinics Account Number** (located on your mailing label above your name), and contact customer service at:

Email: journalscustomerservice-usa@elsevier.com

800-654-2452 (subscribers in the U.S. & Canada)
314-447-8871 (subscribers outside of the U.S. & Canada)

Fax number: 314-447-8029

Elsevier Health Sciences Division
Subscription Customer Service
3251 Riverport Lane
Maryland Heights, MO 63043

*To ensure uninterrupted delivery of your subscription, please notify us at least 4 weeks in advance of move.

Printed and bound by CPI Group (UK) Ltd, Croydon, CR0 4YY

03/10/2024

01040483-0007